Essentials of Public Health Management

Essentials of Public Health Management

Editor: Dwight Parcher

FOSTER ACADEMICS

www.fosteracademics.com

www.fosteracademics.com

FOSTER ACADEMICS

Cataloging-in-Publication Data

Essentials of public health management / edited by Dwight Parcher.
p. cm.
Includes bibliographical references and index.
ISBN 978-1-63242-543-0
1. Public health--Management. 2. Public health administration.
I. Parcher, Dwight.
RA425 .E87 2018
362.1--dc23

Foster Academics,
118-35 Queens Blvd., Suite 400,
Forest Hills, NY 11375, USA

ISBN 978-1-63242-543-0 (Hardback)

Contents

Preface

Public health management is that branch of health care science which deals with the management and development of public health care providers like hospitals, departments of public health, agencies dealing in public health, etc. Public health is an essential part of the development of society. It includes regulating, promoting and monitoring the health of the population, as a whole. This book attempts to understand the multiple branches that fall under the discipline of public health management and how such concepts have practical applications. Most of the topics introduced in it cover new techniques and the applications of this subject. Those in search of information to further their knowledge in the field of public health management will be greatly assisted by this textbook.

A detailed account of the significant topics covered in this book is provided below:

Chapter 1- Public health is concerned with promoting health and knowledge of well-being. Some of the measures promoted are vaccination, hand washing, awareness regarding sexually transmitted diseases, etc. This chapter will provide an integrated understanding of public health management.

Chapter 2- Population health aims to improve the well being of the whole population. Individuals are grouped differently according to income and their health determinants are determined accordingly. Policies and health outcomes are also taken into account. Public health management is best understood in confluence with the major topics listed in the following chapter.

Chapter 3- The measures taken to prevent diseases and generate proper awareness related to hygiene is known as preventive healthcare. Health promotions can be of various sorts like workplace health promotion, health literacy, peer education and breastfeeding promotion. The major components of preventive healthcare are discussed in this chapter.

Chapter 4- The aim of health education is to educate people about the benefits of staying healthy. Health education, as a subject includes topics like physical health, social health, intellectual health, emotional and spiritual health. The major categories of public health education are dealt with great details in the chapter.

Chapter 5- A health care system is a knowledge system that contains all information about the healthcare facilities and services of a nation, town or city. It is also an indicator of the access to medical facilities to a group of people. The exact kind of facilities varies from country to country. Some of themes discussed are first aid, health care ratings, geriatric care management and eHealth. This chapter discusses the methods of public health management in a critical manner providing key analysis to the subject matter.

I would like to make a special mention of my publisher who considered me worthy of this opportunity and also supported me throughout the process. I would also like to thank the editing team at the back-end who extended their help whenever required.

Editor

1

An Introduction to Public Health

Public health is concerned with promoting health and knowledge of well-being. Some of the measures promoted are vaccination, hand washing, awareness regarding sexually transmitted diseases, etc. This chapter will provide an integrated understanding of public health management.

Public Health

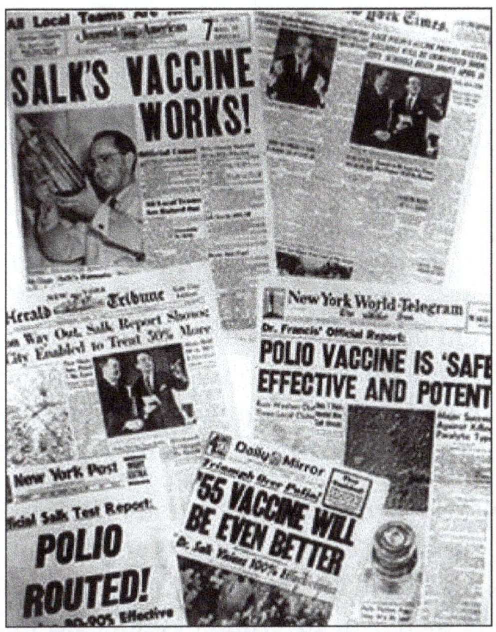

SALK'S VACCINE WORKS!
New York World-Telegram
Dr. Francis' Official Report:
POLIO VACCINE IS 'SAFE EFFECTIVE AND POTENT
New York Post
POLIO ROUTED!
Daily Mirror
'55 VACCINE WILL BE EVEN BETTER

Newspaper headlines from around the world about polio vaccine tests (13 April 1955).

Public health refers to "the science and art of preventing disease, prolonging life and promoting human health through organized efforts and informed choices of society, organizations, public and private, communities and individuals." It is concerned with threats to health based on population health analysis. The population in question can be as small as a handful of people, or as large as all the inhabitants of several continents (for instance, in the case of a pandemic). The dimensions of health can encompass "a state of complete physical, mental and social well-being and not merely the absence of disease or infirmity," as defined by the United Nations' World Health Organization. Public health incorporates the interdisciplinary approaches of epidemiology, biostatistics and health services. Environmental health, community health, behavioral health, health economics, public policy, mental health and occupational safety and health are other important subfields.

The focus of public health intervention is to improve health and quality of life through prevention and treatment of disease and other physical and mental health conditions. This is done through surveillance of cases and health indicators, and through promotion of healthy behaviors. Examples of common public health measures include promotion of hand washing, breastfeeding, delivery of vaccinations, suicide prevention and distribution of condoms to control the spread of sexually transmitted diseases.

Modern public health practice requires multidisciplinary teams of public health workers and professionals including the following: physicians specializing in public health, community medicine, or infectious disease; psychologists; epidemiologists; biostatisticians; medical assistants or Assistant Medical Officers; public health nurses; midwives; medical microbiologists; environmental health officers or public health inspectors; pharmacists; dentists; dietitians and nutritionists; veterinarians; public health engineers; public health lawyers; sociologists; community development workers; communications experts; bioethicists; and others.

There is a great disparity in access to health care and public health initiatives between developed nations and developing nations. In the developing world, public health infrastructures are still forming.

Background

The focus of a public health intervention is to prevent and manage diseases, injuries and other health conditions through surveillance of cases and the promotion of healthy behaviors, communities and environments. Many diseases are preventable through simple, nonmedical methods. For example, research has shown that the simple act of hand washing with soap can prevent many contagious diseases. In other cases, treating a disease or controlling a pathogen can be vital to preventing its spread to others, either during an outbreak of infectious disease or through contamination of food or water supplies. Public health communications programs, vaccination programs and distribution of condoms are examples of common public health measures. Measures such as these have contributed greatly to the health of populations and increases in life expectancy.

Public health plays an important role in disease prevention efforts in both the developing world and in developed countries, through local health systems and non-governmental organizations. The World Health Organization (WHO) is the international agency that coordinates and acts on global public health issues. Most countries have their own government public health agencies, sometimes known as ministries of health, to respond to domestic health issues. For example, in the United States, the front line of public health initiatives are state and local health departments. The United States Public Health Service (PHS), led by the Surgeon General of the United States, and the Centers for Disease Control and Prevention, headquartered in Atlanta, are involved with several international health activities, in addition to their national duties. In Canada, the Public Health Agency of Canada is the national agency responsible for public health, emergency preparedness and response, and infectious and chronic disease control and prevention. The Public health system in India is managed by the Ministry of Health & Family Welfare of the government of India with state-owned health care facilities.

Current Practice

Public Health Programs

There's a push and pull, as you know, between cheap alternatives for industry and public health concerns...We're always looking at retrospectively what the data shows...Unfortunately, for example, take tobacco: It took 50, 60 years of research before policy catches up with what the science is showing— Laura Anderko, professor at Georgetown University and director of the Mid-Atlantic Center for Children's Health and the Environment commenting on public health practices in response to proposal to ban chlorpyrifos pesticide.

Most governments recognize the importance of public health programs in reducing the incidence of disease, disability, and the effects of aging and other physical and mental health conditions, although public health generally receives significantly less government funding compared with medicine. Public health programs providing vaccinations have made strides in promoting health, including the eradication of smallpox, a disease that plagued humanity for thousands of years.

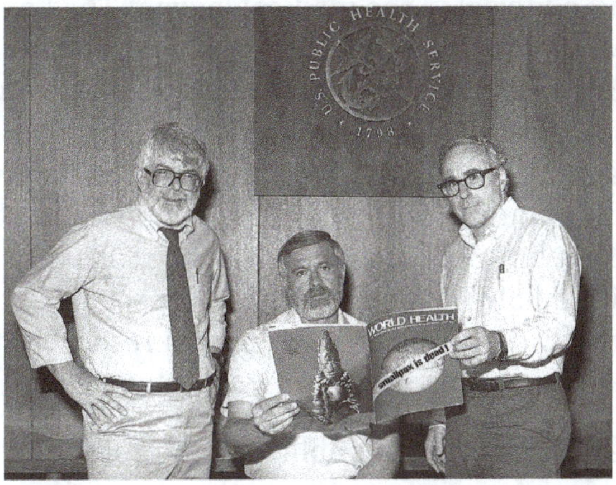

Three former directors of the Global Smallpox Eradication Programme read the news that smallpox had been globally eradicated, 1980.

The World Health Organization (WHO) identifies core functions of public health programs including:

- providing leadership on matters critical to health and engaging in partnerships where joint action is needed;
- shaping a research agenda and stimulating the generation, translation and dissemination of valuable knowledge;
- setting norms and standards and promoting and monitoring their implementation;
- articulating ethical and evidence-based policy options;
- monitoring the health situation and assessing health trends.

In particular, public health surveillance programs can:

- serve as an early warning system for impending public health emergencies;
- document the impact of an intervention, or track progress towards specified goals; and
- monitor and clarify the epidemiology of health problems, allow priorities to be set, and inform health policy and strategies.
- diagnose, investigate, and monitor health problems and health hazards of the community

Public health surveillance has led to the identification and prioritization of many public health issues facing the world today, including HIV/AIDS, diabetes, waterborne diseases, zoonotic diseases, and antibiotic resistance leading to the reemergence of infectious diseases such as tuberculosis. Antibiotic resistance, also known as drug resistance, was the theme of World Health Day 2011. Although the prioritization of pressing public health issues is important, Laurie Garrett argues that there are following consequences. When foreign aid is funnelled into disease-specific programs, the importance of public health in general is disregarded. This public health problem of stovepiping is thought to create a lack of funds to combat other existing diseases in a given country.

For example, the WHO reports that at least 220 million people worldwide suffer from diabetes. Its incidence is increasing rapidly, and it is projected that the number of diabetes deaths will double by the year 2030. In a June 2010 editorial in the medical journal *The Lancet*, the authors opined that "The fact that type 2 diabetes, a largely preventable disorder, has reached epidemic proportion is a public health humiliation." The risk of type 2 diabetes is closely linked with the growing problem of obesity. The WHO's latestestimates highlighted that globally approximately 1.5 billion adults were overweight in 2008, and nearly 43 million children under the age of five were overweight in 2010. The United States is the leading country with 30.6% of its population being obese. Mexico follows behind with 24.2% and the United Kingdom with 23%. Once considered a problem in high-income countries, it is now on the rise in low-income countries, especially in urban settings. Many public health programs are increasingly dedicating attention and resources to the issue of obesity, with objectives to address the underlying causes including healthy diet and physical exercise.

Some programs and policies associated with public health promotion and prevention can be controversial. One such example is programs focusing on the prevention of HIV transmission through safe sex campaigns and needle-exchange programmes. Another is the control of tobacco smoking. Changing smoking behavior requires long-term strategies, unlike the fight against communicable diseases, which usually takes a shorter period for effects to be observed. Many nations have implemented major initiatives to cut smoking, such as increased taxation and bans on smoking in some or all public places. Proponents argue by presenting evidence that smoking is one of the major killers, and that therefore governments have a duty to reduce the death rate, both through limiting passive (second-hand) smoking and by providing fewer opportunities for people to smoke. Opponents say that this undermines individual freedom and personal responsibility, and worry that the state may be emboldened to remove more and more choice in the name of better population health overall.

Simultaneously, while communicable diseases have historically ranged uppermost as a global health priority, non-communicable diseases and the underlying behavior-related risk factors have been at the bottom. This is changing however, as illustrated by the United Nations hosting its first General Assembly Special Summit on the issue of non-communicable diseases in September 2011.

Many health problems are due to maladaptive personal behaviors. From an evolutionary psychology perspective, over consumption of novel substances that are harmful is due to the activation of an evolved reward system for substances such as drugs, tobacco, alcohol, refined salt, fat, and carbohydrates. New technologies such as modern transportation also cause reduced physical activity. Research has found that behavior is more effectively changed by taking evolutionary motivations into consideration instead of only presenting information about health effects. Thus, the increased use of soap and hand-washing to prevent diarrhea is much more effectively promoted if its lack of use is associated with the emotion of disgust. Disgust is an evolved system for avoiding contact with substances that spread infectious diseases. Examples might include films that show how fecal matter contaminates food. The marketing industry has long known the importance of associating products with high status and attractiveness to others. Conversely, it has been argued that emphasizing the harmful and undesirable effects of tobacco smoking on other persons and imposing smoking bans in public places have been particularly effective in reducing tobacco smoking.

Applications in Health Care

As well as seeking to improve population health through the implementation of specific population-level interventions, public health contributes to medical care by identifying and assessing population needs for health care services, including:

- Assessing current services and evaluating whether they are meeting the objectives of the health care system
- Ascertaining requirements as expressed by health professionals, the public and other stakeholders
- Identifying the most appropriate interventions
- Considering the effect on resources for proposed interventions and assessing their cost-effectiveness
- Supporting decision making in health care and planning health services including any necessary changes.
- Informing, educating, and empowering people about health issues

Implementing Effective Improvement Strategies

To improve public health, one important strategy is to promote modern medicine and scientific neutrality to drive the public health policy and campaign, which is recommended by Armanda Solorzana, through a case study of the Rockefeller Foundation's hookworm campaign in Mexico in the 1920s. Soloranza argues that public health policy can't concern only politics or economics. Political concerns can lead government officials to hide the real numbers of people affected by disease in their regions, such as upcoming elections. Therefore, scientific neutrality in making public health policy is critical; it can ensure treatment needs are met regardless of political and economic conditions.

The history of public health care clearly shows the global effort to improve health care for all. However, in modern-day medicine, real, measurable change has not been clearly seen, and critics argue that this lack of improvement is due to ineffective methods that are being implemented. As argued by Paul E. Farmer, structural interventions could possibly have a large impact, and yet there are numerous problems as to why this strategy has yet to be incorporated into the health system. One of the main reasons that he suggests could be the fact that physicians are not properly trained to carry out structural interventions, meaning that the ground level health care professionals cannot implement these improvements. While structural interventions can not be the only area for improvement, the lack of coordination between socioeconomic factors and health care for the poor could be counterproductive, and end up causing greater inequity between the health care services received by the rich and by the poor. Unless health care is no longer treated as a commodity, global public health can ultimately not be achieved. This being the case, without changing the way in which health care is delivered to those who have less access to it, the universal goal of public health care cannot be achieved.

Public Health 2.0

Public Health 2.0 is a movement within public health that aims to make the field more accessible to the general public and more user-driven. The term is used in three senses. In the first sense, "Public Health 2.0" is similar to "Health 2.0" and describes the ways in which traditional public health practitioners and institutions are reaching out (or could reach out) to the public through social media and health blogs.

In the second sense, "Public Health 2.0" describes public health research that uses data gathered from social networking sites, search engine queries, cell phones, or other technologies. A recent example is the proposal of statistical framework that utilizes online user-generated content (from social media or search engine queries) to estimate the impact of an influenza vaccination campaign in the UK.

In the third sense, "Public Health 2.0" is used to describe public health activities that are completely user-driven. An example is the collection and sharing of information about environmental radiation levels after the March 2011 tsunami in Japan. In all cases, Public Health 2.0 draws on ideas from Web 2.0, such as crowdsourcing, information sharing, and user-centred design. While many individual healthcare providers have started making their own personal contributions to "Public Health 2.0" through personal blogs, social profiles, and websites, other larger organizations, such as the American Heart Association (AHA) and United Medical Education (UME), have a larger team of employees centered around online driven health education, research, and training. These private organizations recognize the need for free and easy to access health materials often building libraries of educational articles.

Developing Countries

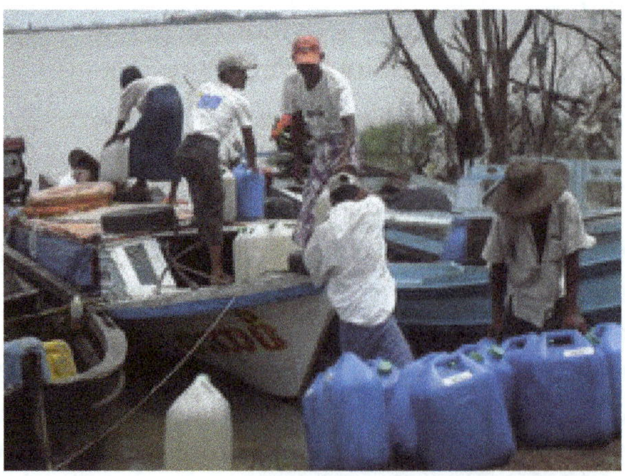

Emergency Response Team in Burma after Cyclone Nargis in 2008

There is a great disparity in access to health care and public health initiatives between developed nations and developing nations. In the developing world, public health infrastructures are still forming. There may not be enough trained health workers or monetary resources to provide even a basic level of medical care and disease prevention. As a result, a large majority of disease and mortality in the developing world results from and contributes to extreme poverty. For example, many African governments spend less than US$10 per person per year on health care, while, in the United States, the federal government spent approximately US$4,500 per capita in 2000. However, expenditures on health care should not be confused with spending on public health. Public health measures may not generally be considered "health care" in the strictest sense. For example, mandating the use of seat belts in cars can save countless lives and contribute to the health of a population, but typically money spent enforcing this rule would not count as money spent on health care.

Large parts of the developing world remained plagued by largely preventable or treatable infectious diseases and poor maternal and child health, exacerbated by malnutrition and poverty. The WHO reports that a lack of exclusive breastfeeding during the first six months of life contributes to over a million avoidable child deaths each year. Intermittent preventive therapy aimed at treating and preventing malaria episodes among pregnant women and young children is one public health measure in endemic countries.

Each day brings new front-page headlines about public health: emerging infectious diseases such as SARS, rapidly making its way from China to Canada, the United States and other geographically distant countries; reducing inequities in health care access through publicly funded health insurance programs; the HIV/AIDS pandemic and its spread from certain high-risk groups to the general population in many countries, such as in South Africa; the increase of childhood obesity and the concomitant increase in type II diabetes among children; the social, economic and health effects of adolescent pregnancy; and the public health challenges related to natural disasters such as the 2004 Indian Ocean tsunami, 2005's Hurricane Katrina in the United States and the 2010 Haiti earthquake.

Since the 1980s, the growing field of population health has broadened the focus of public health from individual behaviors and risk factors to population-level issues such as inequality, poverty, and education. Modern public health is often concerned with addressing determinants of health across a population. There is a recognition that our health is affected by many factors including where we live, genetics, our income, our educational status and our social relationships; these are known as "social determinants of health." A social gradient in health runs through society. The poorest generally suffer the worst health, but even the middle classes will generally have worse health outcomes than those of a higher social stratum. The new public health advocates for population-based policies that improve health in an equitable manner.

Sustainable Development Goals

To address current and future challenges in addressing health issues in the world, the United Nations have developed the Sustainable Development Goals 2015 building off of the Millennium Development Goals of 2000 to be completed by 2030. These goals in their entirety encompass the entire spectrum of development across nations, however Goals 1-6 directly address health disparities, primarily in developing countries. These six goals address key issues in global public health:

Poverty, Hunger and food security, Health, Education, Gender equality and women's empowerment, and water and sanitation. Public health officials can use these goals to set their own agenda and plan for smaller scale initiatives for their organizations. These goals hope to lessen the burden of disease and inequality faced by developing countries and lead to a healthier future.

The links between the various sustainable development goals and public health are numerous and well established:

- Living below the poverty line is attributed to poorer health outcomes and can be even worse for persons living in developing countries where extreme poverty is more common. A child born into poverty is twice as likely to die before the age of five compared to a child from a wealthier family.
- The detrimental effects of hunger and malnutrition that can arise from systemic challenges with food security are enormous. The World Health Organization estimates that 12.9 percent of the population in developing countries is undernourished.
- Health challenges in the developing world are enormous, with "only half of the women in developing nations receiving the recommended amount of healthcare they need.
- Educational equity has yet to be reached in the world. Public health efforts are impeded by this, as a lack of education can lead to poorer health outcomes. This is shown by children of mothers who have no education having a lower survival rate compared to children born to mothers with primary or greater levels of education. Cultural differences in the role of women vary by country, many gender inequalities are found in developing nations. Combating these inequalities has shown to also lead to better public health outcome.
- In studies done by the World Bank on populations in developing countries, it was found that when women had more control over household resources, the children benefit through better access to food, healthcare, and education.
- Basic sanitation resources and access to clean sources of water are a basic human right. However, 1.8 billion people globally use a source of drinking water that is fecally contaminated, and 2.4 billion people lack access to basic sanitation facilities like toilets or pit latrines. A lack of these resources is what causes approximately 1000 children a day to die from diarrhoel diseases that could have been prevented from better water and sanitation infrastructure.

Education and Training

Education and training of public health professionals is available throughout the world in Schools of Public Health, Medical Schools, Veterinary Schools, Schools of Nursing, and Schools of Public Affairs. The training typically requires a university degree with a focus on core disciplines of biostatistics, epidemiology, health services administration, health policy, health education, behavioral science and environmental health. In the global context, the field of public health education has evolved enormously in recent decades, supported by institutions such as the World Health Organization and the World Bank, among others. Operational structures are formulated by strategic principles, with educational and career pathways guided by competency frameworks, all requiring modulation according to local, national and global realities. It is critically important for the health of populations that nations assess their public health human resource needs and develop their ability to deliver this capacity, and not depend on other countries to supply it.

Schools of Public Health - a U.S. Perspective

In the United States, the Welch-Rose Report of 1915 has been viewed as the basis for the critical movement in the history of the institutional schism between public health and medicine because it led to the establishment of schools of public health supported by the Rockefeller Foundation. The report was authored by William Welch, founding dean of the Johns Hopkins Bloomberg School of Public Health, and Wickliffe Rose of the Rockefeller Foundation. The report focused more on research than practical education. Some have blamed the Rockefeller Foundation's 1916 decision to support the establishment of schools of public health for creating the schism between public health and medicine and legitimizing the rift between medicine's laboratory investigation of the mechanisms of disease and public health's nonclinical concern with environmental and social influences on health and wellness.

Even though schools of public health had already been established in Canada, Europe and North Africa, the United States had still maintained the traditional system of housing faculties of public health within their medical institutions. A $25,000 donation from businessman Samuel Zemurray instituted the School of Public Health and Tropical Medicine at Tulane University in 1912 conferring its first doctor of public health degree in 1914. The Johns Hopkins School of Hygiene and Public Health became an independent, degree-granting institution for research and training in public health, and the largest public health training facility in the United States, when it was founded in 1916. By 1922, schools of public health were established at Columbia, Harvard and Yale on the Hopkins model. By 1999 there were twenty nine schools of public health in the US, enrolling around fifteen thousand students.

Over the years, the types of students and training provided have also changed. In the beginning, students who enrolled in public health schools typically had already obtained a medical degree; public health school training was largely a second degree for medical professionals. However, in 1978, 69% of American students enrolled in public health schools had only a bachelor's degree.

Degrees in Public Health

Schools of public health offer a variety of degrees which generally fall into two categories: professional or academic. The two major postgraduate degrees are the Master of Public Health (M.P.H.) or the Master of Science in Public Health (MSPH). Doctoral studies in this field include Doctor of Public Health (DrPH) and Doctor of Philosophy (Ph.D.) in a subspeciality of greater Public Health disciplines. DrPH is regarded as a professional degree and Ph.D. as more of an academic degree.

Professional degrees are oriented towards practice in public health settings. The Master of Public Health, Doctor of Public Health, Doctor of Health Science (DHSc) and the Master of Health Care Administration are examples of degrees which are geared towards people who want careers as practitioners of public health in health departments, managed care and community-based organizations, hospitals and consulting firms among others. Master of Public Health degrees broadly fall into two categories, those that put more emphasis on an understanding of epidemiology and statistics as the scientific basis of public health practice and those that include a more eclectic range of methodologies. A Master of Science of Public Health is similar to an MPH but is considered an academic degree (as opposed to a professional degree) and places more emphasis on scientific methods and research. The same distinction can be made between the DrPH and the DHSc. The DrPH is considered a professional degree and the DHSc is an academic degree.

Academic degrees are more oriented towards those with interests in the scientific basis of public health and preventive medicine who wish to pursue careers in research, university teaching in graduate programs, policy analysis and development, and other high-level public health positions. Examples of academic degrees are the Master of Science, Doctor of Philosophy, Doctor of Science (ScD), and Doctor of Health Science (DHSc). The doctoral programs are distinct from the MPH and other professional programs by the addition of advanced coursework and the nature and scope of a dissertation research project.

In the United States, the Association of Schools of Public Health represents Council on Education for Public Health (CEPH) accredited schools of public health. Delta Omega is the honor society for graduate studies in public health. The society was founded in 1924 at the Johns Hopkins School of Hygiene and Public Health. Currently, there are approximately 68 chapters throughout the United States and Puerto Rico.

History

Early History

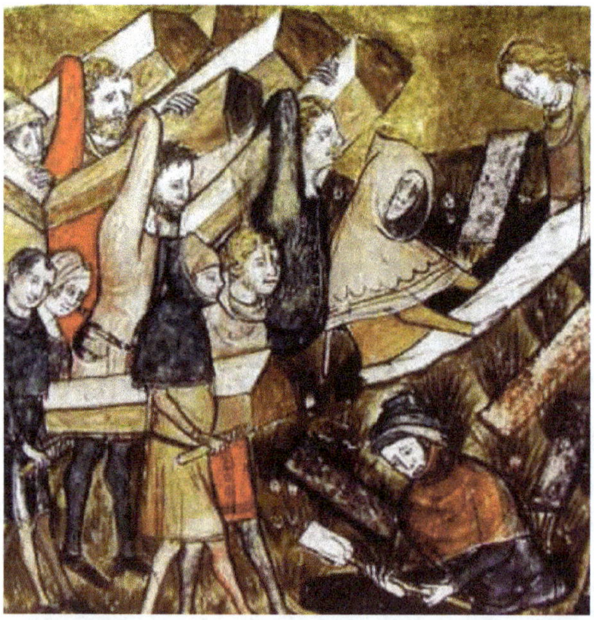

The primitive nature of medieval medicine rendered Europe helpless to the onslaught of the Black Death in the 14th century. Fragment of a miniature from "The Chronicles of Gilles Li Muisis" (1272-1352). Bibliothèque royale de Belgique, MS 13076-77, f. 24v.

Public health has early roots in antiquity. From the beginnings of human civilization, it was recognized that polluted water and lack of proper waste disposal spread communicable diseases (theory of miasma). Early religions attempted to regulate behavior that specifically related to health, from types of food eaten, to regulating certain indulgent behaviors, such as drinking alcohol or sexual relations. Leaders were responsible for the health of their subjects to ensure social stability, prosperity, and maintain order.

By Roman times, it was well understood that proper diversion of human waste was a necessary tenet of public health in urban areas. The ancient Chinese medical doctors developed the practice of variolation following a smallpox epidemic around 1000 BC. An individual without the disease could gain some measure of immunity against it by inhaling the dried crusts that formed around lesions of infected individuals. Also, children were protected by inoculating a scratch on their forearms with the pus from a lesion.

In 1485 the Republic of Venice established a Permanent Court of supervisors of health with special attention to the prevention of the spread of epidemics in the territory from abroad. The three supervisors were initially appointed by the Venetian Senate. In 1537 it was assumed by the Grand Council, and in 1556 added two judges, with the task of control, on behalf of the Republic, the efforts of the supervisors.

However, according to Michel Foucault, the plague model of governmentality was later controverted by the cholera model. A Cholera pandemic devastated Europe between 1829 and 1851, and was first fought by the use of what Foucault called "social medicine", which focused on flux, circulation of air, location of cemeteries, etc. All those concerns, born of the miasma theory of disease, were mixed with urbanistic concerns for the management of populations, which Foucault designated as the concept of "biopower". The German conceptualized this in the *Polizeiwissenschaft* ("Police science").

Modern Public Health

The 18th century saw rapid growth in voluntary hospitals in England. The latter part of the century brought the establishment of the basic pattern of improvements in public health over the next two centuries: a social evil was identified, private philanthropists brought attention to it, and changing public opinion led to government action.

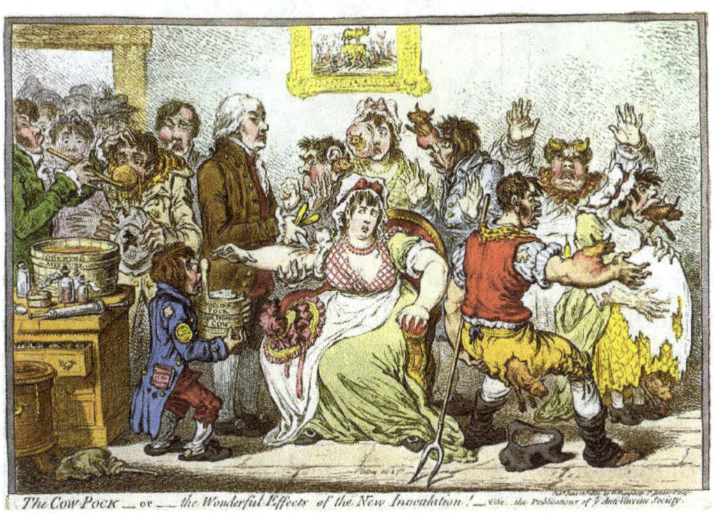
The Cow-Pock — or — the Wonderful Effects of the New Inoculation! — vide. the Publications of y Anti-Vaccine Society.

1802 caricature of Edward Jenner vaccinating patients who feared it would make them sprout cowlike appendages.

The practice of vaccination became prevalent in the 1800s, following the pioneering work of Edward Jenner in treating smallpox. James Lind's discovery of the causes of scurvy amongst sailors and its mitigation via the introduction of fruit on lengthy voyages was published in 1754 and led to the adoption of this idea by the Royal Navy. Efforts were also made to promulgate health matters to the broader public; in 1752 the British physician Sir John Pringle published *Observations on the Diseases of the Army in Camp and Garrison*, in which he advocated for the importance of adequate ventilation in the military barracks and the provision of latrines for the soldiers.

With the onset of the Industrial Revolution, living standards amongst the working population began to worsen, with cramped and unsanitary urban conditions. In the first four decades of the 19th century alone, London's population doubled and even greater growth rates were recorded in the new industrial towns, such as Leeds and Manchester. This rapid urbanisation exacerbated the spread of disease in the large conurbations that built up around the workhouses and factories. These settlements were cramped and primitive with no organized sanitation. Disease was inevitable and its incubation in these areas was encouraged by the poor lifestyle of the inhabitants. Unavailable housing led to the rapid growth of slums and the per capita death rate began to rise alarmingly, almost doubling in Birmingham and Liverpool. Thomas Malthus warned of the dangers of overpopulation in 1798. His ideas, as well as those of Jeremy Bentham, became very influential in government circles in the early years of the 19th century.

Public Health Legislation

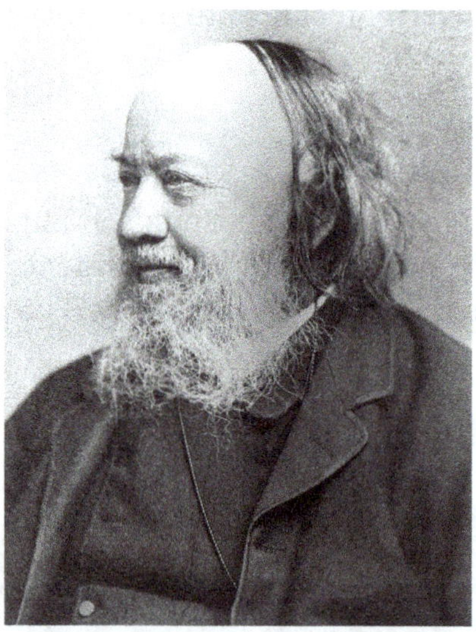

Sir Edwin Chadwick was a pivotal influence on the early public health campaign.

The first attempts at sanitary reform and the establishment of public health institutions were made in the 1840s. Thomas Southwood Smith, physician at the London Fever Hospital, began to write papers on the importance of public health, and was one of the first physicians brought in to give evidence before the Poor Law Commission in the 1830s, along with Neil Arnott and James Phillips Kay. Smith advised the government on the importance of quarantine and sanitary improvement for limiting the spread of infectious diseases such as cholera and yellow fever.

The Poor Law Commission reported in 1838 that "the expenditures necessary to the adoption and maintenance of measures of prevention would ultimately amount to less than the cost of the disease now constantly engendered". It recommended the implementation of large scale government engineering projects to alleviate the conditions that allowed for the propagation of disease. The Health of Towns Association was formed in Exeter on 11 December 1844, and vigorously campaigned for the development of public health in the United Kingdom. Its formation followed the 1843 establishment of the Health of Towns Commission, chaired by Sir Edwin Chadwick, which produced a series of reports on poor and insanitary conditions in British cities.

These national and local movements led to the Public Health Act, finally passed in 1848. It aimed to improve the sanitary condition of towns and populous places in England and Wales by placing the supply of water, sewerage, drainage, cleansing and paving under a single local body with the General Board of Health as a central authority. The Act was passed by the Liberal government of Lord John Russell, in response to the urging of Edwin Chadwick. Chadwick's seminal report on *The Sanitary Condition of the Labouring Population* was published in 1842 and was followed up with a supplementary report a year later.

Vaccination for various diseases was made compulsory in the United Kingdom in 1851, and by 1871 legislation required a comprehensive system of registration run by appointed vaccination officers.

Further interventions were made by a series of subsequent Public Health Acts, notably the 1875 Act. Reforms included latrinization, the building of sewers, the regular collection of garbage followed by incineration or disposal in a landfill, the provision of clean water and the draining of standing water to prevent the breeding of mosquitoes.

The Infectious Disease (Notification) Act 1889 mandated the reporting of infectious diseases to the local sanitary authority, which could then pursue measures such as the removal of the patient to hospital and the disinfection of homes and properties.

In the U.S., the first public health organization based on a state health department and local boards of health was founded in New York City in 1866.

Epidemiology

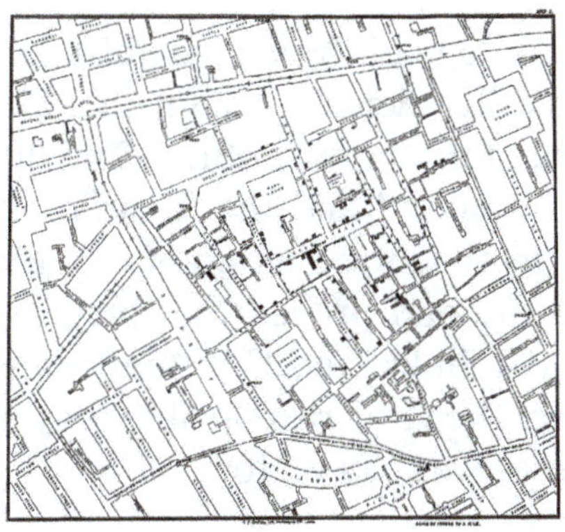

John Snow's dot map, showing the clusters of cholera cases in the London epidemic of 1854.

The science of epidemiology was founded by John Snow's identification of a polluted public water well as the source of an 1854 cholera outbreak in London. Dr. Snow believed in the germ theory of disease as opposed to the prevailing miasma theory. He first publicized his theory in an essay, *On the Mode of Communication of Cholera*, in 1849, followed by a more detailed treatise in 1855 incorporating the results of his investigation of the role of the water supply in the Soho epidemic of 1854.

By talking to local residents (with the help of Reverend Henry Whitehead), he identified the source of the outbreak as the public water pump on Broad Street (now Broadwick Street). Although Snow's chemical and microscope examination of a water sample from the Broad Street pump did not conclusively prove its danger, his studies of the pattern of the disease were convincing enough to persuade the local council to disable the well pump by removing its handle.

Snow later used a dot map to illustrate the cluster of cholera cases around the pump. He also used statistics to illustrate the connection between the quality of the water source and cholera cases. He showed that the Southwark and Vauxhall Waterworks Company was taking water from sewage-polluted sections of the Thames and delivering the water to homes, leading to an increased incidence of cholera. Snow's study was a major event in the history of public health and geography. It is regarded as the founding event of the science of epidemiology.

Disease Control

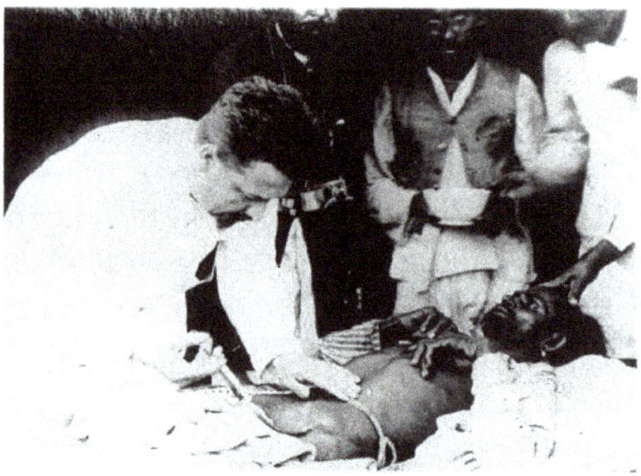

Paul-Louis Simond injecting a plague vaccine in Karachi, 1898.

With the pioneering work in bacteriology of French chemist Louis Pasteur and German scientist Robert Koch, methods for isolating the bacteria responsible for a given disease and vaccines for remedy were developed at the turn of the 20th century. British physician Ronald Ross identified the mosquito as the carrier of malaria and laid the foundations for combating the disease. Joseph Lister revolutionized surgery by the introduction of antiseptic surgery to eliminate infection. French epidemiologist Paul-Louis Simond proved that plague was carried by fleas on the back of rats, and Cuban scientist Carlos J. Finlay and U.S. Americans Walter Reed and James Carroll demonstrated that mosquitoes carry the virus responsible for yellow fever. Brazilian scientist Carlos Chagas identified a tropical disease and its vector.

With onset of the epidemiological transition and as the prevalence of infectious diseases decreased through the 20th century, public health began to put more focus on chronic diseases such as cancer and heart disease. Previous efforts in many developed countries had already led to dramatic reductions in the infant mortality rate using preventative methods. In Britain, the infant mortality rate fell from over 15% in 1870 to 7% by 1930.

Country Examples

France

France 1871-1914 followed well behind Bismarckian Germany, as well as Great Britain, in developing the welfare state including public health. Tuberculosis was the most dreaded disease of the day, especially striking young people in their 20s. Germany set up vigorous measures of public hygiene and public sanatoria, but France let private physicians handle the problem, which left it with a much higher death rate. The French medical profession jealously guarded its prerogatives, and public health activists were not as well organized or as influential as in Germany, Britain or the United States. For example, there was a long battle over a public health law which began in the 1880s as a campaign to reorganize the nation's health services, to require the registration of infectious diseases, to mandate quarantines, and to improve the deficient health and housing legislation of 1850. However the reformers met opposition from bureaucrats, politicians, and physicians. Because it was so threatening to so many interests, the proposal was debated and postponed for 20 years before becoming law in 1902. Success finally came when the government realized that contagious diseases had a national security impact in weakening military recruits, and keeping the population population growth rate well below Germany's.

United States

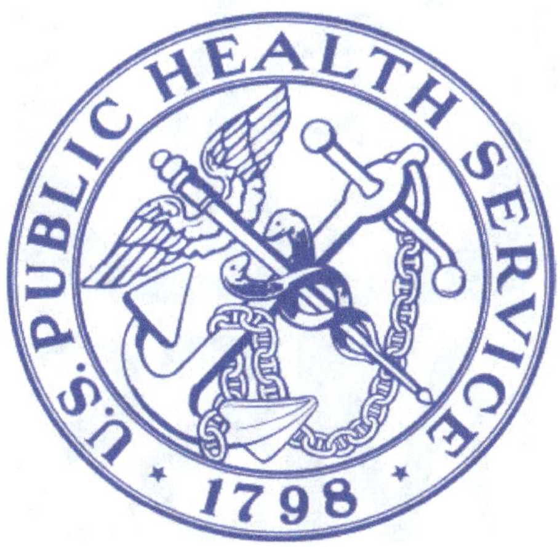

Seal of the United States Public Health Service

Most of the Public health activity in the United States took place at the municipal level before the mid-20th century. There was some activity at the national and state level as well.

In the administration of the second president of the United States John Adams, the Congress authorized the creation of hospitals for mariners. As the U.S. expanded, the scope of the governmental health agency expanded. In the United States, public health worker Sara Josephine Baker, M.D. established many programs to help the poor in New York City keep their infants healthy, leading teams of nurses into the crowded neighborhoods of Hell's Kitchen and teaching mothers how to dress, feed, and bathe their babies.

Another key pioneer of public health in the U.S. was Lillian Wald, who founded the Henry Street Settlement house in New York. The Visiting Nurse Service of New York was a significant organization for bringing health care to the urban poor.

Dramatic increases in average life span in the late 19th century and 20th century, is widely credited to public health achievements, such as vaccination programs and control of many infectious diseases including polio, diphtheria, yellow fever and smallpox; effective health and safety policies such as road traffic safety and occupational safety; improved family planning; tobacco control measures; and programs designed to decrease non-communicable diseases by acting on known risk factors such as a person's background, lifestyle and environment.

Another major public health improvement was the decline in the "urban penalty" brought about by improvements in sanitation. These improvements included chlorination of drinking water, filtration and sewage treatment which led to the decline in deaths caused by infectious waterborne diseases such as cholera and intestinal diseases. The federal Office of Indian Affairs (OIA) operated a large-scale field nursing program. Field nurses targeted native women for health education, emphasizing personal hygiene and infant care and nutrition.

Mexico

Logo for the Mexican Social Security Institute, a governmental agency dealing with public health.

Public health issues were important for the Spanish empire during the colonial era. Epidemic disease was the main factor in the decline of indigenous populations in the era immediately following the sixteenth-century conquest era and was a problem during the colonial era. The Spanish crown took steps in eighteenth-century Mexico to bring in regulations to make populations healthier.

In the late nineteenth century, Mexico was in the process of modernization, and public health issues were again tackled from a scientific point of view. Even during the Mexican Revolution (1910–20), public health was an important concern, with a text on hygiene published in 1916. During the Mexican Revolution, feminist and trained nurse Elena Arizmendi Mejia founded the Neutral White Cross, treating wounded soldiers no matter for what faction they fought.

In the post-revolutionary period after 1920, improved public health was a revolutionary goal of the Mexican government. The Mexican state promoted the health of the Mexican population, with most resources going to cities. Concern about disease conditions and social impediments to the improvement of Mexicans' health were important in the formation of the Mexican Society for Eugenics. The movement flourished from the 1920s to the 1940s. Mexico was not alone in Latin America or the world in promoting eugenics. Government campaigns against disease and alcoholism were also seen as promoting public health.

The Mexican Social Security Institute was established in 1943, during the administration of President Manuel Avila Camacho to deal with public health, pensions, and social security.

Cuba

Since the 1959 Cuban Revolution the Cuban government has devoted extensive resources to the improvement of health conditions for its entire population via universal access to health care. Infant mortality has plummeted. Cuban medical internationalism as a policy has seen the Cuban government sent doctors as a form of aid and export to countries in need in Latin America, especially Venezuela, as well as Oceania and Africa countries.

Colombia and Bolivia

Public health was important elsewhere in Latin America in consolidating state power and integrating marginalized populations into the nation-state. In Colombia, public health was a means for creating and implementing ideas of citizenship. In Bolivia, a similar push came after their 1952 revolution.

Health Marketing

Health marketing is a new approach to public health that applies traditional marketing principles and theories alongside science-based strategies to prevention, health promotion and health protection. Health marketing is one of the ways through which advancements in medicine and in health-protecting services like insurance are made widely known. A good example is the current drive in Kenya to promote circumcision among communities that do not customarily circumcise. Medical researchers have recently documented that circumcision is 65% effective in preventing HIV infection among men.

The marketing strategy would follow the traditional 4 "P's" of marketing namely:

- The "product" in question in this case the surgical procedure.
- The "place" which refers to the access to this procedure.
- "Promotion" refers to creating awareness and hence demand.
- "Price" refers to the cost of the procedure e.g. money, time, reputation etc.

"Health marketing" is a term rarely used in public health and related disciplines. "Social marketing" or "integrated marketing communication" are more commonly used in public health and other disciplines to refer to marketing-based planning frameworks for public health communication.

Social Determinants of Health

The social determinants of health (SDOH) are the economic and social conditions and their distribution among the population that influence individual and group differences in health status. They are health promoting factors found in one's living and working conditions (such as the distribution of income, wealth, influence, and power), rather than individual risk factors (such as behavioural risk factors or genetics) that influence the risk for a disease, or vulnerability to disease or injury. According to some viewpoints, the distributions of social determinants are shaped by public policies that reflect the influence of prevailing political ideologies of those governing a jurisdiction. The World Health Organization says, "This unequal distribution of health-damaging experiences is not in any sense a 'natural' phenomenon but is the result of a toxic combination of poor social policies, unfair economic arrangements [where the already well-off and healthy become even richer and the poor who are already more likely to be ill become even poorer], and bad politics."

Commonly Accepted Determinants

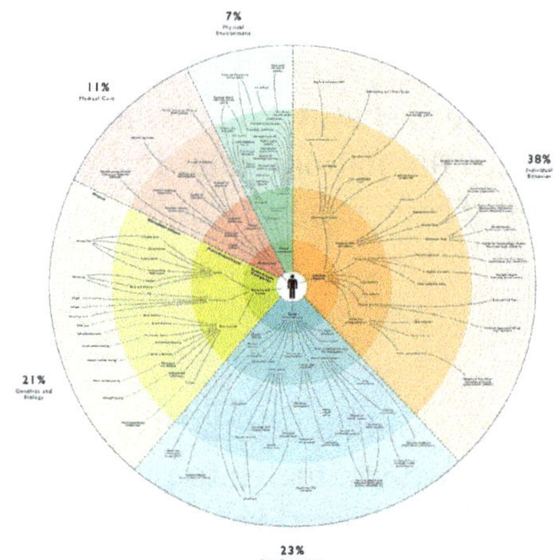

Social Determinants of Health Map

There is no single definition of the social determinants of health, but there are commonalities, and many governmental and non-governmental organizations recognize that there are social factors which impact the health of individuals.

In 2003, the World Health Organisation (WHO) Europe suggested that the social determinants of health included:

- The Social gradient
- Stress
- Early Life
- Social exclusion
- work
- Unemployment

- Social support
- Addiction
- Food
- Transportation

In Canada, these social determinants of health have gained wide usage.

1. Income and income distribution
2. Education
3. Unemployment and job security
4. Employment and working conditions
5. Early childhood development
6. Food insecurity
7. Housing
8. Social exclusion
9. Social safety network
10. Health services
11. Aboriginal status
12. Gender
13. Race
14. Disability

These SDOH are clearly related to health outcomes, are closely tied to public policy, and are clearly understandable by the public. They tend to cluster together – for example, those living in poverty also experience numerous other adverse social determinants. The quality and equitable distribution of these social determinants in Canada and the USA are clearly well below the standards seen in other developed nations.

The WHO later developed a Commission on Social Determinants of Health, which in 2008 published a report entitled "Closing the Gap in a Generation". This report identified two broad areas of social determinants of health that needed to be addressed. The first area was daily living conditions, which included healthy physical environments, fair employment and decent work, social protection across the lifespan, and access to health care. The second major area was distribution of power, money, and resources, including equity in health programs, public financing of action on the social determinants, economic inequalities, resource depletion, healthy working conditions, gender equity, political empowerment, and a balance of power and prosperity of nations.

The 2011 World Conference on Social Determinants of Health brought together delegations from 125 member states and resulted in the Rio Political Declaration on Social Determinants of Health. This declaration involved an affirmation that health inequities are unacceptable, and noted that these inequities arise from the societal conditions in which people are born, grow, live, work, and age, including early childhood development, education, economic status, employment and decent work, housing environment, and effective prevention and treatment of health problems.

The United States Centers for Disease Control defines social determinants of health as "life-enhancing resources, such as food supply, housing, economic and social relationships, transportation, education, and health care, whose distribution across populations effectively determines length and quality of life". These include access to care and resources such as food, insurance coverage, income, housing, and transportation. Social determinants of health influence health-promoting behaviours, and health equity among the population is not possible without equitable distribution of social determinants among groups.

Woolf states, "The degree to which social conditions affect health is illustrated by the association between education and mortality rates". Reports in 2005 revealed the mortality rate was 206.3 per 100,000 for adults aged 25 to 64 years with little education beyond high school, but was twice as great (477.6 per 100,000) for those with only a high school education and 3 times as great (650.4 per 100,000) for those less educated. Based on the data collected, the social conditions such as education, income, and race were very much dependent on one another, but these social conditions also apply independent health influences.

Marmot and Bell found that in wealthy countries, income and mortality are correlated as a marker of relative position within society, and this relative position is related to social conditions that are important for health including good early childhood development, access to good quality education, rewarding work with some degree of autonomy, decent housing, and a clean and safe living environment. The social condition of autonomy, control, and empowerment turns are important influences on health and disease, and individuals who lack social participation and control over their lives are at a greater risk for heart disease and mental illness.

International Health Inequalities

Even in the wealthiest countries, there are economic inequalities in health between the rich and the poor. Canadian authors Labonte and Schrecker from the University of Ottawa note that globalization is a key context for the study of the social determinants of health, and as Bushra (2011) the impacts of globalization are asymmetric. As a result, there is an uneven distribution of wealth and influence both within and across national borders, leading to negative impacts on the social determinants of health. The Organization for Economic Cooperation and Development found significant differences among developed nations in health status indicators such as life expectancy, infant mortality, incidence of disease, and death from injuries. International labor migration and the policies that attempt to regulate it can also impact the health of only those that migrate but their family members who stay behind.

These inequalities may exist in the context of the health care system, or in broader social approaches. According to the WHO's Commission on Social Determinants of Health, access to health care is essential for equitable health, and it argued that health care should be a common good rather than a market commodity. However, there is substantial variation in health care systems and coverage from country to country. The Commission also calls for government action on such things as access to clean water and safe, equitable working conditions, and it notes that dangerous working conditions exist even in some wealthy countries. In the Rio Political Declaration on Social Determinants of Health, several key areas of action were identified to address inequalities, including promotion of participatory policy-making processes, strengthening global governance and collaboration, and encouraging developed countries to reach a target of 0.7% of gross national product (GNP) for official development assistance.

Theoretical Approaches

The UK *Black* and *The Health Divide* reports considered two primary mechanisms for understanding the process by which the social determinants influence health: cultural/ behavioural and materialist/structuralist. The cultural/behavioural explanation was that individuals' behavioural choices (e.g., tobacco and alcohol use, diet, physical activity, etc.) were responsible for their developing and dying from a variety of diseases. However, both the Black and Health divide reports found that behavioural choices are heavily structured by one's material conditions of life, and these behavioural risk factors account for a relatively small proportion of variation in the incidence and death from various diseases.

The materialist/structuralist explanation emphasizes the material conditions under which people live. These conditions include availability of resources to access the amenities of life, working conditions, and quality of available food and housing among others. Within this view, three frameworks have been developed to explain how social determinants influence health. These frameworks are: (a) materialist; (b) neo-materialist; and (c) psychosocial comparison. The materialist explanation is about how living conditions – and the social determinants of health that constitute these living conditions – shape health. The neo-materialist explanation extends the materialist analysis by asking how these living conditions come about. The psychosocial comparison explanation considers whether people compare themselves to others and how these comparisons affect health and wellbeing.

The wealth of nations is a strong indicator of population health. But within nations, socio-economic position is a powerful predictor of health as it is an indicator of material advantage or disadvantage over the lifespan. Material conditions of life determine health by influencing the quality of individual development, family life and interaction, and community environments. Material conditions of life lead to differing likelihood of physical (infections, malnutrition, chronic disease, and injuries), developmental (delayed or impaired cognitive, personality, and social development), educational (learning disabilities, poor learning, early school leaving), and social (socialization, preparation for work, and family life) problems. Overall wealth of nations is a strong indicator of population health. But within nations, socio-economic position is a powerful predictor of health as it is an indicator of material advantage or disadvantage over the lifespan. Material conditions of life also lead to differences in psychosocial stress. The fight-or-flight reaction – chronically elicited in response to threats such as income, housing, and food insecurity, among others – weakens the immune system, leads to increased insulin resistance, greater incidence of lipid and clotting disorders, and other biomedical insults that are precursors to adult disease.

Adoption of health-threatening behaviours is also influenced by material deprivation and stress. Environments influence whether individuals take up tobacco, use alcohol, experience poor diets, and have low levels of physical activity. Tobacco and excessive alcohol use, and carbohydrate-dense diets are also means of coping with difficult circumstances. The materialist approach offers insight into the sources of health inequalities among individuals and nations and the role played by the social determinants of health.

The neo-materialist approach is concerned with how nations, regions, and cities differ on how economic and other resources are distributed among the population. This distribution of resources can vary widely from country to country. The neo-materialist view therefore, directs attention to both the effects of living conditions – the social determinants of health – on individuals' health and the societal factors that determine the quality of the distribution of these social determinants of health. How a society decides to distribute resources among citizens is especially important.

The social comparison approach holds that the social determinants of health play their role through citizens' interpretations of their standings in the social hierarchy. There are two mechanisms by which this occurs. At the individual level, the perception and experience of one's status in unequal societies lead to stress and poor health. Feelings of shame, worthlessness, and envy can lead to harmful effects upon neuro-endocrine, autonomic and metabolic, and immune systems. Comparisons to those of a higher social class can also lead to attempts to alleviate such feelings by overspending, taking on additional employment that threaten health, and adopting health-threatening coping behaviours such as overeating and using alcohol and tobacco. At the communal level, widening and strengthening of hierarchy weakens social cohesion, which is a determinant of health. The social comparison approach directs attention to the psychosocial effects of public policies that weaken the social determinants of health. However, these effects may be secondary to how societies distribute material resources and provide security to its citizens, which are described in the materialist and neo-materialist approaches.

Life-course Perspective

Life-course approaches emphasize the accumulated effects of experience across the life span in understanding the maintenance of health and the onset of disease. The economic and social conditions – the social determinants of health – under which individuals live their lives have a cumulative effect upon the probability of developing any number of diseases, including heart disease and stroke Studies into the childhood and adulthood antecedents of adult-onset diabetes show that adverse economic and social conditions across the life span predispose individuals to this disorder.

Hertzman outlines three health effects that have relevance for a life-course perspective. Latent effects are biological or developmental early life experiences that influence health later in life. Low birth weight, for instance, is a reliable predictor of incidence of cardiovascular disease and adult-onset diabetes in later life. Experience of nutritional deprivation during childhood has lasting health effects.

Pathway effects are experiences that set individuals onto trajectories that influence health, well-being, and competence over the life course. As one example, children who enter school with delayed vocabulary are set upon a path that leads to lower educational expectations, poor employment prospects, and greater likelihood of illness and disease across the lifespan. Deprivation associated with poor-quality neighbourhoods, schools, and housing sets children off on paths that are not conducive to health and well-being.

Cumulative effects are the accumulation of advantage or disadvantage over time that manifests itself in poor health. These involve the combination of latent and pathways effects. Adopting a life-course perspective directs attention to how social determinants of health operate at every level of development – early childhood, childhood, adolescence, and adulthood – to both immediately influence health and provide the basis for health or illness later in life.

Chronic Stress and Health

Stress is hypothesised to be a major influence in the social determinants of health. There is a relationship between experience of chronic stress and negative health outcomes. There are two ways that this relationship is explained, through both direct and indirect effects of chronic stress on health outcomes.

One possible reason for the relationship between chronic stress and health outcomes is the effect that stress has on the physiology of a person. This is referred to as a direct relationship between chronic stress and health. The long term stress hormone, cortisol, is believed to be the key driver in this relationship. Chronic stress has been found to be significantly associated with chronic low grade inflammation, slower wound healing, increased susceptibility to infections, and poorer responses to vaccines. For example, a study of otherwise healthy adult males found that those with high levels of perceived stress in their lives had significantly longer wound healing times, and that elevated cortisol levels, rather than health behaviour responses, appeared to be the main reason for this relationship. Meta-analysis of healing studies has found that there is a robust relationship between elevated stress levels and slower healing for many different acute and chronic conditions However, it is also important to note that certain factors, such as coping styles and social support, can mitigate the relationship between chronic stress and health outcomes.

Stress can also be seen to have an indirect effect on health status. One way this happens is due to the strain on the psychological resources of the stressed individual. Chronic stress is common in those of a low socio-economic status, who are having to balance worries about financial security, how they will feed their families, housing status, and many other concerns. Therefore, individuals with these kinds of worries may lack the emotional resources to adopt positive health behaviours. Chronically stressed individuals may therefore be less likely to be able to prioritise their health.

In addition to this, the way that an individual responds to stress can influence their health status. Often, individuals responding to chronic stress will develop coping behaviours, some of which have a positive influences on health and others which have a negative influence. People who cope with stress through positive behaviours such as exercise or social connections may not be as affected by the relationship between stress and health, whereas those with a coping style more prone to over consumption (i.e. emotional eating, drinking, smoking or drug use) are more likely to be see negative health effects of stress. For example, a laboratory study has shown that, while stress did not alter calorie intake or food type eaten when averaged across the sample as a whole, when looking at a subset of the sample who were classed as emotional eaters, high stress levels were associated with eating more high fat and sweet food and a more calorie dense meal overall. Therefore, the authors conclude that stress may compromise the health of certain susceptible individuals (I.e those with an emotional eating coping style).

The detrimental effects of stress on health outcomes are hypothesised to partly explain why countries that have high levels of income inequality have poorer health outcomes compared to more equal countries. Wilkinson and Picket hypothesise in their book The Spirit Level that the stressors associated with low social status are amplified in societies where others are clearly far better off.

Improving Health Conditions Worldwide

Reducing the health gap in a generation requires that governments build systems that allow a healthy standard of living where no one should fall below due to circumstances beyond his or her control. Social protection schemes can be instrumental in realizing developmental goals rather than being dependent on achieving those goals. They can be effective ways to reduce poverty and local economies can benefit.

Policies to reduce child poverty are particularly important, as elevated stress hormones in children interfere with the development of brain circuitry and connections, causing long term chemical damage. Studies showed that the immune system of participants were stronger if their parents had the security of home ownership while the participants were growing up. In most wealthy countries, the relative child poverty rate is 10 percent or less; in the United States, it is 21.9 percent. The lowest poverty rates are more common in smaller well-developed and high-spending welfare states like Sweden and Finland, with about 5 or 6 percent. Middle-level rates are found in major European countries where unemployment compensation is more generous and social policies provide more generous support to single mothers and working women (through paid family leave, for example), and where social assistance minimums are high. For instance, the Netherlands, Austria, Belgium and Germany have poverty rates that are in the 7 to 8 percent range.

The Commission on Social Determinants of Health (CSDH) in 2005 made recommendations for action to promote health equity based on 3 principles of action: "improve the circumstances in which people are born, grow, live, work, and age; tackle the inequitable distribution of power, money, and resources, the structural drivers of conditions of daily life, globally, nationally, and locally; and measure the problem, evaluate action, and expand the knowledge base." These recommendations would involve providing resources such as quality education, decent housing, access to affordable health care, access to healthy food, and safe places to exercise for everyone despite gaps in affluence. Expansion of knowledge of the social determinants of health, including among healthcare workers, can improve the quality and standard of care for people who are marginalized, poor or living in developing nations by preventing early death and disability while working to improve quality of life.

Public Policy

The Rio Political Declaration on Social Determinants of Health embraces a transparent, participatory model of policy development that, among other things, addresses the social determinants of health leading to persistent health inequalities for indigenous peoples.

The United States Department of Health and Human Services includes social determinants in its model of population health, and one of its missions is to strengthen policies which are backed by the best available evidence and knowledge in the field Social determinants of health do not exist in a vacuum. Their quality and availability to the population are usually a result of public policy decisions made by governing authorities. For example, early life is shaped by availability of sufficient material resources that assure adequate educational opportunities, food and housing among others. Much of this has to do with the employment security and the quality of working conditions and wages. The availability of quality, regulated childcare is an especially important policy option in support of early life. These are not issues that usually come under individual control but rather they are socially constructed conditions which require institutional responses. A policy-oriented approach places such findings within a broader policy context. In this context, Health in All Policies has seen as a response to incorporate health and health equity into all public policies as means to foster synergy between sectors and ultimately promote health.

Yet it is not uncommon to see governmental and other authorities individualize these issues. Governments may view early life as being primarily about parental behaviours towards their children. They then focus upon promoting better parenting, assist in having parents read to their children, or urge schools to foster exercise among children rather than raising the amount of financial or housing resources available to families. Indeed, for every social determinant of health, an individualized manifestation of each is available. There is little evidence to suggest the efficacy of such approaches in improving the health status of those most vulnerable to illness in the absence of efforts to modify their adverse living conditions.

One of the recommendations by the CSDH is expanding knowledge – particularly to health care workers.

Power

A recent article outlines the role that "raw power" plays in shaping the distribution of the social determinants of health through public policy action. Here the business sector is seen as shaping public policy to increase profits at the expense of the population's health. This is a political economy approach that is typically ignored in discussions of the social determinants of health.

References

- "Healthy People 2020 Framework" (PDF). United States Department of Health and Human Services. 2010. Retrieved 2013-03-27
- Kumar, Rajiv; Goel, Naveen K. (2008). "Current Status Of Cardiovascular Risk Due To Stress". Internet Journal of Health. 7 (1): 19. doi:10.5580/1e7c
- Raphael, Dennis (2010). Staying Alive: Critical Perspectives on Health, Illness, and Health Care. Canada: Canadian Scholars' Press. p. 159. ISBN 9781551303703
- Gouin, J.-P. (2011). "Chronic Stress, Immune Dysregulation, and Health". American Journal of Lifestyle Medicine. 5 (6): 476–85. doi:10.1177/1559827610395467
- Raphael, D. (2001). Inequality is Bad for our Hearts: Why Low Income and Social Exclusion are Major Causes of Heart Disease in Canada. ISBN 0-9689444-0-X
- Kajang, Y.G (2015). "INDICES THAT CAN ENSURE THE HEALTH SECURITY OF CHILDREN IN NIGERIA" (PDF). International Journal of Information Research and Review. 2: 371–375

- Esping-Andersen, Gøsta (2002). "A Child-Centred Social Investment Strategy". In Esping-Andersen, Gøsta. Why We Need a New Welfare State. pp. 26–67. ISBN 978-0-19-925642-6
- World Conference on Social Determinants of Health (2011). "Rio Political Declaration on Social Determinants of Health" (PDF). World Health Organization. Retrieved 2013-03-27
- Smeeding, Timothy (2006). "Poor People in Rich Nations: The United States in Comparative Perspective" (PDF). Journal of Economic Perspectives. 20: 69–90
- Wilkinson, Richard; Marmot, Michael, eds. (2003). The Social Determinants of Health: The Solid Facts (PDF) (2nd ed.). World Health Organization Europe. ISBN 978-92-890-1371-0
- Smeeding, Timothy (2006). "Poor People in Rich Nations: The United States in Comparative Perspective". Journal of Economic Perspectives. 20 (1): 69–90. doi:10.1257/089533006776526094. JSTOR 30033634

2

Population Health: An Integrated Study

Population health aims to improve the well being of the whole population. Individuals are grouped differently according to income and their health determinants are determined accordingly. Policies and health outcomes are also taken into account. Public health management is best understood in confluence with the major topics listed in the following chapter.

Population Health

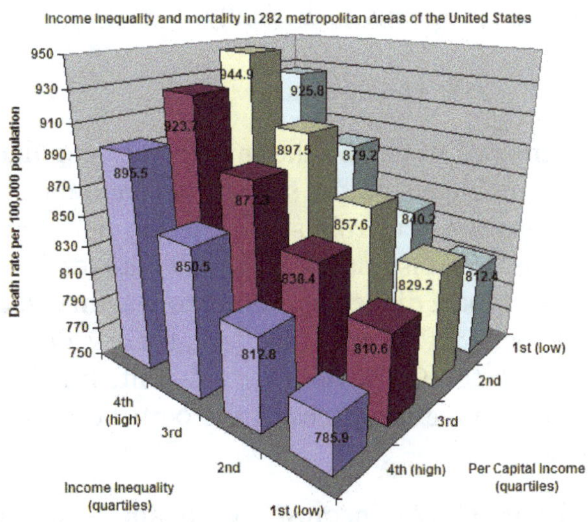

Income inequality and mortality in 282 metropolitan areas of the United States.
Mortality is correlated with both income and inequality.

Population health has been defined as"the health outcomes of a group of individuals, including the distribution of such outcomes within the group". It is an approach to health that aims to improve the health of an entire human population. This concept does not refer to animal or plant populations. It has been described as consisting of three components. These are "health outcomes, patterns of health determinants, and policies and interventions". A priority considered important in achieving the aim of Population Health is to reduce health inequities or disparities among different population groups due to, among other factors, the social determinants of health, SDOH. The SDOH include all the factors: social, environmental, cultural and physical the different populations are born into, grow up and function with throughout their lifetimes which potentially have a measurable impact on the health of human populations. The Population Health concept represents a change in the focus from the individual-level, characteristic of most mainstream medicine. It also seeks to complement the classic efforts of public health agencies by addressing a broader range of factors shown to impact the health of different populations. The World Health Organization's

Commission on Social Determinants of Health, reported in 2008, that the SDOH factors were responsible for the bulk of diseases and injuries and these were the major causes of health inequities in all countries. In the US, SDOH were estimated to account for 70% of avoidable mortality.

From a population health perspective, health has been defined not simply as a state free from disease but as "the capacity of people to adapt to, respond to, or control life's challenges and changes". The World Health Organization (WHO) defined health in its broader sense in 1946 as "a state of complete physical, mental, and social well-being and not merely the absence of disease or infirmity."

Healthy People 2020

Healthy People 2020 is a web site sponsored by the US Department of Health and Human Services, representing the cumulative effort of 34 years of interest by the Surgeon General's office and others. It identifies 42 topics considered social determinants of health and approximately 1200 specific goals considered to improve population health. It provides links to the current research available for selected topics and identifies and supports the need for community involvement considered essential to address these problems realistically.

The Human Role of Economic Inequality

Recently, human role has been encouraged by the influence of population growth there has been increasing interest from epidemiologists on the subject of economic inequality and its relation to the health of populations. There is a very robust correlation between socioeconomic status and health. This correlation suggests that it is not only the poor who tend to be sick when everyone else is healthy, heart disease, ulcers, type 2 diabetes, rheumatoid arthritis, certain types of cancer, and premature aging. Despite the reality of the SES Gradient, there is debate as to its cause. A number of researchers (A. Leigh, C. Jencks, A. Clarkwest) see a definite link between economic status and mortality due to the greater economic resources of the better-off, but they find little correlation due to social status differences.

Other researchers such as Richard G. Wilkinson, J. Lynch, and G.A. Kaplan have found that socioeconomic status strongly affects health even when controlling for economic resources and access to health care. Most famous for linking social status with health are the Whitehall studies—a series of studies conducted on civil servants in London. The studies found that, despite the fact that all civil servants in England have the same access to health care, there was a strong correlation between social status and health. The studies found that this relationship stayed strong even when controlling for health-affecting habits such as exercise, smoking and drinking. Furthermore, it has been noted that no amount of medical attention will help decrease the likelihood of someone getting type 1 diabetes or rheumatoid arthritis—yet both are more common among populations with lower socioeconomic status. Lastly, it has been found that amongst the wealthiest quarter of countries on earth (a set stretching from Luxembourg to Slovakia) there is no relation between a country's wealth and general population health—suggesting that past a certain level, absolute levels of wealth have little impact on population health, but relative levels within a country do. The concept of psychosocial stress attempts to explain how psychosocial phenomenon such as status and social stratification can lead to the many diseases associated with the SES gradient. Higher levels of economic inequality tend to intensify social hierarchies and generally degrades the quality of social relations—leading to greater levels of stress and stress related diseases. Richard Wilkinson found this to be true not only for the poorest members of society, but also for the wealthiest. Economic inequality is bad for everyone's health. Inequality does not only affect the health of human populations. David H. Abbott at the Wisconsin National Primate Research Center found that among many primate species, less egalitarian social structures correlated with higher levels of stress hormones among socially subordinate individuals. Research by Robert Sapolsky of Stanford University provides similar findings.

Research

There is well-documented variation in health outcomes and health care utilization & costs by geographic variation in the U.S., down to the level of Hospital Referral Regions (defined as a regional health care market, which may cross state boundaries, of which there are 306 in the U.S.). There is ongoing debate as to the relative contributions of race, gender, poverty, education level and place to these variations. The Office of Epidemiology of the Maternal and Child Health Bureau recommends using an analytic approach (Fixed Effects or hybrid Fixed Effects) to research on health disparities to reduce the confounding effects of neighborhood (geographic) variables on the outcomes.

The Importance of Family Planning Programs

Family planning programs (including contraceptives, sexuality education, and promotion of safe sex) play a major role in population health. Family planning is one of the most highly cost-effective interventions in medicine. Family planning saves lives and money by reducing unintended pregnancy and the transmission of sexually transmitted infections.

For example, the United States Agency for International Development lists as benefits of its international family planning program:

- "Protecting the health of women by reducing high-risk pregnancies"
- "Protecting the health of children by allowing sufficient time between pregnancies"
- "Fighting HIV/AIDS through providing information, counseling, and access to male and female condoms"
- "Reducing abortions"
- "Supporting women's rights and opportunities for education, employment, and full participation in society"
- "Protecting the environment by stabilizing population growth"

Population Health Management (PHM)

One method to improve population health is population health management (PHM), which has been defined as "the technical field of endeavor which utilizes a variety of individual, organizational and cultural interventions to help improve the morbidity patterns (i.e., the illness and injury burden) and the health care use behavior of defined populations". PHM is distinguished from disease management by including more chronic conditions and diseases, by use of "a single point of contact and coordination", and by "predictive modeling across multiple clinical conditions". PHM is considered broader than disease management in that it also includes "intensive care management for individuals at the highest level of risk" and "personal health management... for those at lower levels of predicted health risk". Many PHM-related articles are published in *Population Health Management*, the official journal of DMAA: The Care Continuum Alliance.

The following road map has been suggested for helping healthcare organizations navigate the path toward implementing effective population health management:

- Establish precise patient registries
- Determine patient-provider attribution
- Define precise numerators in the patient registries
- Monitor and measure clinical and cost metrics
- Adhere to basic clinical practice guidelines
- Engage in risk-management outreach
- Acquire external data
- Communicate with patients
- Educate patients and engage with them
- Establish and adhere to complex clinical practice guidelines
- Coordinate effectively between care team and patient
- Track specific outcomes

Healthcare Reform and Population Health

Healthcare reform is driving change to traditional hospital reimbursement models. Prior to the introduction of the Patient Protection and Affordable Care Act (PPACA), hospitals were reimbursed based on the volume of procedures through fee-for-service models. Under the PPACA, reimbursement models are shifting from volume to value. New reimbursement models are built around pay for performance, a value-based reimbursement approach, which places financial incentives around patient outcomes and has drastically changed the way US hospitals must conduct business to remain financially viable. In addition to focusing on improving patient experience of care and reducing costs, hospitals must also focus on improving the health of populations (IHI Triple Aim).

As participation in value-based reimbursement models such as accountable care organizations (ACOs) increases, these initiatives will help drive population health. Within the ACO model, hospitals have to meet specific quality benchmarks, focus on prevention, and carefully manage patients with chronic diseases. Providers get paid more for keeping their patients healthy and out of the hospital. Studies have shown that inpatient admission rates have dropped over the past ten years in communities that were early adopters of the ACO model and implemented population health measures to treat "less sick" patients in the outpatient setting. A study conducted in the Chicago area showed a decline in inpatient utilization rates across all age groups, which was an average of a 5% overall drop in inpatient admissions.

Hospitals are finding it financially advantageous to focus on population health management and keeping people in the community well. The goal of population health management is to improve patient outcomes and increase health capital. Other goals include preventing disease, closing care gaps, and cost savings for providers. In the last few years, more effort has been directed towards developing telehealth services, community-based clinics in areas with high proportion of residents using the emergency department as primary care, and patient care coordinator roles to coordinate healthcare services across the care continuum.

Health can be considered a capital good; health capital is part of human capital as defined by the Grossman model. Health can be considered both an investment good and consumption good. Factors such as obesity and smoking have negative effects on health capital, while education, wage rate, and age may also impact health capital. When people are healthier through preventative care, they have the potential to live a longer and healthier life, work more and participate in the economy, and produce more based on the work done. These factors all have the potential to increase earnings. Some states, like New York, have implemented statewide initiatives to address population health. In New York state there are 11 such programs. One example is the Mohawk Valley Population Health Improvement Program. These programs work to address the needs of the people in their region, as well as assist their local community based organizations and social services to gather data, address health disparities, and explore evidence-based interventions that will ultimately lead to better health for everyone.

Global Health

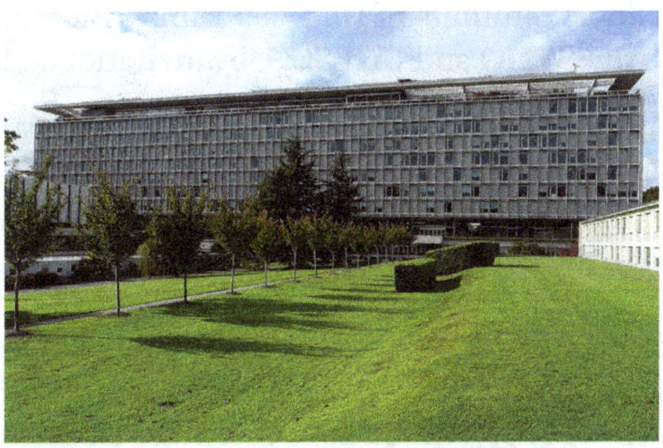

Headquarters of the World Health Organization in Geneva, Switzerland.

Global health is the health of populations in the global context; it has been defined as "the area of study, research and practice that places a priority on improving health and achieving equity in health for all people worldwide". Problems that transcend national borders or have a global political and economic impact are often emphasized. Thus, global health is about worldwide health improvement (including mental health), reduction of disparities, and protection against global threats that disregard national borders. Global health is not international health, which is defined as the branch of public health focusing on developing nations and foreign aid efforts by industrialized countries. Global health can be measured as a function of various global diseases and their prevalence in the world and threat to decrease life in the present day.

The predominant agency associated with global health (and international health) is the World Health Organization (WHO). Other important agencies impacting global health include UNICEF, World Food Programme, and the World Bank. The United Nations has also played a part with declaration of the Millennium Development Goals and the more recent Sustainable Development Goals.

Definition

Global health employs several perspectives that focus on the determinants and distribution of health in international contexts:

- Medicine describes the pathology of diseases and promotes prevention, diagnosis, and treatment.
- Public health emphasizes the health of populations.
- Epidemiology helps identify risk factors and causes of health problems.
- Demography provides data for policy decisions.
- Economics emphasizes the cost-effectiveness and cost-benefit approaches for the optimal allocation of health resources.
- Other social sciences such as sociology, development studies, psychology, anthropology, cultural studies, and law can help understand the determinants of health in societies.

Both individuals and organizations working in the domain of global health often face many questions regarding ethical and human rights. Critical examination of the various causes and justifications of health inequities is necessary for the success of proposed solutions. Such issues are discussed at the bi-annual Global Summits of National Ethics/Bioethics Councils, next in March 2016 in Berlin, with experts from WHO and UNESCO, by invitation of the German Ethics Council.

History

The 19th century held major discoveries in medicine and public health. The Broad Street cholera outbreak of 1854 was central to the development of modern epidemiology. The microorganisms responsible for malaria and tuberculosis were identified in 1880 and 1882, respectively. The 20th century saw the development of preventive and curative treatments for many diseases, including the BCG vaccine (for tuberculosis) and penicillin in the 1920s. The eradication of smallpox, with the last naturally occurring case recorded in 1977, raised hope that other diseases could be eradicated as well.

Important steps were taken towards global cooperation in health with the formation of the United Nations (UN) and the World Bank Group in 1945, after World War II. In 1948, the member states of the newly formed United Nations gathered to create the World Health Organization. A cholera epidemic that took 20,000 lives in Egypt in 1947 and 1948 helped spur the international community to action. The WHO published its Model List of Essential Medicines, and the 1978 Alma Ata declaration underlined the importance of primary health care.

At a United Nations Summit in 2000, member nations declared eight Millennium Development Goals (MDGs), which reflected the major challenges facing human development globally, to be achieved by 2015. The declaration was matched by unprecedented global investment by donor and recipient countries. According to the UN, these MDGs provided an important framework for development and significant progress has been made in a number of areas. However, progress has been uneven and some of the MDGs were not fully realized including maternal, newborn and child health and reproductive health. Building on the MDGs, a new Sustainable Development Agenda with 17 Sustainable Development Goals (SDGs) has been established for the years 2016-2030. The first goal being an ambitious and historic pledge to end poverty. On 25 September 2015, the 193 countries of the UN General Assembly adopted the 2030 Development Agenda titled *Transforming our world: the 2030 Agenda for Sustainable Development.*

In 2015 a book titled "To Save Humanity" was published, with nearly 100 essays regarding today's most pressing global health issues. The essays were authored by global figures in politics, science, and advocacy ranging from Bill Clinton to Peter Piot, and addressed a wide range of issues including vaccinations, antimicrobial resistance, health coverage, tobacco use, research methodology, climate change, equity, access to medicine, and media coverage of health research.

Measures

Measures of global health include disability-adjusted life year (DALY), quality-adjusted life years (QALYs), and mortality rate.

Disability-adjusted Life Years

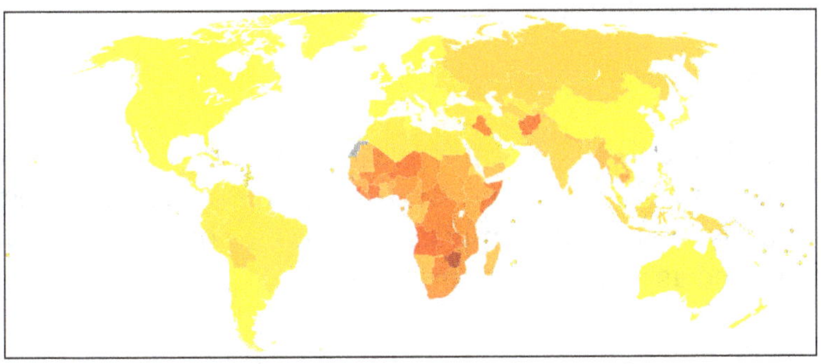

Disability-adjusted life years per 100,000 people in 2004.

No data
Less than 9,250
9,250–16,000
16,000–22,750
22,750–29,500
29,500–36,250
36,250–43,000
43,000–49,750
49,750–56,500
56,500–63,250
63,250–70,000
70,000–80,000
Over 80000

The DALY is a summary measure that combines the impact of illness, disability, and mortality by measuring the time lived with disability and the time lost due to premature mortality. One DALY can be thought of as one lost year of "healthy" life. The DALY for a disease is the sum of the years of life lost due to premature mortality and the years lost due to disability for incident cases of the health condition.

Quality-adjusted Life Years

QALYs combine expected survival with expected quality of life into a single number: if an additional year of healthy life is worth a value of one (year), then a year of less healthy life is worth less than one (year). QALY calculations are based on measurements of the value that individuals place on expected years of survival. Measurements can be made in several ways: by techniques that simulate gambles about preferences for alternative states of health, with surveys or analyses that infer willingness to pay for alternative states of health, or through instruments that are based on trading off some or all likely survival time that a medical intervention might provide in order to gain less survival time of higher quality.

Infant and Child Mortality

Infant mortality and child mortality for children under age 5 are more specific than DALYs or QALYs in representing the health in the poorest sections of a population, and are thus especially useful when focusing on health equity.

Morbidity

Morbidity measures include incidence rate, prevalence, and cumulative incidence, with incidence rate referring to the risk of developing a new health condition within a specified period of time. Although sometimes loosely expressed simply as the number of new cases during a time period, morbidity is better expressed as a proportion or a rate.

Health Conditions

The diseases and health conditions targeted by global health initiatives are sometimes grouped under "diseases of poverty" versus "diseases of affluence", although the impact of globalization is increasingly blurring the lines between the two.

Respiratory Infections

Infections of the respiratory tract and middle ear are major causes of morbidity and mortality worldwide. Some respiratory infections of global significance include tuberculosis, measles, influenza, and pneumonias caused by pneumococci and *Haemophilus influenzae*. The spread of respiratory infections is exacerbated by crowded conditions, and poverty is associated with more than a 20-fold increase in the relative burden of lung infections.

Diarrheal Diseases

Diarrhea is the second most common cause of child mortality worldwide, responsible for 17% of deaths of children under age 5. Poor sanitation can increase transmission of bacteria and viruses through water, food, utensils, hands, and flies. Dehydration due to diarrhea can be effectively treated through oral rehydration therapy with dramatic reductions in mortality. Important nutritional measures include the promotion of breastfeeding and zinc supplementation. While hygienic measures alone may be insufficient for the prevention of rotavirus diarrhea, it can be prevented by a safe and potentially cost-effective vaccine.

Maternal Health

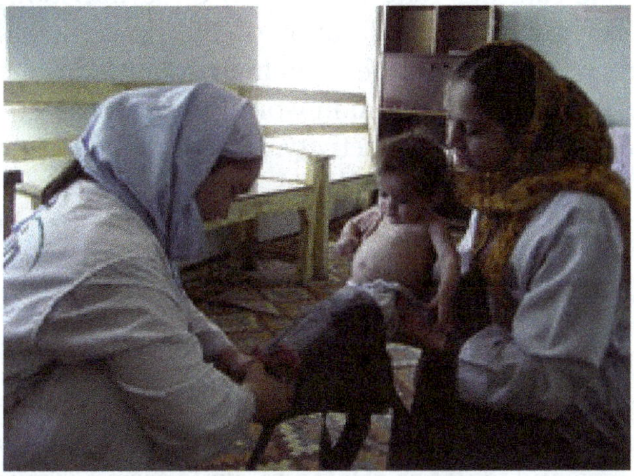

Maternal health clinic in Afghanistan

Complications of pregnancy and childbirth are the leading causes of death among women of reproductive age in many developing countries: a woman dies from complications from childbirth approximately every minute. According to the World Health Organization's 2005 World Health Report, poor maternal conditions are the fourth leading cause of death for women worldwide, after HIV/AIDS, malaria, and tuberculosis. Most maternal deaths and injuries can be prevented, and such deaths have been largely eradicated in the developed world. Targets for improving maternal health include increasing the number of deliveries accompanied by skilled birth attendants.

68 low-income countries tracked by the WHO- and UNICEF-led collaboration *Countdown to 2015* are estimated to hold for 97% of worldwide maternal and child deaths.

HIV/AIDS

Human immunodeficiency virus (HIV) is transmitted through unprotected sex, unclean needles, blood transfusions, and from mother to child during birth or lactation. Globally, HIV is primarily spread through sexual intercourse. The infection damages the immune system, leading to acquired immunodeficiency syndrome (AIDS) and eventually, death. Antiretroviral drugs prolong life and delay the onset of AIDS by minimizing the amount of HIV in the body.

Malaria

Malaria is a mosquito-borne infectious disease caused by the parasites of the genus *Plasmodium*. Symptoms may include fever, headaches, chills, and nausea. Each year, there are approximately 500 million cases of malaria worldwide, most commonly among children and pregnant women in developing countries. The use of insecticide-treated bednets is a cost-effective way to reduce deaths from malaria, as is prompt artemisin-based combination therapy, supported by intermittent preventive therapy in pregnancy.

Nutrition

In 2010, about 104 million children were underweight, and undernutrition contributes to about one third of child deaths around the world. (Undernutrition is not *malnutrition*, which refers to poor *proportion* of food intake and can thus refer to obesity.) Undernutrition impairs the immune system, increasing the frequency, severity, and duration of infections (including measles, pneumonia, and diarrhea). Infection can further contribute to malnutrition. Deficiencies of micronutrient, such as vitamin A, iron, iodine, and zinc, are common worldwide and can compromise intellectual potential, growth, development, and adult productivity. Interventions to prevent malnutrition include micronutrient supplementation, fortification of basic grocery foods, dietary diversification, hygienic measures to reduce spread of infections, and the promotion of breastfeeding.

Violence Against Women

Violence against women has been defined as: "physical, sexual and psychological violence occurring in the family and in the general community, including battering, sexual abuse of children, dowry-related violence, rape, female genital mutilation and other traditional practices harmful to women, non-spousal violence and violence related to exploitation, sexual harassment and intimidation at work, in educational institutions and elsewhere, trafficking in women, forced prostitution and violence perpetrated or condoned by the state." In addition to causing injury, violence may increase "women's long-term risk of a number of other health problems, including chronic pain, physical disability, drug and alcohol abuse, and depression".

Although statistics can be difficult to obtain as many cases go unreported, it is estimated that one in every five women faces some form of violence during her lifetime, in some cases leading to serious injury or even death. Risk factors for being a perpetrator include low education, past exposure to child maltreatment or witnessing violence between parents, harmful use of alcohol, attitudes accepting of violence and gender inequality. Equality of women has been addressed in the Millennium development goals.

Chronic Disease

Approximately 80% of deaths linked to non-communicable diseases occur in developing countries. Increases in refugee urbanization, has led to a growing number of people diagnosed with chronic noncommunicable diseases.

In September 2011, the United Nations is hosting its first General Assembly Special Summit on the issue of non-communicable diseases. Noting that non-communicable diseases are the cause of some 35 million deaths each year, the international community is being increasingly called to take measures for the prevention and control of chronic diseases and mitigate their impacts on the world population, especially on women, who are usually the primary caregivers.

For example, the rate of type 2 diabetes, associated with obesity, has been on the rise in countries previously plagued by hunger. In low-income countries, the number of individuals with diabetes is expected to increase from 84 million to 228 million by 2030. Obesity, a preventable condition, is associated with numerous chronic diseases, including cardiovascular conditions, stroke, certain cancers, and respiratory disease. About 16% of the global burden of disease, measured as DALYs, has been accounted for by obesity.

Neglected Tropical Diseases

More than one billion people were treated for at least one neglected tropical disease in 2015. Neglected tropical diseases are a diverse group of infectious diseases that are endemic in tropical and subtropical regions of 149 countries, primarily effecting low and middle income populations in Africa, Asia, and Latin America. They are variously caused by bacteria (Trachoma, Leprosy), viruses (Dengue, Rabies), protozoa (Human African trypanosomiasis, Chagas), and helminths (Schistosomiasis, Onchocerciasis, Soil transmitted helminths). The Global Burden of Disease Study concluded that neglected tropical diseases comprehensively contributed to approximately 26.06 million disability-adjusted life years in 2010, as well as significant deleterious economic effects. In 2011, the World Health Organization launched a 2020 Roadmap for neglected tropical diseases, aiming for the control or elimination of 10 common diseases. The 2012 London Declaration builds on this initiative, and called on endemic countries and the international community to improve access to clean water and basic sanitation, improved living conditions, vector control, and health education, to reach the 2020 goals. In 2017, a WHO report cited 'unprecedented progress' against neglected tropical diseases since 2007, especially due to mass drug administration of drugs donated by pharmaceutical companies.

Health Interventions

Global interventions for improved child health and survival include the promotion of breastfeeding, zinc supplementation, vitamin A fortification, salt iodization, hygiene interventions such as hand-washing, vaccinations, and treatments of severe acute malnutrition. The Global Health Council suggests a list of 32 treatments and health interventions that could potentially save several million lives each year.

Many populations face an "outcome gap", which refers to the gap between members of a population who have access to medical treatment versus those who do not. Countries facing outcome gaps lack sustainable infrastructure. In Guatemala, a subset of the public sector, the *Programa de Accessibilidad a los Medicamentos* ("Program for Access to Medicines"), had the lowest average availability (25%) compared to the private sector (35%). In the private sector, highest- and lowest-priced medicines were 22.7 and 10.7 times more expensive than international reference prices respectively. Treatments were generally unaffordable, costing as much as 15 days wages for a course of the antibiotic ceftriaxone. The public sector in Pakistan, while having access to medicines at a lower price than international reference prices, has a chronic shortage of and lack of access to basic medicines.

Journalist Laurie Garrett argues that the field of global health is not plagued by a lack of funds, but that more funds do not always translate into positive outcomes. The problem lies in the way these funds are allocated, as they are often disproportionately allocated to alleviating a single disease.

In its 2006 World Health Report, the WHO estimated a shortage of almost 4.3 million doctors, midwives, nurses, and support workers worldwide, especially in sub-Saharan Africa.

Community Health

Community health is a major field of study within the medical and clinical sciences which focuses on the maintenance, protection and improvement of the health status of population groups and communities as opposed to the health of individual patients. It is a distinct field of study that may be taught within a separate school of public health or environmental health.

It is a discipline which concerns itself with the study and improvement of the health characteristics of biological communities. While the term community can be broadly defined, community health tends to focus on geographical areas rather than people with shared characteristics. The health characteristics of a community are often examined using geographic information system (GIS) software and public health datasets. Some projects, such as InfoShare or GEOPROJ combine GIS with existing datasets, allowing the general public to examine the characteristics of any given community in participating countries.

Because 'health III' (broadly defined as well-being) is influenced by a wide array of socio-demographic characteristics, relevant variables range from the proportion of residents of a given age group to the overall life expectancy of the neighborhood/community. Medical interventions aimed at improving the health of a community range from improving access to medical care to public health communications campaigns. Recent research efforts have focused on how the built environment and socio-economic status affect health.

Community health may be studied within three broad categories:

- Primary healthcare which refers to interventions that focus on the individual or family such as hand-washing, immunization, circumcision, personal dietary choices, and lifestyle improvement.
- Secondary healthcare refers to those activities which focus on the environment such as draining puddles of water near the house, clearing bushes, and spraying insecticides to control vectors like mosquitoes.
- Tertiary healthcare on the other hand refers to those interventions that take place in a hospital setting, such as intravenous rehydration or surgery.

The success of community health programmes relies upon the transfer of information from health professionals to the general public using one-to-one or one to many communication (mass communication). The latest shift is towards health marketing.

Academic Resources

- *Journal of Urban Health*, Springer. ISSN 1468-2869 (electronic) ISSN 1099-3460 (paper).

Environmental Health

Environmental health is the branch of public health that is concerned with all aspects of the natural and built environment that may affect human health. Other terms referring to or concerning environmental health are environmental public health, and public health protection / environmental health protection. Environmental health and environmental protection are very much related. Environmental health is focused on the natural and built environments for the benefit of human health, whereas environmental protection is concerned with protecting the natural environment for the benefit of human health and the ecosystem.

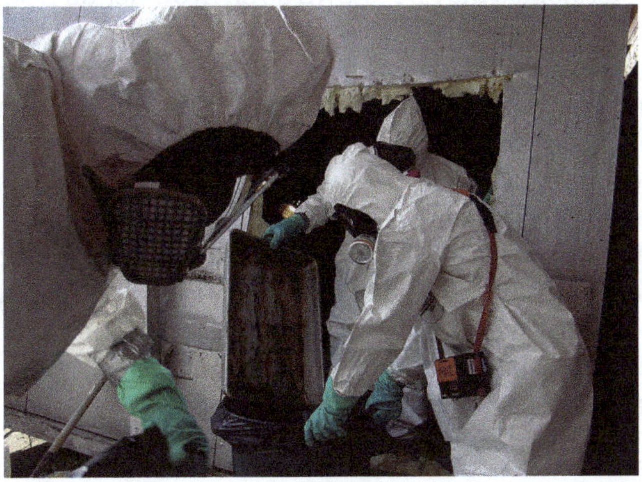

FEMA/EPA Hazardous Materials Team removing hazards left in the wake of Hurricane Katrina, 2005.

Definitions

Environmental health has been defined in a 1999 document by the World Health Organization (WHO) as:

> Those aspects of the human health and disease that are determined by factors in the environment. It also refers to the theory and practice of assessing and controlling factors in the environment that can potentially affect health.
>
> Environmental health as used by the WHO Regional Office for Europe, includes both the direct pathological effects of chemicals, radiation and some biological agents, and the effects (often indirect) on health and well being of the broad physical, psychological, social and cultural environment, which includes housing, urban development, land use and transport.

As of 2016 the WHO website on environmental health states "Environmental health addresses all the physical, chemical, and biological factors external to a person, and all the related factors impacting behaviours. It encompasses the assessment and control of those environmental factors that can potentially affect health. It is targeted towards preventing disease and creating health-supportive environments. This definition excludes behaviour not related to environment, as well as behaviour related to the social and cultural environment, as well as genetics."

The WHO has also defined environmental health services as "those services which implement environmental health policies through monitoring and control activities. They also carry out that role by promoting the improvement of environmental parameters and by encouraging the use of environmentally friendly and healthy technologies and behaviors. They also have a leading role in developing and suggesting new policy areas."

The term environmental medicine may be seen as a medical specialty, or branch of the broader field of environmental health. Terminology is not fully established, and in many European countries they are used interchangeably.

Environmental Health Profession

Environmental health professionals may be known as environmental health officers, public health inspectors, environmental health specialists, environmental health practitioners, or sanitarians. Researchers and policy-makers also play important roles in how environmental health is practiced in the field. In many European countries, physicians and veterinarians are involved in environmental health. In the United Kingdom, practitioners must have a graduate degree in environmental health and be certified and registered with the Chartered Institute of Environmental Health or the Royal Environmental Health Institute of Scotland. In Canada, practitioners in environmental health are required to obtain an approved bachelor's degree in environmental health along with the national professional certificate, the Certificate in Public Health Inspection (Canada) CPHI(C). Many states in the United States also require that individuals have a bachelor's degree and professional licenses in order to practice environmental health. California state law defines the scope of practice of environmental health as follows:

> "Scope of practice in environmental health" means the practice of environmental health by registered environmental health specialists in the public and private sector within the meaning of this article and includes, but is not limited to, organization, management, education, enforcement, consultation, and emergency response for the purpose of prevention of environmental health hazards and the promotion and protection of the public health and the environment in the following areas: food protection; housing; institutional environmental health; land use; community noise control; recreational swimming areas and waters; electromagnetic radiation control; solid, liquid, and hazardous materials management; underground storage tank control; onsite septic systems; vector control; drinking water quality; water sanitation; emergency preparedness; and milk and dairy sanitation pursuant to Section 33113 of the Food and Agricultural Code.

The environmental health profession had its modern-day roots in the sanitary and public health movement of the United Kingdom. This was epitomized by Sir Edwin Chadwick, who was instrumental in the repeal of the poor laws, and in 1884 was the founding president of the Association of Public Sanitary Inspectors, now called the Chartered Institute of Environmental Health.

Disciplines

Five basic disciplines generally contribute to the field of environmental health: environmental epidemiology, toxicology, exposure science, environmental engineering, and environmental law. Each of these disciplines contributes different information to describe problems and solutions in environmental health, but there is some overlap among them.

- Environmental epidemiology studies the relationship between environmental exposures (including exposure to chemicals, radiation, microbiological agents, etc.) and human health. Observational studies, which simply observe exposures that people have already experienced, are common in environmental epidemiology because humans cannot ethically be exposed to agents that are known or suspected to cause disease. While the inability to use experimental study designs is a limitation of environmental epidemiology, this discipline directly observes effects on human health rather than estimating effects from animal studies.

- Toxicology studies how environmental exposures lead to specific health outcomes, generally in animals, as a means to understand possible health outcomes in humans. Toxicology has the advantage of being able to conduct randomized controlled trials and other experimental studies because they can use animal subjects. However there are many differences in animal and human biology, and there can be a lot of uncertainty when interpreting the results of animal studies for their implications for human health.

- Exposure science studies human exposure to environmental contaminants by both identifying and quantifying exposures. Exposure science can be used to support environmental epidemiology by better describing environmental exposures that may lead to a particular health outcome, identify common exposures whose health outcomes may be better understood through a toxicology study, or can be used in a risk assessment to determine whether current levels of exposure might exceed recommended levels. Exposure science has the advantage of being able to very accurately quantify exposures to specific chemicals, but it does not generate any information about health outcomes like environmental epidemiology or toxicology.

- Environmental engineering applies scientific and engineering principles for protection of human populations from the effects of adverse environmental factors; protection of environments from potentially deleterious effects of natural and human activities; and general improvement of environmental quality.

- Environmental law includes the network of treaties, statutes, regulations, common and customary laws addressing the effects of human activity on the natural environment.

Information from epidemiology, toxicology, and exposure science can be combined to conduct a risk assessment for specific chemicals, mixtures of chemicals or other risk factors to determine whether an exposure poses significant risk to human health (exposure would likely result in the development of pollution-related diseases). This can in turn be used to develop and implement environmental health policy that, for example, regulates chemical emissions, or imposes standards for proper sanitation. Actions of engineering and law can be combined to provide risk management to minimize, monitor, and otherwise manage the impact of exposure to protect human health to achieve the objectives of environmental health policy.

Concerns

Environmental health addresses all human-health-related aspects of the natural environment and the built environment. Environmental health concerns include:

- Air quality, including both ambient outdoor air and indoor air quality, which also comprises concerns about environmental tobacco smoke.

- Climate change and its effects on health.
- Disaster preparedness and response.
- Food safety, including in agriculture, transportation, food processing, wholesale and retail distribution and sale.
- Hazardous materials management, including hazardous waste management, contaminated site remediation, the prevention of leaks from underground storage tanks and the prevention of hazardous materials releases to the environment and responses to emergency situations resulting from such releases.
- Housing, including substandard housing abatement and the inspection of jails and prisons.
- Childhood lead poisoning prevention.
- Land use planning, including smart growth.
- Liquid waste disposal, including city waste water treatment plants and on-site waste water disposal systems, such as septic tank systems and chemical toilets.
- Medical waste management and disposal.
- Noise pollution control.
- Occupational health and industrial hygiene.
- Radiological health, including exposure to ionizing radiation from X-rays or radioactive isotopes.
- Recreational water illness prevention, including from swimming pools, spas and ocean and freshwater bathing places.
- Safe drinking water.
- Solid waste management, including landfills, recycling facilities, composting and solid waste transfer stations.
- Toxic chemical exposure whether in consumer products, housing, workplaces, air, water or soil.
- Vector control, including the control of mosquitoes, rodents, flies, cockroaches and other animals that may transmit pathogens.

According to recent estimates, about 5 to 10% of Disability-adjusted life years (DALYs) lost are due to environmental causes in Europe. By far the most important factor is fine particulate matter pollution in urban air. Similarly, environmental exposures have been estimated to contribute to 4.9 million (8.7%) deaths and 86 million (5.7%) DALYs globally. In the United States, Superfund sites created by various companies have been found to be hazardous to human and environmental health in nearby communities. It was this perceived threat, raising the specter of miscarriages, mutations, birth defects, and cancers that most frightened the public.

Information

The Toxicology and Environmental Health Information Program (TEHIP) is a comprehensive toxicology and environmental health web site, that includes open access to resources produced by US government agencies and organizations, and is maintained under the umbrella of the Specialized Information Service at the United States National Library of Medicine. TEHIP includes links to technical databases, bibliographies, tutorials, and consumer-oriented resources. TEHIP is responsible for the Toxicology Data Network (TOXNET), an integrated system of toxicology and environmental health databases including the Hazardous Substances Data Bank, that are open access, i.e. available free of charge.

Mapping

There are many environmental health mapping tools. TOXMAP is a geographic information system (GIS) from the Division of Specialized Information Services of the United States National Library of Medicine (NLM) that uses maps of the United States to help users visually explore data from the United States Environmental Protection Agency's (EPA) Toxics Release Inventory and Superfund Basic Research Programs. TOXMAP is a resource funded by the US federal government. TOXMAP's chemical and environmental health information is taken from the NLM's Toxicology Data Network (TOXNET) and PubMed, and from other authoritative sources.

Epidemiology

Epidemiology is the study and analysis of the patterns, causes, and effects of health and disease conditions in defined populations. It is the cornerstone of public health, and shapes policy decisions and evidence-based practice by identifying risk factors for disease and targets for preventive healthcare. Epidemiologists help with study design, collection, and statistical analysis of data, amend interpretation and dissemination of results (including peer review and occasional systematic review). Epidemiology has helped develop methodology used in clinical research, public health studies, and, to a lesser extent, basic research in the biological sciences.

Major areas of epidemiological study include disease causation, transmission, outbreak investigation, disease surveillance, forensic epidemiology and screening, biomonitoring, and comparisons of treatment effects such as in clinical trials. Epidemiologists rely on other scientific disciplines like biology to better understand disease processes, statistics to make efficient use of the data and draw appropriate conclusions, social sciences to better understand proximate and distal causes, and engineering for exposure assessment.

Etymology

Epidemiology, literally meaning "the study of what is upon the people", is derived from Greek *epi*, meaning 'upon, among', *demos*, meaning 'people, district', and *logos*, meaning 'study, word, discourse', suggesting that it applies only to human populations. However, the term is widely used in studies of zoological populations (veterinary epidemiology), although the term "epizoology" is available, and it has also been applied to studies of plant populations (botanical or plant disease epidemiology).

The distinction between "epidemic" and "endemic" was first drawn by Hippocrates, to distinguish between diseases that are "visited upon" a population (epidemic) from those that "reside within" a population (endemic). The term "epidemiology" appears to have first been used to describe the study of epidemics in 1802 by the Spanish physician Villalba in *Epidemiología Española*. Epidemiologists also study the interaction of diseases in a population, a condition known as a syndemic.

The term epidemiology is now widely applied to cover the description and causation of not only epidemic disease, but of disease in general, and even many non-disease, health-related conditions, such as high blood pressure and obesity. Therefore, this epidemiology is based upon how the pattern of the disease cause changes in the function of everyone.

History

The Greek physician Hippocrates is known as the father of medicine, sought a logic to sickness; he is the first person known to have examined the relationships between the occurrence of disease and environmental influences. Hippocrates believed sickness of the human body to be caused by an imbalance of the four humors (air, fire, water and earth "atoms"). The cure to the sickness was to remove or add the humor in question to balance the body. This belief led to the application of bloodletting and dieting in medicine. He coined the terms *endemic* (for diseases usually found in some places but not in others) and *epidemic* (for diseases that are seen at some times but not others).

Modern Era

In the middle of the 16th century, a doctor from Verona named Girolamo Fracastoro was the first to propose a theory that these very small, unseeable, particles that cause disease were alive. They were considered to be able to spread by air, multiply by themselves and to be destroyable by fire. In this way he refuted Galen's miasma theory (poison gas in sick people). In 1543 he wrote a book *De contagione et contagiosis morbis*, in which he was the first to promote personal and environmental hygiene to prevent disease. The development of a sufficiently powerful microscope by Antonie van Leeuwenhoek in 1675 provided visual evidence of living particles consistent with a germ theory of disease.

Wu Youke (1582–1652) developed the concept that some diseases were caused by transmissible agents, which he called liqi (pestilential factors). His book Wenyi Lun (Treatise on Acute Epidemic Febrile Diseases) can be regarded as the main etiological work that brought forward the concept, ultimately attributed to Westerners, of germs as a cause of epidemic diseases. His concepts are still considered in current scientific research in relation to Traditional Chinese Medicine studies.

Another pioneer, Thomas Sydenham (1624–1689), was the first to distinguish the fevers of Londoners in the later 1600s. His theories on cures of fevers met with much resistance from traditional physicians at the time. He was not able to find the initial cause of the smallpox fever he researched and treated.

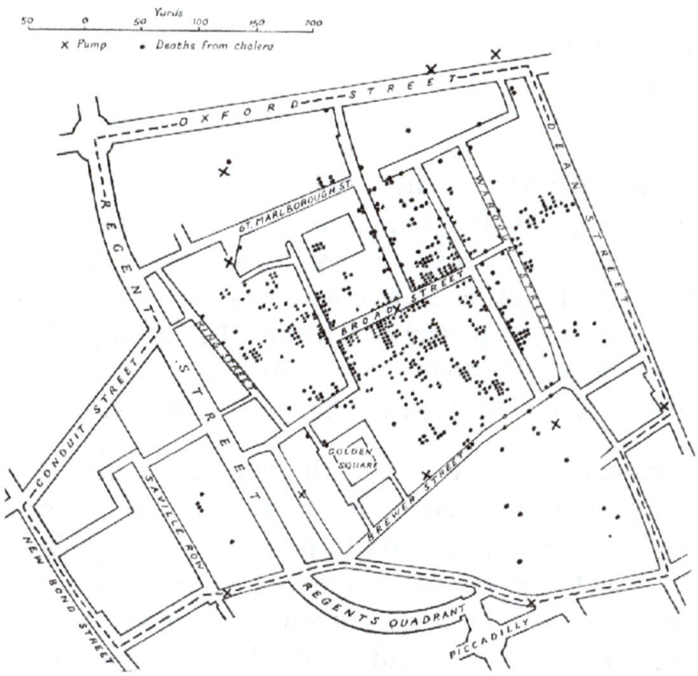

Original map by John Snow showing the clusters of cholera cases in the London epidemic of 1854.

John Graunt, a haberdasher and amateur statistician, published *Natural and Political Observations ... upon the Bills of Mortality* in 1662. In it, he analysed the mortality rolls in London before the Great Plague, presented one of the first life tables, and reported time trends for many diseases, new and old. He provided statistical evidence for many theories on disease, and also refuted some widespread ideas on them.

John Snow is famous for his investigations into the causes of the 19th century cholera epidemics, and is also known as the father of (modern) epidemiology. He began with noticing the significantly higher death rates in two areas supplied by Southwark Company. His identification of the Broad Street pump as the cause of the Soho epidemic is considered the classic example of epidemiology. Snow used chlorine in an attempt to clean the water and removed the handle; this ended the outbreak. This has been perceived as a major event in the history of public health and regarded as the founding event of the science of epidemiology, having helped shape public health policies around the world. However, Snow's research and preventive measures to avoid further outbreaks were not fully accepted or put into practice until after his death.

Other pioneers include Danish physician Peter Anton Schleisner, who in 1849 related his work on the prevention of the epidemic of neonatal tetanus on the Vestmanna Islands in Iceland. Another important pioneer was Hungarian physician Ignaz Semmelweis, who in 1847 brought down infant mortality at a Vienna hospital by instituting a disinfection procedure. His findings were published in 1850, but his work was ill-received by his colleagues, who discontinued the procedure. Disinfection did not become widely practiced until British surgeon Joseph Lister 'discovered' antiseptics in 1865 in light of the work of Louis Pasteur.

In the early 20th century, mathematical methods were introduced into epidemiology by Ronald Ross, Janet Lane-Claypon, Anderson Gray McKendrick, and others.

Another breakthrough was the 1954 publication of the results of a British Doctors Study, led by Richard Doll and Austin Bradford Hill, which lent very strong statistical support to the link between tobacco smoking and lung cancer.

In the late 20th century, with advancement of biomedical sciences, a number of molecular markers in blood, other biospecimens and environment were identified as predictors of development or risk of a certain disease. Epidemiology research to examine the relationship between these biomarkers analyzed at the molecular level, and disease was broadly named "molecular epidemiology". Specifically, "genetic epidemiology" has been used for epidemiology of germline genetic variation and disease. Genetic variation is typically determined using DNA from peripheral blood leukocytes. Since the 2000s, genome-wide association studies (GWAS) have been commonly performed to identify genetic risk factors for many diseases and health conditions.

While most molecular epidemiology studies are still using conventional disease diagnosis and classification systems, it is increasingly recognized that disease evolution represents inherently heterogeneous processes differing from person to person. Conceptually, each individual has a unique disease process different from any other individual ("the unique disease principle"), considering uniqueness of the exposome (a totality of endogenous and exogenous / environmental exposures) and its unique influence on molecular pathologic process in each individual. Studies to examine the relationship between an exposure and molecular pathologic signature of disease (particularly cancer) became increasingly common throughout the 2000s. However, the use of molecular pathology in epidemiology posed unique challenges including lack of research guidelines and standardized statistical methodologies, and paucity of interdisciplinary experts and training programs. Furthermore, the concept of disease heterogeneity appears to conflict with the long-standing premise in epidemiology that individuals with the same disease name have similar etiologies and disease processes. To resolve these issues and advance population health science in the era of molecular precision medicine, "molecular pathology" and "epidemiology" was integrated to create a new interdisciplinary field of "molecular pathological epidemiology" (MPE), defined as "epidemiology of molecular pathology and heterogeneity of disease". In MPE, investigators analyze the relationships between; (A) environmental, dietary, lifestyle and genetic factors; (B) alterations in cellular or extracellular molecules; and (C) evolution and progression of disease. A better understanding of heterogeneity of disease pathogenesis will further contribute to elucidate etiologies of disease. The MPE approach can be applied to not only neoplastic diseases but also non-neoplastic diseases. The concept and paradigm of MPE have become widespread in the 2010s.

Types of Studies

Epidemiologists employ a range of study designs from the observational to experimental and generally categorized as descriptive, analytic (aiming to further examine known associations or hypothesized relationships), and experimental (a term often equated with clinical or community trials of treatments and other interventions). In observational studies, nature is allowed to "take its course," as epidemiologists observe from the sidelines. Conversely, in experimental studies, the epidemiologist is the one in control of all of the factors entering a certain case study. Epidemiological studies are aimed, where possible, at revealing unbiased relationships between exposures such as alcohol or smoking, biological agents, stress, or chemicals to mortality or morbidity. The identification of causal relationships between these exposures and outcomes is an important aspect of epidemiology. Modern epidemiologists use informatics as a tool.

Observational studies have two components, descriptive and analytical. Descriptive observations pertain to the "who, what, where and when of health-related state occurrence". However, analytical observations deal more with the 'how' of a health-related event. Experimental epidemiology contains three case types: randomized controlled trials (often used for new medicine or drug testing), field trials (conducted on those at a high risk of conducting a disease), and community trials (research on social originating diseases).

The term 'epidemiologic triad' is used to describe the intersection of *Host*, *Agent*, and *Environment* in analyzing an outbreak.

Case Series

Case-series may refer to the qualitative study of the experience of a single patient, or small group of patients with a similar diagnosis, or to a statistical factor with the potential to produce illness with periods when they are unexposed.

The former type of study is purely descriptive and cannot be used to make inferences about the general population of patients with that disease. These types of studies, in which an astute clinician identifies an unusual feature of a disease or a patient's history, may lead to formulation of a new hypothesis. Using the data from the series, analytic studies could be done to investigate possible causal factors. These can include case control studies or prospective studies. A case control study would involve matching comparable controls without the disease to the cases in the series. A prospective study would involve following the case series over time to evaluate the disease's natural history.

The latter type, more formally described as self-controlled case-series studies, divide individual patient follow-up time into exposed and unexposed periods and use fixed-effects Poisson regression processes to compare the incidence rate of a given outcome between exposed and unexposed periods. This technique has been extensively used in the study of adverse reactions to vaccination, and has been shown in some circumstances to provide statistical power comparable to that available in cohort studies.

Case-control Studies

Case-control studies select subjects based on their disease status. It is a retrospective study. A group of individuals that are disease positive (the "case" group) is compared with a group of disease negative individuals (the "control" group). The control group should ideally come from the same population that gave rise to the cases. The case-control study looks back through time at potential exposures that both groups (cases and controls) may have encountered. A 2×2 table is constructed, displaying exposed cases (A), exposed controls (B), unexposed cases (C) and unexposed controls (D). The statistic generated to measure association is the odds ratio (OR), which is the ratio of the odds of exposure in the cases (A/C) to the odds of exposure in the controls (B/D), i.e. OR = (AD/BC).

	Cases	Controls
Exposed	A	B
Unexposed	C	D

If the OR is significantly greater than 1, then the conclusion is "those with the disease are more likely to have been exposed," whereas if it is close to 1 then the exposure and disease are not likely associated. If the OR is far less than one, then this suggests that the exposure is a protective factor in the causation of the disease. Case-control studies are usually faster and more cost effective than cohort studies, but are sensitive to bias (such as recall bias and selection bias). The main challenge is to identify the appropriate control group; the distribution of exposure among the control group should be representative of the distribution in the population that gave rise to the cases. This can be achieved by drawing a random sample from the original population at risk. This has as a consequence that the control group can contain people with the disease under study when the disease has a high attack rate in a population.

A major drawback for case control studies is that, in order to be considered to be statistically significant, the minimum number of cases required at the 95% confidence interval is related to the odds ratio by the equation:

$$\text{total cases} = A + C = 1.96^2(1+N)\left(\frac{1}{\ln(OR)}\right)^2\left(\frac{OR+2\sqrt{OR}+1}{\sqrt{OR}}\right) \approx 15.5(1+N)\left(\frac{1}{\ln(OR)}\right)^2$$

where N is the ratio of cases to controls. As the odds ratio approached 1, approaches 0; rendering case control studies all but useless for low odds ratios. For instance, for an odds ratio of 1.5 and cases = controls, the table shown above would look like this:

	Cases	Controls
Exposed	103	84
Unexposed	84	103

For an odds ratio of 1.1:

	Cases	Controls
Exposed	1732	1652
Unexposed	1652	1732

Cohort Studies

Cohort studies select subjects based on their exposure status. The study subjects should be at risk of the outcome under investigation at the beginning of the cohort study; this usually means that they should be disease free when the cohort study starts. The cohort is followed through time to assess their later outcome status. An example of a cohort study would be the investigation of a cohort of smokers and non-smokers over time to estimate the incidence of lung cancer. The same 2×2 table is constructed as with the case control study. However, the point estimate generated is the relative risk (RR), which is the probability of disease for a person in the exposed group, $P_e = A / (A + B)$ over the probability of disease for a person in the unexposed group, $P_u = C / (C + D)$, i.e. $RR = P_e / P_u$.

.....	Case	Non-case	Total
Exposed	*A*	*B*	$(A + B)$
Unexposed	*C*	*D*	$(C + D)$

As with the OR, a RR greater than 1 shows association, where the conclusion can be read "those with the exposure were more likely to develop disease."

Prospective studies have many benefits over case control studies. The RR is a more powerful effect measure than the OR, as the OR is just an estimation of the RR, since true incidence cannot be calculated in a case control study where subjects are selected based on disease status. Temporality can be established in a prospective study, and confounders are more easily controlled for. However, they are more costly, and there is a greater chance of losing subjects to follow-up based on the long time period over which the cohort is followed.

Cohort studies also are limited by the same equation for number of cases as for cohort studies, but, if the base incidence rate in the study population is very low, the number of cases required is reduced by ½.

Causal Inference

Although epidemiology is sometimes viewed as a collection of statistical tools used to elucidate the associations of exposures to health outcomes, a deeper understanding of this science is that of discovering *causal* relationships.

"Correlation does not imply causation" is a common theme for much of the epidemiological literature. For epidemiologists, the key is in the term inference. Correlation is a necessary but not sufficient criteria for inference of causation. Epidemiologists use gathered data and a broad range of biomedical and psychosocial theories in an iterative way to generate or expand theory, to test hypotheses, and to make educated, informed assertions about which relationships are causal, and about exactly how they are causal.

Epidemiologists emphasize that the "one cause – one effect" understanding is a simplistic mis-belief. Most outcomes, whether disease or death, are caused by a chain or web consisting of many component causes (Rothman et al., 2008). Causes can be distinguished as necessary, sufficient or probabilistic conditions. If a necessary condition can be identified and controlled (e.g., antibodies to a disease agent, energy in an injury), the harmful outcome can be avoided (Robertson, 2015).

Bradford Hill Criteria

In 1965, Austin Bradford Hill proposed a series of considerations to help assess evidence of causation, which have come to be commonly known as the "Bradford Hill criteria". In contrast to the explicit intentions of their author, Hill's considerations are now sometimes taught as a checklist to be implemented for assessing causality. Hill himself said "None of my nine viewpoints can bring indisputable evidence for or against the cause-and-effect hypothesis and none can be required *sine qua non.*"

1. Strength of Association: A small association does not mean that there is not a causal effect, though the larger the association, the more likely that it is causal.

2. Consistency of Data: Consistent findings observed by different persons in different places with different samples strengthens the likelihood of an effect.
3. Specificity: Causation is likely if a very specific population at a specific site and disease with no other likely explanation. The more specific an association between a factor and an effect is, the bigger the probability of a causal relationship.
4. Temporality: The effect has to occur after the cause (and if there is an expected delay between the cause and expected effect, then the effect must occur after that delay).
5. Biological gradient: Greater exposure should generally lead to greater incidence of the effect. However, in some cases, the mere presence of the factor can trigger the effect. In other cases, an inverse proportion is observed: greater exposure leads to lower incidence.
6. Plausibility: A plausible mechanism between cause and effect is helpful (but Hill noted that knowledge of the mechanism is limited by current knowledge).
7. Coherence: Coherence between epidemiological and laboratory findings increases the likelihood of an effect. However, Hill noted that "... lack of such [laboratory] evidence cannot nullify the epidemiological effect on associations".
8. Experiment: "Occasionally it is possible to appeal to experimental evidence".
9. Analogy: The effect of similar factors may be considered.

Legal Interpretation

Epidemiological studies can only go to prove that an agent could have caused, but not that it did cause, an effect in any particular case:

"Epidemiology is concerned with the incidence of disease in populations and does not address the question of the cause of an individual's disease. This question, sometimes referred to as specific causation, is beyond the domain of the science of epidemiology. Epidemiology has its limits at the point where an inference is made that the relationship between an agent and a disease is causal (general causation) and where the magnitude of excess risk attributed to the agent has been determined; that is, epidemiology addresses whether an agent can cause a disease, not whether an agent did cause a specific plaintiff's disease."

In United States law, epidemiology alone cannot prove that a causal association does not exist in general. Conversely, it can be (and is in some circumstances) taken by US courts, in an individual case, to justify an inference that a causal association does exist, based upon a balance of probability.

The subdiscipline of forensic epidemiology is directed at the investigation of specific causation of disease or injury in individuals or groups of individuals in instances in which causation is disputed or is unclear, for presentation in legal settings.

Population-based Health Management

Epidemiological practice and the results of epidemiological analysis make a significant contribution to emerging population-based health management frameworks.

Population-based health management encompasses the ability to:

- Assess the health states and health needs of a target population;
- Implement and evaluate interventions that are designed to improve the health of that population; and
- Efficiently and effectively provide care for members of that population in a way that is consistent with the community's cultural, policy and health resource values.

Modern population-based health management is complex, requiring a multiple set of skills (medical, political, technological, mathematical etc.) of which epidemiological practice and analysis is a core component, that is unified with management science to provide efficient and effective health care and health guidance to a population. This task requires the forward looking ability of modern risk management approaches that transform health risk factors, incidence, prevalence and mortality statistics (derived from epidemiological analysis) into management metrics that not only guide how a health system responds to current population health issues, but also how a health system can be managed to better respond to future potential population health issues.

Examples of organizations that use population-based health management that leverage the work and results of epidemiological practice include Canadian Strategy for Cancer Control, Health Canada Tobacco Control Programs, Rick Hansen Foundation, Canadian Tobacco Control Research Initiative.

Each of these organizations use a population-based health management framework called Life at Risk that combines epidemiological quantitative analysis with demographics, health agency operational research and economics to perform:

- *Population Life Impacts Simulations*: Measurement of the future potential impact of disease upon the population with respect to new disease cases, prevalence, premature death as well as potential years of life lost from disability and death;
- *Labour Force Life Impacts Simulations*: Measurement of the future potential impact of disease upon the labour force with respect to new disease cases, prevalence, premature death and potential years of life lost from disability and death;
- *Economic Impacts of Disease Simulations*: Measurement of the future potential impact of disease upon private sector disposable income impacts (wages, corporate profits, private health care costs) and public sector disposable income impacts (personal income tax, corporate income tax, consumption taxes, publicly funded health care costs).

Validity: Precision and Bias

Different fields in epidemiology have different levels of validity. One way to assess the validity of findings is the ratio of false-positives (claimed effects that are not correct) to false-negatives (studies which fail to support a true effect). To take the field of genetic epidemiology, candidate-gene studies produced over 100 false-positive findings for each false-negative. By contrast genome-wide association appear close to the reverse, with only one false positive for every 100 or more false-negatives. This ratio has improved over time in genetic epidemiology as the field has adopted stringent criteria. By contrast other epidemiological fields have not required such rigorous reporting and are much less reliable as a result.

Random Error

Random error is the result of fluctuations around a true value because of sampling variability. Random error is just that: random. It can occur during data collection, coding, transfer, or analysis. Examples of random error include: poorly worded questions, a misunderstanding in interpreting an individual answer from a particular respondent, or a typographical error during coding. Random error affects measurement in a transient, inconsistent manner and it is impossible to correct for random error.

There is random error in all sampling procedures. This is called sampling error.

Precision in epidemiological variables is a measure of random error. Precision is also inversely related to random error, so that to reduce random error is to increase precision. Confidence intervals are computed to demonstrate the precision of relative risk estimates. The narrower the confidence interval, the more precise the relative risk estimate.

There are two basic ways to reduce random error in an epidemiological study. The first is to increase the sample size of the study. In other words, add more subjects to your study. The second is to reduce the variability in measurement in the study. This might be accomplished by using a more precise measuring device or by increasing the number of measurements.

If sample size or number of measurements are increased, or a more precise measuring tool is purchased, the costs of the study are usually increased. There is usually an uneasy balance between the need for adequate precision and the practical issue of study cost.

Systematic Error

A systematic error or bias occurs when there is a difference between the true value (in the population) and the observed value (in the study) from any cause other than sampling variability. An example of systematic error is if, unknown to you, the pulse oximeter you are using is set incorrectly and adds two points to the true value each time a measurement is taken. The measuring device could be precise but not accurate. Because the error happens in every instance, it is systematic. Conclusions you draw based on that data will still be incorrect. But the error can be reproduced in the future (e.g., by using the same mis-set instrument).

A mistake in coding that affects *all* responses for that particular question is another example of a systematic error.

The validity of a study is dependent on the degree of systematic error. Validity is usually separated into two components:

- Internal validity is dependent on the amount of error in measurements, including exposure, disease, and the associations between these variables. Good internal validity implies a lack of error in measurement and suggests that inferences may be drawn at least as they pertain to the subjects under study.

- External validity pertains to the process of generalizing the findings of the study to the population from which the sample was drawn (or even beyond that population to a more universal statement). This requires an understanding of which conditions are relevant (or irrelevant) to the generalization. Internal validity is clearly a prerequisite for external validity.

Selection Bias

Selection bias occurs when study subjects are selected or become part of the study as a result of a third, unmeasured variable which is associated with both the exposure and outcome of interest. For instance, it has repeatedly been noted that cigarette smokers and non smokers tend to differ in their study participation rates. (Sackett D cites the example of Seltzer et al., in which 85% of non smokers and 67% of smokers returned mailed questionnaires.) It is important to note that such a difference in response will not lead to bias if it is not also associated with a systematic difference in outcome between the two response groups.

Information Bias

Information bias is bias arising from systematic error in the assessment of a variable. An example of this is recall bias. A typical example is again provided by Sackett in his discussion of a study examining the effect of specific exposures on fetal health: "in questioning mothers whose recent pregnancies had ended in fetal death or malformation (cases) and a matched group of mothers whose pregnancies ended normally (controls) it was found that 28% of the former, but only 20% of the latter, reported exposure to drugs which could not be substantiated either in earlier prospective interviews or in other health records". In this example, recall bias probably occurred as a result of women who had had miscarriages having an apparent tendency to better recall and therefore report previous exposures.

Confounding

Confounding has traditionally been defined as bias arising from the co-occurrence or mixing of effects of extraneous factors, referred to as confounders, with the main effect(s) of interest. A more recent definition of confounding invokes the notion of *counterfactual* effects. According to this view, when one observes an outcome of interest, say Y=1 (as opposed to Y=0), in a given population A which is entirely exposed (i.e. exposure $X = 1$ for every unit of the population) the risk of this event will be R_{A1}. The counterfactual or unobserved risk R_{A0} corresponds to the risk which would have been observed if these same individuals had been unexposed (i.e. $X = 0$ for every unit of the population). The true effect of exposure therefore is: $R_{A1} - R_{A0}$ (if one is interested in risk differences) or R_{A1}/R_{A0} (if one is interested in relative risk). Since the counterfactual risk R_{A0} is unobservable we approximate it using a second population B and we actually measure the following relations: $R_{A1} - R_{B0}$ or R_{A1}/R_{B0}. In this situation, confounding occurs when $R_{A0} \neq R_{B0}$. (NB: Example assumes binary outcome and exposure variables.)

Some epidemiologists prefer to think of confounding separately from common categorizations of bias since, unlike selection and information bias, confounding stems from real causal effects.

The Profession

To date, few universities offer epidemiology as a course of study at the undergraduate level. One notable undergraduate program exists at Johns Hopkins University, where students who major in public health can take graduate level courses, including epidemiology, their senior year at the Bloomberg School of Public Health.

Many epidemiologists are physicians, or hold graduate degrees such as a Master of Public Health (MPH), Master of Science of Epidemiology (MSc.). Doctorates include the Doctor of Public Health (DrPH), Doctor of Pharmacy (PharmD), Doctor of Philosophy (PhD), Doctor of Science (ScD), Doctor of Social Work (DSW), Doctor of Clinical Practice (DClinP), Doctor of Podiatric Medicine (DPM), Doctor of Veterinary Medicine (DVM), Doctor of Nursing Practice (DNP), Doctor of Physical Therapy (DPT), or for clinically trained physicians, Doctor of Medicine (MD) or Bachelor of Medicine and Surgery (MBBS or MBChB) and Doctor of Osteopathic Medicine (DO).

As public health/health protection practitioners, epidemiologists work in a number of different settings. Some epidemiologists work 'in the field'; i.e., in the community, commonly in a public health/health protection service, and are often at the forefront of investigating and combating disease outbreaks. Others work for non-profit organizations, universities, hospitals and larger government entities such as state and local health departments, various Ministries of Health, Doctors without Borders, the Centers for Disease Control and Prevention (CDC), the Health Protection Agency, the World Health Organization (WHO), or the Public Health Agency of Canada. Epidemiologists can also work in for-profit organizations such as pharmaceutical and medical device companies in groups such as market research or clinical development.

Health Impact Assessment

Health impact assessment (HIA) is defined as "a combination of procedures, methods, and tools by which a policy, program, or project may be judged as to its potential effects on the health of a population, and the distribution of those effects within the population." (ECHP 1999, p. 4)

Overview

HIA is intended to produce a set of evidence-based recommendations to inform decision-making (Taylor & Quigley 2002, p. 2). HIA seeks to maximise the positive health impacts and minimise the negative health impacts of proposed policies, programs or projects.

The procedures of HIA are similar to those used in other forms of impact assessment, such as environmental impact assessment or social impact assessment. HIA is usually described as following the steps listed, though many practitioners break these into sub-steps or label them differently:

1. *Screening* - determining if an HIA is warranted/required
2. *Scoping* - determining which impacts will be considered and the plan for the HIA
3. *Identification and assessment of impacts* - determining the magnitude, nature, extent and likelihood of potential health impacts, using a variety of different methods and types of information

4. *Decision-making and recommendations* - making explicit the trade-offs to be made in decision-making and formulating evidence-informed recommendations
5. *Evaluation, monitoring and follow-up* - process and impact evaluation of the HIA and the monitoring and management of health impacts

The main objective of HIA is to apply existing knowledge and evidence about health impacts, to specific social and community contexts, to develop evidence-based recommendations that inform decision-making in order to protect and improve community health and wellbeing. Because of financial and time constraints, HIAs do not generally involve new research or the generation of original scientific knowledge. However, the findings of HIAs, especially where these have been monitored and evaluated over time, can be used to inform other HIAs in contexts that are similar. An HIA's recommendations may focus on both design and operational aspects of a proposal.

HIA has also been identified as a mechanism by which potential health inequalities can be identified and redressed prior to the implementation of proposed policy, program or project (Acheson 1998).

A number of manuals and guidelines for HIA's use have been developed.

Determinants of Health

The proposition that policies, programs and projects have the potential to change the determinants of health underpins HIA's use. Changes to health determinants then leads to changes in health outcomes or the health status of individuals and communities. The determinants of health are largely environmental and social, so that there are many overlaps with environmental impact assessment and social impact assessment.

Levels of HIA

Three forms of HIA exist:

- Desk-based HIA, which takes 2–6 weeks for one assessor to complete and provides a broad overview of potential health impacts;
- Rapid HIA, which takes approximately 12 weeks for one assessor to complete and provides more detailed information on potential health impacts; and
- Comprehensive HIA, which takes approximately 6 months for one assessor and provides a in-depth assessment of potential health impacts. (IMPACT 2004, p. 7)

It has been suggested that HIAs can be prospective (done before a proposal is implemented), concurrent (done while the proposal is being implemented) or retrospective (done after a proposal has been implemented) (Taylor, Gorman & Quigley 2003, p. 1). This remains controversial, however, with a number of HIA practitioners suggesting that concurrent HIA is better regarded as a monitoring activity and that retrospective HIA is more akin to evaluation with a health focus, rather than being assessment per se (Kemm 2003, p. 387). Prospective HIA is preferred as it allows the maximum practical opportunity to influence decision-making and subsequent health impacts.

HIA Practitioners

HIA practitioners can be found in the private and public sectors, but are relatively few in number. There are no universally accepted competency frameworks or certification processes. It is suggested that a lead practitioner should have extensive education and training in a health related field, experience of participating in HIAs, and have attended an HIA training course. It has been suggested and widely accepted that merely having a medical or health degree should not be regarded as an indication of competency.

The International Association for Impact Assessment has an active health section.

A HIA People Directory can be found on the HIA GATEWAY.

HIA Worldwide

HIA is currently being used or developed around the world, most notably in Europe, North America, Australia, New Zealand, Africa and Thailand.

The new safeguard policies and standards of the International Finance Corporation (IFC), part of the World Bank, were established in 2006. These contain a requirement for health impact assessment in large projects. The standards have been accepted by most of the leading lending banks who are parties to the Equator Principles. Health impact assessments are becoming routine in many large development projects in both public and private sectors of developing countries. There is also a long history of health impact assessment in the water resource development sector - large dams and irrigation systems.

HIA Conferences

The 13th International HIA Conference was held in Geneva in 2013.

The 12th International HIA Conference was held in Québec City in 2012.

Public Health Informatics

Public health informatics has been defined as the systematic application of information and computer science and technology to public health practice, research, and learning. It is one of the subdomains of health informatics.

Definition

Public health informatics is defined as the use of computers, clinical guidelines, communication and information systems, which apply to vast majority of public health, related professions, such as nursing, clinical/ hospital care/ public health and medical research.

United States

In developed countries like the United States, public health informatics is practiced by individuals in public health agencies at the federal and state levels and in the larger local health jurisdictions. Additionally, research and training in public health informatics takes place at a variety of academic institutions.

At the federal Centers for Disease Control and Prevention in US states like Atlanta, Georgia, the Public Health Surveillance and Informatics Program Office (PHSIPO) focuses on advancing the state of information science and applies digital information technologies to aid in the detection and management of diseases and syndromes in individuals and populations.

The bulk of the work of public health informatics in the United States, as with public health generally, takes place at the state and local level, in the state departments of health and the county or parish departments of health. At a state health department the activities may include: collection and storage of *vital statistics* (birth and death records); collection of reports of communicable disease cases from doctors, hospitals, and laboratories, used for infectious disease surveillance; display of infectious disease statistics and trends; collection of child immunization and lead screening information; daily collection and analysis of emergency room data to detect early evidence of biological threats; collection of hospital capacity information to allow for planning of responses in case of emergencies. Each of these activities presents its own information processing challenge.

Collection of Public Health Data

(TODO: describe CDC-provided DOS/desktop-based systems like TIMSS (TB), STDMIS (Sexually transmitted diseases); Epi-Info for epidemiology investigations; and others)

Since the beginning of the World Wide Web, public health agencies with sufficient information technology resources have been transitioning to web-based collection of public health data, and, more recently, to automated messaging of the same information. In the years roughly 2000 to 2005 the Centers for Disease Control and Prevention, under its National Electronic Disease Surveillance System (NEDSS), built and provided free to states a comprehensive web and message-based reporting system called the NEDSS Base System (NBS). Due to the funding being limited and it not being wise to have fiefdom-based systems, only a few states and larger counties have built their own versions of electronic disease surveillance systems, such as Pennsylvania's PA-NEDSS. These do not provide timely full intestate notification services causing an increase in disease rates versus the NEDSS federal product.

To promote interoperability, the CDC has encouraged the adoption in public health data exchange of several standard vocabularies and messaging formats from the health care world. The most prominent of these are: the Health Level 7 (HL7) standards for health care messaging; the LOINC system for encoding laboratory test and result information; and the Systematized Nomenclature of Medicine (SNOMED) vocabulary of health care concepts.

Since about 2005, the CDC has promoted the idea of the Public Health Information Network to facilitate the transmission of data from various partners in the health care industry and elsewhere (hospitals, clinical and environmental laboratories, doctors' practices, pharmacies) to local health agencies, then to state health agencies, and then to the CDC. At each stage the entity must be capable of receiving the data, storing it, aggregating it appropriately, and transmitting it to the next level. A typical example would be infectious disease data, which hospitals, labs, and doctors are legally required to report to local health agencies; local health agencies must report to their state public health department; and which the states must report in aggregate form to the CDC. Among other uses, the CDC publishes the Morbidity and Mortality Weekly Report (MMWR) based on these data acquired systematically from across the United States.

Major issues in the collection of public health data are: awareness of the need to report data; lack of resources of either the reporter or collector; lack of interoperability of data interchange formats, which can be at the purely syntactic or at the semantic level; variation in reporting requirements across the states, territories, and localities.

Public health informatics can be thought or divided into three categories.

Study Models of Different Systems

The first category is to discover and study models of complex systems, such as disease transmission. This can be done through different types of data collections, such as hospital surveys, or electronic surveys submitted to the organization (such as the CDC). Transmission rates or disease incidence rates/surveillance can be obtained through government organizations, such as the CDC, or global organizations, such as WHO. Not only disease transmission/rates can be looked at. Public health informatics can also delve into people with/without health insurance and the rates at which they go to the doctor. Before the advent of the internet, public health data in the United States, like other healthcare and business data, were collected on paper forms and stored centrally at the relevant public health agency. If the data were to be computerized they required a distinct data entry process, were stored in the various file formats of the day and analyzed by mainframe computers using standard batch processing.

Storage of Public Health Data

The second category is to find ways to improve the efficiency of different public health systems. This is done through various collections methods, storage of data and how the data is used to improve current health problems. In order to keep everything standardized, vocabulary and word usage needs to be consistent throughout all systems. Finding new ways to link together and share new data with current systems is important to keep everything up to date.

Storage of public health data shares the same data management issues as other industries. And like other industries, the details of how these issues play out are affected by the nature of the data being managed.

Due to the complexity and variability of public health data, like health care data generally, the issue of data modeling presents a particular challenge. While a generation ago flat data sets for statistical analysis were the norm, today's requirements of interoperability and integrated sets of data across the public health enterprise require more sophistication. The relational database is increasingly the norm in public health informatics. Designers and implementers of the many sets of data required for various public health purposes must find a workable balance between very complex and abstract data models such as HL7's Reference Information Model (RIM) or CDC's Public Health Logical Data Model, and simplistic, ad hoc models that untrained public health practitioners come up with and feel capable of working with.

Due to the variability of the incoming data to public health jurisdictions, data quality assurance is also a major issue.

Analysis of Public Health Data

Finally, the last category can be thought as maintaining and enriching current systems and models to adapt to overflow of data and storing/sorting of this new data. This can be as simple as connecting directly to an electronic data collection source, such as health records from the hospital, or can go public information (CDC) about disease rates/transmission. Finding new algorithms that will sort through large quantities of data quickly and effectively is necessary as well.

The need to extract usable public health information from the mass of data available requires the public health informaticist to become familiar with a range of analysis tools, ranging from business intelligence tools to produce routine or ad hoc reports, to sophisticated statistical analysis tools such as DAP/SAS and PSPP/SPSS, to Geographical Information Systems (GIS) to expose the geographical dimension of public health trends.Such analyses usually require methods that appropriately secure the privacy of the health data. One approach is to separate the individually identifiable variables of the data from the rest

Applications in Health Surveillance and Epidemiology

There are a few organizations out there that provide useful information for those professionals that want to be more involved in public health informatics. Such as the American Medical Informatics Association (AMIA). AMIA is for professions that are involved in health care, informatics research, biomedical research, including physicians, scientists, researchers, and students. The main goals of AMIA are to move from 'bench to bedside', help improve the impact of health innovations and advance the public health informatics field. They hold annual conferences, online classes and webinars, which are free to their members. There is also a career center specific for the biomedical and health informatics community.

Many jobs or fellowships in public health informatics are offered. The CDC (Center for Disease Control) has various fellowship programs, while multiple colleges/companies offer degree programs or training in this field.

- SAPPHIRE (Health care) or *Situational Awareness and Preparedness for Public Health Incidences and Reasoning Engines* is a semantics-based health information system capable of tracking and evaluating situations and occurrences that may affect public health.

References

- Howe, Rufus, and Christopher Spence. Population health management: Healthways' PopWorks. HCT Project 2004-07-17, volume 2, chapter 5, pages 291-297. Retrieved 2008-10-12
- Kindig D, Stoddart G (Mar 2003). "What is population health?" (PDF). American Journal of Public Health. 93 (3): 380–3. doi:10.2105/ajph.93.3.380
- White F, Nanan DJ (2008). "International and Global Health". In Maxcy-Rosenau-Last. Public Health and Preventive Medicine (15th ed.). McGraw Hill. pp. 1252–8. ISBN 9780071441988
- Frankish, CJ et al. "Health Impact Assessment as a Tool for Population Health Promotion and Public Policy". Vancouver: Institute of Health Promotion Research, University of British Columbia, 1996. Retrieved 2008-10-12

- Kindig, David; Stoddart, Greg (2016-10-15). "What Is Population Health?". American Journal of Public Health. 93 (3): 380–383. ISSN 0090-0036. PMC 1447747. PMID 12604476
- Birn, A., Pillay; Yogan, Holtz, T. (2009). Textbook of International Health (3rd ed.). Oxford University Press. p. 273. ISBN 9780199719853
- Hillman, Michael. Testimony before the Subcommittee on Health of the House Committee on Ways and Means, hearing on promoting disease management in Medicare. 2002-04-16. Retrieved 2008-10-12
- Schaible UE, Kaufmann SH; Kaufmann (May 2007). "Malnutrition and infection: complex mechanisms and global impacts". PLoS Med. 4 (5): e115. doi:10.1371/journal.pmed.0040115. PMC 1858706. PMID 17472433
- "Transforming our world: the 2030 Agenda for Sustainable Development .:. Sustainable Development Knowledge Platform". sustainabledevelopment.un.org. Retrieved 2016-02-26

3

Public Health Education: An Essential Aspect

The aim of health education is to educate people about the benefits of staying healthy. Health education, as a subject includes topics like physical health, social health, intellectual health, emotional and spiritual health. The major categories of public health education are dealt with great details in the chapter.

Health Education

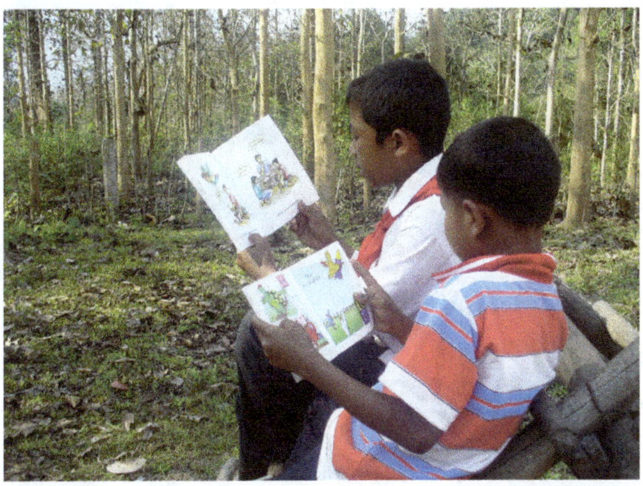

Two boys in rural Laos take a clear interest in a book about intestinal parasites.

Health education is a profession of educating people about health. Areas within this profession encompass environmental health, physical health, social health, emotional health, intellectual health, and spiritual health.

Health education can be defined as the principle by which individuals and groups of people, learn to behave in a manner conducive to the promotion, maintenance, or restoration of health. However, as there are multiple definitions of health, there are also multiple definitions of health education. The Joint Committee on Health Education and Promotion Terminology of 2001 defined Health Education as "any combination of planned learning experiences based on sound theories that provide individuals, groups, and communities the opportunity to acquire information and the skills needed to make quality health decisions."

The World Health Organization defined Health Education as "comprising of consciously constructed opportunities for learning involving some form of communication designed to improve health literacy, including improving knowledge, and developing life skills which are conducive to individual and community health."

The Role of Health Education Specialists

From the late nineteenth to the mid-twentieth century, the aim of public health was controlling the harm from infectious diseases, which were largely under control by the 1950s. By the mid 1970s it was clear that reducing illness, death, and rising health care costs could best be achieved through a focus on health promotion and disease prevention. At the heart of the new approach was the role of a health educator A health educator is "a professionally prepared individual who serves in a variety of roles and is specifically trained to use appropriate educational strategies and methods to facilitate the development of policies, procedures, interventions, and systems conducive to the health of individuals, groups, and communities" (Joint Committee on Terminology, 2001, p. 100). In January 1978 the Role Delineation Project was put into place, in order to define the basic roles and responsibilities for the health educator. The result was a Framework for the Development of Competency-Based Curricula for Entry Level Health Educators (NCHEC, 1985). A second result was a revised version of A Competency-Based Framework for the Professional Development of Certified Health Education Specialists (NCHEC,1996). These documents outlined the seven areas of responsibilities which are shown below.

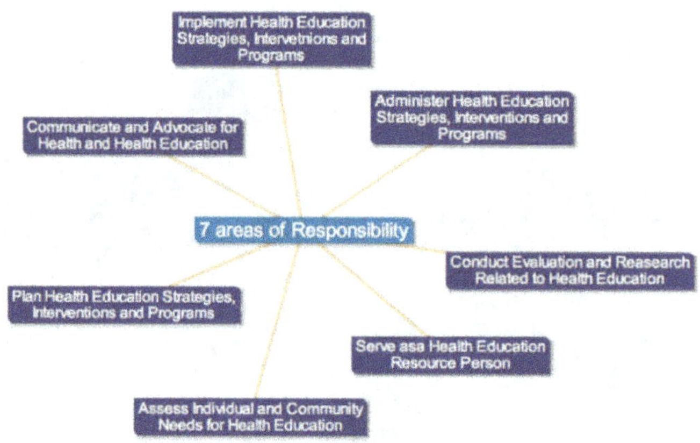

Responsibility I: Assessing Individual and Community Needs for Health Education

-Provides the foundation for program planning

-Determines what health problems might exist in any given groups

-Includes determination of community resources available to address the problem

-Community Empowerment encourages the population to take ownership of their health problems

-Includes careful data collection and analysis

-It is essential for healthy life

Responsibility II: Plan Health Education Strategies, Interventions, and Programs

-Actions are based on the needs assessment done for the community (Responsibility I)

-Involves the development of goals and objectives which are specific and measurable

-Interventions are developed that will meet the goals and objectives

-According to Rule of Sufficiency, strategies are implemented which are sufficiently robust, effective enough, and have a reasonable chance of meeting stated objectives

Responsibility III: Implement Health Education Strategies, Interventions, and Programs

-Implementation is based on a thorough understanding of the priority population

-Utilize a wide range of educational methods and techniques

Responsibility IV: Conduct Evaluation and Research Related to Health Education

-Depending on the setting, utilize tests, surveys, observations, tracking epidemiologicaldata, or other methods of data collection

-Health Educators make use of research to improve their practices.

Responsibility V: Administer Health Education Strategies, Interventions, and Programs

-Administration is generally a function of the more experienced practitioner

-Involves facilitating cooperation among personnel, both within and between programs

Responsibility VI: Serve as a Health Education Resource Person

-Involves skills to access needed resources, and establish effective consultative relationships.

Responsibility VII: Communicate and Advocate for Health and Health Education

-Translates scientific language into understandable information

-Address diverse audience in diverse settings

-Formulates and support rules, policies and legislation

-Advocate for the profession of health education

Motivation

Education for health begins with people. It hopes to motivate them with whatever interests they may have in improving their living conditions. Its aim come is to develop in them a sense of responsibility for health conditions for themselves as individuals, as members of families, and as communities. In communicable disease control, health education commonly includes an appraisal of what is known by a population about a disease, an assessment of habits and attitudes of the people as they relate to spread and frequency of the disease, and the presentation of specific means to remedy observed deficiencies.

Health education is also an effective tool that helps improve health in developing nations. It not only teaches prevention and basic health knowledge but also conditions ideas that re-shape everyday habits of people with unhealthy lifestyles in developing countries. This type of conditioning not only affects the immediate recipients of such education but also future generations will benefit from an improved and properly cultivated ideas about health that will eventually be ingrained with widely spread health education. Moreover, besides physical health prevention, health education can also provide more aid and help people deal healthier with situations of extreme stress, anxiety, depression or other emotional disturbances to lessen the impact of these sorts of mental and emotional constituents, which can consequently lead to detrimental physical effects.,

Credentialing

Credentialing is the process by which the qualifications of licensed professionals, organizational members or an organization are determined by assessing the individuals or group background and legitimacy through a standardized process. Accreditation, licensure, or certifications are all forms of credentialing.

In 1978, Helen Cleary, the president of the Society for Public Health Education (SOPHE) started the process of certification of health educators. Prior to this, there was no certification for individual health educators, with exception to the licensing for school health educators. The only accreditation available in this field was for school health and public health professional preparation programs.

Her initial response was to incorporate experts in the field and to promote funding for the process. The director if the Division of Associated Health Professions in the Bureau of Health Manpower of the Department of Health, Education, and Welfare, Thomas Hatch, became interested in the project. To ensure that the commonalities between health educators across the spectrum of professions would be sufficient enough to create a set of standards, Dr. Cleary spent a great amount of time to create the first conference called the Bethesda Conference. In attendance were interested professionals who covered the possibility of creating credentialing within the profession.

With the success of the conference and the consensus that the standardization of the profession was vital, those who organized the conference created the National Task Force in the Preparation and Practice of Health Educators. Funding for this endeavor became available in January 1979, and role delineation became a realistic vision for the future. They presented the framework for the system in 1981 and published entry-level criteria in 1983. Seven areas of responsibility, 29 areas of competency and 79 sub-competencies were required of health education professionals for approximately 20 years for entry-level educators.

In 1986 a second conference was held in Bethesda, Maryland to further the credentialing process. In June 1988, the National Task Force in the Preparation and Practice of Health Educators became the National Commission for Health Education Credentialing, Inc. (NCHEC). Their mission was to improve development of the field by promoting, preparing and certifying health education specialists. The NCHEC has three division boards that included preparation, professional development and certification of health educator professionals. The third board, which is called the Division Board of Certification of Health Education Specialist (DBCHES), has the responsibility of developing and administering the CHES exam. An initial certification process allowed 1,558 individuals to be chartered into the program through a recommendation and application process. The first exam was given in 1990.

In order for a candidate to sit for an exam they must have either a bachelor's, master's, or doctoral degree from an accredited institution, and an official transcript that shows a major in health education, Community Health Education, Public Health Education, or School Health Education, etc. The transcript will be accepted if it reflects 25 semester hours or 37 quarter hours in health education preparation and covers the 7 responsibilities covered in the framework.

In 1998 a project called the Competencies Update Project (CUP) began. The purpose of the CUP project was to up-date entry-level requirements and to develop advanced-level competences. Through research the CUP project created the requirements for three levels, which included entry-level, Advanced I and Advanced II educators.

Recently the Master Certified Health Education Specialist (MCHES) was created. The MCHES exam measures the knowledge of the advanced levels and sub levels of the Seven Areas of Responsibilities. The first MCHES exam was given in October 2011.

In order to be eligible to take the MCHES exam you must have at least a master's degree in health education or related discipline along with a least 25 credit hours related to health education. In addition, five years of documented information of practice in health education and two recommendations of past/present supervisors must be provided. A vitae/resume must also be submitted.

The Competency Update Project (CUP), 1998-2004 revealed that there were higher levels of health education practitioners, which is the reasoning for the advancements for the MCHES. Many health educators felt that the current CHES credential was an entry-level exam.

Teaching

In the United States some forty states require the teaching of health education. A comprehensive health education curriculum consists of planned learning experiences which will help students achieve desirable attitudes and practices related to critical health issues. Some of these are: emotional health and a positive self image; appreciation, respect for, and care of the human body and its vital organs; physical fitness; health issues of alcohol, tobacco, drug use and abuse; health misconceptions and myths; effects of exercise on the body systems and on general well being; nutrition and weight control; sexual relationships and sexuality, the scientific, social, and economic aspects of community and ecological health; communicable and degenerative diseases including sexually transmitted diseases; disaster preparedness; safety and driver education; factors in the environment and how those factors affect an individual's or population's Environmental health (ex: air quality, water quality, food sanitation); life skills; choosing professional medical and health services; and choices of health careers.

The National Center for Education Statistics share that 99% of public schools conduct some type of nutrition education. For each grade from kindergarten through eighth, 50 percent or more of all schools have district or state requirements for students to receive nutrition education. However, only 40 percent have these requirements for ninth and tenth grades; and about 20 percent for eleventh and twelfth grades. The issue still lies with the content and thoroughness that is being taught. Topics taught in a most all of the schools are: the relationship between diet and health, finding and choosing healthy foods, nutrients and their food sources, the Food Guide Pyramid, and the Dietary Guidelines and goals. However, with the exception of the Food Guide Pyramid, less than half of schools cover these topics thoroughly. Overall, schools focus on increasing students' knowledge about what is meant by good nutrition, with less emphasis on influencing students' motivation, attitudes, and eating behaviors. Four of the five topics covered by more than 90 percent of all schools are related to knowledge. With the exception of finding and choosing healthy foods, less than one-third of schools provide thorough coverage of topics related to motivation, attitudes, and eating behaviors. Not often are there teachers specific for nutrition. Most of the time the nutrition content is taught by the primary teacher.

Health Education Code of Ethics

The Health Education Code of Ethics has been a work in progress since approximately 1976, begun by the Society of Public Health Education (SOPHE). Various Public Health and Health Education organizations such as the American Association of Health Education (AAHE), the Coalition of National Health Education Organizations (CNHEO), SOPHE, and others collaborated year after year to devise a unified standard of ethics that health educators would be held accountable to professionally. In 1995, the National Commission for Health Education Credentialing, Inc. (NCHEC) proposed a profession-wide standard at the conference: Health Education Profession in the Twenty-First Century: Setting the Stage. Post-conference, an ethics task force was developed with the purpose of solidifying and unifying proposed ethical standards. The document was eventually unanimously approved and ratified by all involved organizations in November 1999 and has since then been used as the standard for practicing health educators.

"The Code of Ethics that has evolved from this long and arduous process is not seen as a completed project. Rather, it is envisioned as a living document that will continue to evolve as the practice of Health Education changes to meet the challenges of the new millennium."

Health Education Code of Ethics Full Text

PREAMBLE The Health Education profession is dedicated to excellence in the practice of promoting individual, family, organizational, and community health. The Code of Ethics provides a framework of shared values within which Health Education is practiced. The responsibility of each Health Educator is to aspire to the highest possible standards of conduct and to encourage the ethical behavior of all those with whom they work.

Article I: Responsibility to the Public A Health Educator's ultimate responsibility is to educate people for the purpose of promoting, maintaining, and improving individual, family, and community health. When a conflict of issues arises among individuals, groups, organizations, agencies, or institutions, health educators must consider all issues and give priority to those that promote wellness and quality of living through principles of self-determination and freedom of choice for the individual.

Article II: Responsibility to the Profession Health Educators are responsible for their professional behavior, for the reputation of their profession, and for promoting ethical conduct among their colleagues.

Article III: Responsibility to Employers Health Educators recognize the boundaries of their professional competence and are accountable for their professional activities and actions.

Article IV: Responsibility in the Delivery of Health Education Health Educators promote integrity in the delivery of health education. They respect the rights, dignity, confidentiality, and worth of all people by adapting strategies and methods to the needs of diverse populations and communities.

Article V: Responsibility in Research and Evaluation Health Educators contribute to the health of the population and to the profession through research and evaluation activities. When planning and conducting research or evaluation, health educators do so in accordance with federal and state laws and regulations, organizational and institutional policies, and professional standards.

Article VI: Responsibility in Professional Preparation Those involved in the preparation and training of Health Educators have an obligation to accord learners the same respect and treatment given other groups by providing quality education that benefits the profession and the public.

The National Health Education Code of Ethics is the property of the Coalition of National Health Education.

National Organizations for Public Health/Health Education

American Public Health Association (APHA) APHA is the main voice for public health advocacy that is the oldest organization of public health since 1872. The American Public Health Association aims to "protect all Americans and their communities from preventable, serious health threats and strives to assure community-based health promotion and disease preventions." Any individual can become a member and benefit in online access and monthly printed issues of The Nation's Health and the American Journal of Public Health.

Society for Public Health Education (SOPHE) The mission of SOPHE is to provide global leadership to the profession of health education and health promotion and to promote the health of society through advances in health education theory and research, excellence in professional preparation and practice, and advocacy for public policies conducive to health, and the achievement of health equity for all. Membership is open to all who have an interest in health education and or work in health education in schools, medical care settings, worksites, community-based organizations, state/local government, and international agencies. Founded in 1950, SOPHE publishes 2 indexed, peer-reviewed journals, *Health Education & Behavior* and *Health Promotion Practice.*

American School Health Association (ASHA) The American School Health Association was founded in 1972 by a group of physicians that already belonged to the American Public Health Association. This group specializes in school-aged health specifically. Over the years it has snowballed and now includes any person that can be a part of a child's life, from dentists, to counselors and school nurses. The American School Health Association mission "is to protect and promote the health of children and youth by supporting coordinated school health programs as a foundation for school success."

American Association of Health Education/American Alliance for Health, Physical Education, Recreation, and Dance (AAHE/AAHPERD) The AAHE/AAHPERD is said to be the largest organization of professionals that supports physical education; which includes leisure, fitness, dance, and health promotion. That is only a few; this incorporates all that is physical movement. This organization is an alliance with five national associations and six districts and is there to provide a comprehensive and coordinated array of resources to help support practitioners to improve their skills and always be learning new things. This organization was first stated in November 1885. William Gilbert Anderson had been out of medical school for two years and was working with many other people that were in the gymnastic field. He wanted them to get together to discuss their field and this organization was created. Today AAHPERD serves 25,000 members and has its headquarters in Reston, Virginia.

Eta Sigma Gamma (ESG) Eta Sigma Gamma is a national health education organization founded in 1967 by three professor from Ball State University. The mission of ESG is to promote public health education by improving the standards, ideals, capability, and ethics of public health education professionals. The three key points of the organization are to teach, research, and provide service to the members of the public health professionals. Some of the goals that the Eta Stigma Gamma targets are support planning and evaluation of future and existing health education programs, support and promote scientific research, support advocacy of health education issues, and promote professional ethics.

American College Health Association (ACHA) The American College Health Association originally began as a student health association in 1920, but then in 1948 the association changed the name to what its known today. The principal interest of the ACHA is to promote advocacy and leadership to colleges and universities around the country. Other part of the mission's association is to encourage education, communication, and services to students and campus community in general. The association also promotes advocacy and research. The American College Health Association has three types of membership: institutions of higher education, individual members who are interested in the public health profession, and susbtain members which are profitable and non-profitable organization. The ACHA is connected to 11 organizations located in six regions around the country. Currently, the American College Health Association serves 900 educative institutions and about 2400 individual members in the United States.

Directors of Health Promotion and Education (DHPE) Founded in 1946 as one of the professional groups of the Health Education Profession. The main goal of the HEPE is to improve the health education standards in any public health agency. As well, build networking opportunities among all public health professionals as a media to communicate ideas for implementing health programs, and to keep accurate information about the latest health news. The DHPE also focus to increase public awareness of health education and promotion by creating and expanding methods of existing health programs that will improve the quality of health. The Directors of Health Promotion and Education is linked to the Association of State and Territorial Health Officials (ASTHO) to "work on health promotion and disease prevention".

National Commission for Health Education Credentialing (NCHEC)

The National Commission for Health Education Credentialing NCHEC is the national accrediting organization for health educators, promoting the certified and master certified health education specialist (CHES and MCHES, respectively) credential. Many government and private sector jobs require that the health educator have at least the CHES credential as a prerequisite qualification for work. NCHEC also administers the affirmation of approved continuing education to maintain these credentials. Both CHES and MCHES are required to take at least 75 continuing education contact hours (CECH) every five years to be recertified. The provision and administration of the CHES credential represents the major strategy of NCHEC to fulfill its mission to "improve the practice of health education and to serve the public and profession of health education by certifying health education specialists, promoting professional development, and strengthening professional preparation and practice." NCHEC's quarterly newsletter is "The CHES Bulletin."

Health Education Career Opportunities

The terms Public Health Educator, Community Health Educator or Health Educator are all used interchangeable to describe an individual who plans implements and evaluates health education and promotion programs. These individuals play a crucial role in many organizations in various settings to improve our nations health. Just as a Community health educator works work toward population health, a school Health educator generally teaches in our Schools. A community health educator is typically focused on their immediate community striving to serve the public.

Health Care Settings: these include hospitals (for-profit and public), medical care clinics, home health agencies, HMOs and PPOs. Here, a health educator teaches employees how to be healthy. Patient education positions are far and few between because insurance companies do not cover the costs.

Public Health Agencies: are official, tax funded, government agencies. They provide police protection, educational systems, as well as clean air and water. Public health departments provide health services and are organized by a city, county, state, or federal government.

School Health Education: involves all strategies, activities, and services offered by, in, or in association with schools that are designed to promote students' physical, emotional, and social development. School health involves teaching students about health and health related behaviors. Curriculum and programs are based on the school's expectations and health.

Non Profit Voluntary Health Agencies: are created by concerned citizens to deal with health needs not met by governmental agencies. Missions include public education, professional education, patient education, research, direct services and support to or for people directly affected by a specific health or medical problem. Usually funded by such means as private donations, grants, and fund-raisers.

Higher Education: typically two types of positions health educators hold including academic, or faculty or health educator in a student health service or wellness center. As a faculty member, the health educator typically has three major responsibilities: teaching, community and professional service, and scholarly research. As a health educator in a university health service or wellness center, the major responsibility is to plan, implement, and evaluate health promotion and education programs for program participants.

Work site Health Promotion: is a combination of educational, organizational and environmental activities designed to improve the health and safety of employees and their families. These work site wellness programs offer an additional setting for health educators and allow them to reach segments of the population that are not easily reached through traditional community health programs. Some work site health promotion activities include: smoking cessation, stress management, bulletin boards, newsletters, and much more.

Independent Consulting and Government Contracting: international, national, regional, state, and local organizations contract with independent consultants for many reasons. They may be hired to assess individual and community needs for health education; plan, implement, administer and evaluate health education strategies; conduct research; serve as health education resource person; and or communicate about and advocate for health and health education. Government contractors are often behind national health education programs, government reports, public information web sites and telephone lines, media campaigns, conferences, and health education materials.

Influential Individuals in Health Education: Past and Present

Dorothy Bird Nyswander

Dr. Nyswander was born September 29, 1894. She earned her bachelor's and master's degree at the University of Nevada and received her Doctorate in educational psychology at Berkeley. She is a founder of the School of Public Health at the University of California at Berkeley. Dr. Nysawnder pursued her interest in public health at the Works Progress Administration during the depression. She served with the Federal Works Agency contributing to the establishment of nursery schools and child care centers to accommodate young mothers working in defense plants. She set up these centers in 15 northeastern states. This did not happen quickly so she advocated all over the nation to train people to act as foster parents for the children of working women. Dr. Nyswander became the director of the City health Center in Astoria, Queens in 1939. She spent her time as director promoting the idea of New York City keeping an eye on the health of children. They would do this by keeping records that would follow them to whatever school they might move to. She wrote "Solving School Health Problems" which is an analysis of the health issues in New York children. This is still used in public health education courses today.

Mayhew Derryberry

Dr. Derryberry was born December 25, 1902 and earned his bachelor's degree in chemistry and mathematics at the University of Tennessee. He began his career in 1926 with the American Child Health Association as the director of one of the first large-scale studies of the health status of the nation's schoolchildren. A year after his work with the American Child Health Association he earned his master's degree in education and psychology at Columbia University. He then went on to earn his doctorate and moved to the New York City Health Department as the secretary to the sanitary superintendent. He finally moved to Washington DC and joined the US Public Health Service as a senior public health analyst. He became chief of the Public Health Service and began assembling a team of behavioral scientists. They studied the nexus of behavior, social factors, and disease. Two scientists and Derryberry conducted the study of the role of health beliefs in explaining utilization of public health screening services. This work contributed to the development of the Health Belief Model. This provided an important theoretical foundation for modern health education. His legacy was very important because he engaged behavioral and social scientists in the problems of public health and gave importance to the role of that health education plays on human health.

Elena Sliepcevich

Elena Sliepcevich was a leading figure in the development of health education both as an academic discipline and a profession. She graduated from the University of Ireland in 1939 and received her master's degree from the University of Michigan in 1949. She received her doctorate in physical education from Springfield College in 1955. After completing her schooling, Elena Sliepcevich worked at Ohio State University in 1961 as a professor of health education. There she helped direct the School Health Education Study from 1961 to 1969, and most health education curricula used in schools today are based on the ten conceptual areas identified by the School Health Education Study. These ten areas of focus include community health, consumer health, environmental health, family life, mental and emotional health, injury prevention and safety, nutrition, personal health, prevention and control of disease, and drug use and abuse.

Helen Agnes Cleary

Helen Cleary was born March 28, 1914, at Petersburg, South Australia. She trained as a nurse at the Broken Hill and District Hospital in New South Wales. She became a general nurse in 1941, and an obstetric nurse in 1942. She joined the Royal Australian Air Force Nursing Service as a sister on November 15, 1943. Along with other RAAF nurses, she would partake in evacuations throughout New Guinea and Borneo, which earned the nurses the nickname "the flying angels", and were also known as the "glamor girls" of the air force. In April 1945, she was ranked No. 2 Medical Air Evacuation Transport Unit, and began bringing thousands of Australian and British servicemen from prisoner-of-war camps after Japan had surrendered. She and other nurses cared for many patients who suffered from malnutrition and dysentery. During the Korean War, Cleary was charge sister on the RAAF, where she organized medical evacuations of Australians from Korea, fought for better treatment and conditions of the critically wounded, and nursed recently exchanged Prisoners of War. On August 18, 1967, Ms. Cleary was made honorary nursing sister to Queen Elizabeth II. She had been appointed an associate of the Royal Red Cross in 1960, and became a leading member in 1968 for her contributions to the training of medical staff, and for maintaining "the high ideals of the nursing profession". She retired on March 28, 1969, and later died on August 26, 1987.

Delbert Oberteuffer

A long time health educator, Delbert Oberteuffer definitely made his mark on the physical education and health education world. He was born in Portland, Oregon in 1902 where he remained through college, attending the University of Oregon receiving his bachelor's degree. His next step took him to the prestigious Columbia University where he obtained his Masters of Arts and Doctor of Philosophy Degree. He furthered his education by becoming a professor at Ohio State University where he taught from 1932 until 1966. During his time there, he was head of the Men's Physical Education Department for 25 years. After years of hard work, he was rewarded with numerous jobs including the President of the American School Health Association and The College of Physical Education Association. He died in 1981 at the age of 79. He was survived by his wife, Katherine, and his son, Theodore K. Oberteuffer.

Howard Hoyman

Howard Hoyman is mainly recognized for his work in sex education and introductions of ecology concepts. He is credited for developing the original sex education program for students in grades 1 through 12. The model Hoyman created heavily influenced the thinking of many health educators. Hoyman received his bachelor's degree from Ohio State University in 1931. He then went on to earn his master's degree in 1932 and Doctorate in 1945 from the University of Colombia. Throughout his career he wrote over 200 articles and was honored many times by multiple organizations such as Phi Beta Kappa and the American Public Health Association. Dr. Hoyman retired in 1970 as A Professor Emeritus.

Lloyd Kolbe

Lloyd Kolbe received his B.S. form Towson University and then received his Ph.D. and M.Ed. from the University of Toledo during the 1970s. Dr. Kolbe played a huge role in the development of many health programs applied to the daily life of different age groups. He received the award for Excellence in Prevention and Control of Chronic Disease, which is the highest recognition in his department of work, for his work forming the Division of Adolescent and School Health. Dr. Kolbe was the Director of this program for 15 years. He has also taken time to write and publish numerous books such as *Food marketing to Children and Youth and School* as well as *Terrorism Related to Advancing and Improving the Nation's Health.*

Robert Morgan Pigg

University of Florida professor, Robert Morgan Pigg, started his health career in 1969 when he received his bachelor's degree in Health, Physical Education, and Recreation from Middle Tennessee State University. A year later he received his M.Ed; also from Middle Tennessee University before moving on to Indian University where he obtained his H.S.D. in 1974 and his M.P.H. in 1980. He held many jobs at numerous Universities including Western Kentucky University, University of Georgia, Indiana University, and the University of Florida where he currently resides today. Pigg's main focus of interest is the promotion of health towards children and adolescents. After spending 20 years as Editor for the Journal of Health, he was given the job as Department Chair in 2007 for The University of Florida.

Linda Rae Murray

Linda Rae Murray holds her MD, and MPH. Currently she is the Chief Officer for the Ambulatory & Community Health Network. She was elected president November 2009. Dr. Murray has served in a number of Medical settings her most recent being Medical Director of the federally funded health center, Winfield Moody, serving the Cabrini–Green public housing project in Chicago. She has also been an active member of the board of national organizations. Along with this she served as Chief Medical Officer in primary care for the twenty three primary care and community health centers. Today Murray serves as the Chief Medical Officer for the Cook County Health & Hospital system. Dr. Murray has also been a voice for social justice and health care as a basic human right for over forty years.

Mark J. Kittleson

Mark J. Kittleson is a professor at New Mexico State University for Public Health Education. His interests include Educational Technology and Behaviorism; he attended the University of Akron and received his PhD in Health Education. Dr. Kittleson has experience as owner and founder of the HEDIR a place where people can hold discussions related to health and health education. His honors and awards consist of Scholar of the Year, American Association of Health Education 2008 and he is a member of the American Association of Health Education.

Elaine Auld

Elaine Auld has been a leading figure for over more than 30 years in the health education field. She attended the University of Michigan, MPH, and Health Behavior/Health Education, from 1976 to 1978 Elaine is the chief executive officer for the Society for Public Health Education (SOPHE) and has had many contributions in health promotion and health communications. She has been a certified health specialist since 1989 and in 1996 was an adviser to the first Health Education Graduate Standards. Elaine was involved with the Competency Update Project (CUP), which provided standards for the health education profession. Elaine's interest and work are related to health education credentialing and standards, workforce development, public policy, and health equity. For the last decade Elaine has been a site visitor for the Council on Education for Public Health, and also strengthened the accreditation and preparation of future health specialists, which is key to an overall healthy well-being. Elaine has received two awards U of MI SPH Alumni of the Year Award in 2010 and SOPHE Distinguished Fellow in 2008.

Susan Wooley

Susan Wooley received her bachelor's degree from Case Western Reserve University, a master's degree in health education from the University of North Carolina at Greensboro, and a Ph.D. in health education from Temple University. Susan is the executive director of the American School Health Association and has been a member to ASHA for 31 years. She co-edited Health Is Academic: A Guide to Coordinated School Health Programs and co-authored Give It a Shot, a Toolkit for Nurses and Other Immunization Champions Working with Secondary Schools. Susan has had many previous jobs such as CDC's Division of Adolescent and School Health, Delaware State College, American Association for Health Education and Delaware Department of Public Instruction and is also a certified health specialist. Wooley spent four years on a curriculum development project for elementary schools, Science for Life and Living: Integrating Science, Technology and Health. Now Susan oversees the day-to-day operations of a national professional association and provides consultation and technical assistance to others working toward health education.

Health Education Worldwide

There are many countries which developed a Health Education curriculum. For example:

Romania

Since 2001, the Ministry of Education, Research, Youth and Sports developed a national curriculum on Health Education. The National Health Education Programme in Romanian Schools was considered as being a priority for the intervention of the GFATM (Global Fund) and UN Agencies.

Japan

Shokuiku (Kanji) is the Japanese term for "food education". The law defines it as the "acquisition of knowledge about food and nutrition, as well as the ability to make appropriate decisions through practical experience with food, with the aim of developing people's ability to live on a healthy diet".

It was initiated by Sagen Ishizuka, a famous military doctor and pioneer of the macrobiotic diet. Following the introduction of Western fast food in the late 20th century, the Japanese government mandated education in nutrition and food origins, starting with the Basic Law of Shokuiku in 2005, and followed with the School Health Law in 2008. Universities have established programs to teach shokuiku in public schools, as well as investigating its effectiveness through academic study.

Major concerns that led to the development of shokuiku law include:

- Schoolchildren skipping breakfast.
- Children purchasing meals at a convenience store instead of eating with their parents.
- Families not eating meals together.

Classes in shokuiku will study the processes of making food, such as farming or fermentation; how additives create flavor; and where food comes from.

Poland

Health education in Poland is not mandatory, but research has shown that even with implantation of health education that the adolescents of Poland were still not choosing to live a health lifestyle. Health education is still needed in Poland, but the factor of what is actually available, especially in rural areas, and what is affordable affects the decisions more than what is healthy.

Taiwan

The Health education in Taiwan focus on multiple topic, this included but not limit to

- Education for student to enhance its health satue
- assists parents to use health resources,information
- Teach student to understand specific diseases & known basic medical knowledge
- help adolescents to handle currency problem,those such as menstruation, erection

Health Campaign

A Health campaign is a type of media campaign which attempts to promote public health by making new health interventions available. The organizers of a health campaign frequently use education along with an opportunity to participate further, such as when a vaccination campaign seeks both to educate the public about a vaccine and provide the vaccine to people who want it. When a health campaign has international relevance it may be called a global health campaign.

Examples

Health Education

Many diseases and medical problems have a "health education campaign" or "awareness campaign" associated with them. The goal of such a campaign is to make people conscious of the impact of diseases and to provide them information about the disease if they want to learn more about it.

Eradication of Infectious Diseases

Various health campaigns have taken the goal of eradicating infectious diseases. In such campaigns the organizers recruit the public to participate in the campaign by talking about it with others and encouraging others to participate.

Behavior Modification Campaign

An organization may organize a campaign which asks for participants to change their behavior in some way. Examples of such projects are smoking cessation campaigns which ask people to quit smoking, HIV prevention campaigns which ask people to do things such as use condoms to reduce HIV infection risk, or exercise campaigns which encourage people to engage in physical activity for health.

Organizations as Campaigns

In some cases the work of an organization may itself be a health campaign. This may happen when, for example, an organization exists to provide health information or medical resources to anyone who requests them. The organization itself may conduct a series of health campaigns, and its entire operation may be called a health campaign.

Management of Obesity

Management of obesity can include lifestyle changes, medications, or surgery. The main treatment for obesity consists of dieting and physical exercise. Diet programs may produce weight loss over the short term, but maintaining this weight loss is frequently difficult and often requires making exercise and a lower calorie diet a permanent part of an individual's lifestyle. Success rates of long-term weight loss maintenance with lifestyle changes are low, ranging from 2 to 20%. Dietary and lifestyle changes are effective in limiting excessive weight gain in pregnancy and improve outcomes for both the mother and the child. The National Institutes of Health recommend a weight loss goal of 5% to 10% of the person's current weight over six months.

One medication, orlistat, is current widely available and approved for long term use. Weight loss however is modest with an average of 2.9 kg (6.4 lb) at 1 to 4 years and there is little information on how these drugs affect longer-term complications of obesity. Its use is associated with high rates of gastrointestinal side effects.

The most effective treatment for obesity is bariatric surgery. Surgery for severe obesity is associated with long-term weight loss and decreased overall mortality. One study found a weight loss of between 14% and 25% (depending on the type of procedure performed) at 10 years, and a 29% reduction in all cause mortality when compared to standard weight loss measures. However, due to its cost and the risk of complications, researchers are searching for other effective yet less invasive treatments.

A 2007 review concluded that certain subgroups such as those with type 2 diabetes and women show long term benefits in all cause mortality, while outcomes for men do not seem to be improved with weight loss. A subsequent study found benefits in mortality from intentional weight loss in those who have severe obesity.

Dieting

Diets to promote weight loss are generally divided into four categories: low-fat, low-carbohydrate, low-calorie, and very low calorie. A meta-analysis of six randomized controlled trials found no difference between three of the main diet types (low calorie, low carbohydrate, and low fat), with a 2–4 kilogram (4.4–8.8 lb) weight loss in all studies. At two years these three methods resulted in similar weight loss irrespective of the macronutrients emphasized. High protein diets do not appear to make any difference. A diet high in simple sugars such as those in soft drinks increases weight.

Very low calorie diets provide 200–800 kcal/day, maintaining protein intake but limiting calories from both fat and carbohydrates. They subject the body to starvation and produce an average weekly weight loss of 1.5–2.5 kilograms (3.3–5.5 lb). These diets are not recommended for general use as they are associated with adverse side effects such as loss of lean muscle mass, increased risks of gout, and electrolyte imbalances. People attempting these diets must be monitored closely by a physician to prevent complications.

Exercise

With use, muscles consume energy derived from both fat and glycogen. Due to the large size of leg muscles, walking, running, and cycling are the most effective means of exercise to reduce body fat. Exercise affects macronutrient balance. During moderate exercise, equivalent to a brisk walk, there is a shift to greater use of fat as a fuel. To maintain health, the American Heart Association recommends a minimum of 30 minutes of moderate exercise at least 5 days a week.

The Cochrane Collaboration found that exercising alone led to limited weight loss. In combination with diet, however, it resulted in a 1 kilogram weight loss over dieting alone. A 1.5 kilogram (3.3 lb) loss was observed with a greater degree of exercise. Even though exercise as carried out in the general population has only modest effects, a dose response curve is found, and very intense exercise can lead to substantial weight loss. During 20 weeks of basic military training with no dietary restriction, obese military recruits lost 12.5 kg (27.6 lb). High levels of physical activity seem to be necessary to maintain weight loss. A pedometer appears useful for motivation. Over an average of 18-weeks of use physical activity increased by 27% resulting in a 0.38 decreased in BMI.

Signs that encourage the use of stairs as well as community campaigns have been shown to be effective in increasing exercise in a population. The city of Bogota, Colombia for example blocks off 113 kilometers (70 mi) of roads every Sunday and on holidays to make it easier for its citizens to get exercise. These pedestrian zones are part of an effort to combat chronic diseases, including obesity.

In an effort to combat the issue, a primary school in Australia instituted a standing classroom in 2013.

Weight Loss Programs

Weight loss programs often promote lifestyle changes and diet modification. This may involve eating smaller meals, cutting down on certain types of food, and making a conscious effort to exercise more. These programs also enable people to connect with a group of others who are attempting to lose weight, in the hopes that participants will form mutually motivating and encouraging relationships.

A number of popular programs exist, including Weight Watchers, Overeaters Anonymous, and Jenny Craig. These appear to provide modest weight loss (2.9 kg, 6.4 lb) over dieting on one's own (0.2 kg, 0.4 lb) over a two-year period. Internet-based programs appear to be ineffective. The Chinese government has introduced a number of "fat farms" where obese children go for reinforced exercise, and has passed a law which requires students to exercise or play sports for an hour a day at school.

In a structured setting, 67% of people who lost greater than 10% of their body mass maintained or continued to lose weight one year later. An average maintained weight loss of more than 3 kg (6.6 lb) or 3% of total body mass could be sustained for five years.

Medication

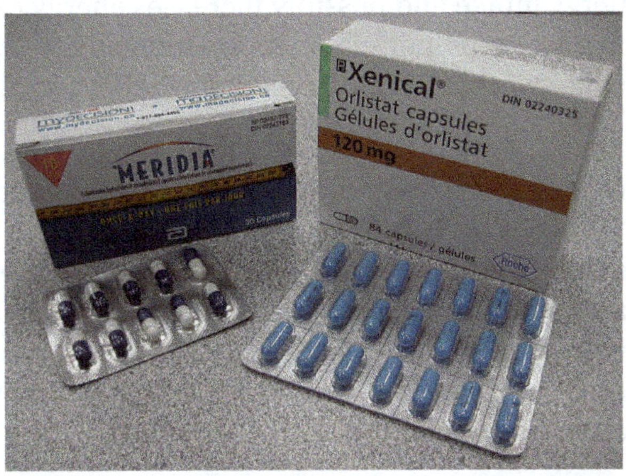

Orlistat (Xenical) the most commonly used medication to treat obesity and sibutramine (Meridia) a withdrawn medication due to cardiovascular side effects

Several anti-obesity medications are currently approved by the FDA for long term use. Orlistat reduces intestinal fat absorption by inhibiting pancreatic lipase.

Lorcaserin has been found to be effective in the treatment of obesity with a weight loss of 5.8 kg at one year as opposed to 2.2 kg with placebo and it is approved by the Food and Drug Administration for use in the treatment of obesity. Side effects may include serotonin syndrome.

The combination drug phentermine/topiramate (Qsymia) is approved by the FDA as an addition to a reduced-calorie diet and exercise for chronic weight management.

Rimonabant (Acomplia), another drug, had been withdrawn from the market. It worked via a specific blockade of the endocannabinoid system. It has been developed from the knowledge that cannabis smokers often experience hunger, which is often referred to as "the munchies". It had been approved in Europe for the treatment of obesity but has not received approval in the United States or Canada due to safety concerns. European Medicines Agency in October 2008 recommended the suspension of the sale of rimonabant as the risk seem to be greater than the benefits. Sibutramine (Meridia), which acts in the brain to inhibit deactivation of the neurotransmitters, thereby decreasing appetite was withdrawn from the UK market in January 2010 and United States and Canadian markets in October 2010 due to cardiovascular concerns.

Weight loss with these drugs is modest. Over the longer term, average weight loss on orlistat is 2.9 kg (6.4 lb), sibutramine is 4.2 kg (9.3 lb) and rimonabant is 4.7 kg (10.4 lb). Orlistat and rimonabant lead to a reduced incidence of diabetes, and all three drugs have some effect on cholesterol. However, there is little information on how these drugs affect the longer-term complications or outcomes of obesity. In 2010 it was found that sibutramine increases the risk of heart attacks and strokes in people with a history of cardiovascular disease.

There are a number of less commonly used medications. Some are only approved for short term use, others are used off-label, and still others are used illegally. Most are appetite suppressants that act on one or more neurotransmitters. Phendimetrazine (Bontril), diethylpropion (Tenuate), and phentermine (Adipex-P) are approved by the FDA for short term use, while bupropion (Wellbutrin), topiramate (Topamax), and zonisamide (Zonegran) are sometimes used off-label. Recombinant human leptin is very effective in those with obesity due to congenital complete leptin deficiency via decreasing energy intake and possibly increases energy expenditure. This condition is, however, rare and this treatment is not effective for inducing weight loss in the majority of people with obesity. It is being investigated to determine whether or not it helps with weight loss maintenance.

The usefulness of certain drugs depends upon the comorbidities present. Metformin (Glucophage) is preferred in overweight diabetics, as it may lead to mild weight loss in comparison to sulfonylureas or insulin. The thiazolidinediones, on the other hand, may cause weight gain, but decrease central obesity. Diabetics also achieve modest weight loss with fluoxetine (Prozac), orlistat and sibutramine over 12–57 weeks. Preliminary evidence has however found higher number of cardiovascular events in people taking sibutramine verses control (11.4% vs. 10.0%). The long-term health benefits of these treatments remain unclear.

Fenfluramine and dexfenfluramine were withdrawn from the market in 1997, while ephedrine (found in the traditional Chinese herbal medicine *má huáng* made from the *Ephedra sinica*) was removed from the market in 2004. Racemic amphetamine is FDA-approved for the treatment of obesity.

Though hypothesized that supplementation of vitamin D may be an effective treatment for obesity, studies do not support this.

Surgery

Bariatric surgery ("weight loss surgery") is the use of surgical intervention in the treatment of obesity. As every operation may have complications, surgery is only recommended for severely obese people (BMI > 40) who have failed to lose weight following dietary modification and pharmacological treatment. Weight loss surgery relies on various principles: the two most common approaches are reducing the volume of the stomach (e.g. by adjustable gastric banding and vertical banded gastroplasty), which produces an earlier sense of satiation, and reducing the length of bowel that comes into contact with food (e.g. by gastric bypass surgery or endoscopic duodenal-jejunal bypass surgery), which directly reduces absorption. Band surgery is reversible, while bowel shortening operations are not. Some procedures can be performed laparoscopically. Complications from weight loss surgery are frequent.

Surgery for severe obesity is associated with long-term weight loss and decreased overall mortality. One study found a weight loss of between 14% and 25% (depending on the type of procedure performed) at 10 years, and a 29% reduction in all cause mortality when compared to standard weight loss measures. A marked decrease in the risk of diabetes mellitus, cardiovascular disease and cancer has also been found after bariatric surgery. Marked weight loss occurs during the first few months after surgery, and the loss is sustained in the long term. In one study there was an unexplained increase in deaths from accidents and suicide, but this did not outweigh the benefit in terms of disease prevention. When the two main techniques are compared, gastric bypass procedures are found to lead to 30% more weight loss than banding procedures one year after surgery.

Ileojejunal bypass, in which the digestive tract is rerouted to bypass the small intestine, was an experimental surgery designed as a remedy for morbid obesity.

The effects of liposuction on obesity are less well determined. Some small studies show benefits while others show none. A treatment involving the placement of an intragastric balloon via gastroscopy has shown promise. One type of balloon led to a weight loss of 5.7 BMI units over 6 months or 14.7 kg (32.4 lb). Regaining lost weight is common after removal, however, and 4.2% of people were intolerant of the device.

An implantable nerve simulator which improves the feeling of fullness was approved by the FDA in 2015.

In 2016 the FDA approved an aspiration therapy device that siphons food from the stomach to the outside and decreases caloric intake. As of 2015 one trial shows promising results.

Clinical Protocols

Much of the Western world has created clinical practice guidelines in an attempt to address rising rates of obesity. Australia, Canada, the European Union, and the United States have all published statements since 2004.

In a clinical practice guideline by the American College of Physicians, the following five recommendations are made:

1. People with a BMI of over 30 should be counseled on diet, exercise and other relevant behavioral interventions, and set a realistic goal for weight loss.
2. If these goals are not achieved, pharmacotherapy can be offered. The person needs to be informed of the possibility of side-effects and the unavailability of long-term safety and efficacy data.
3. Drug therapy may consist of sibutramine, orlistat, phentermine, diethylpropion, fluoxetine, and bupropion. For more severe cases of obesity, stronger drugs such as amphetamine and methamphetamine may be used on a selective basis. Evidence is not sufficient to recommend sertraline, topiramate, or zonisamide.
4. In people with a BMI over 40 who fail to achieve their weight loss goals (with or without medication) and who develop obesity-related complications, referral for bariatric surgery may be indicated. The person needs to be aware of the potential complications.
5. Those requiring bariatric surgery should be referred to high-volume referral centers, as the evidence suggests that surgeons who frequently perform these procedures have fewer complications.

A clinical practice guideline by the US Preventive Services Task Force (USPSTF) concluded that the evidence is insufficient to recommend for or against routine behavioral counseling to promote a healthy diet in unselected people in primary care settings, but that intensive behavioral dietary counseling is recommended in those with hyperlipidemia and other known risk factors for cardiovascular and diet-related chronic disease. Intensive counseling can be delivered by primary care clinicians or by referral to other specialists, such as nutritionists or dietitians.

Canada developed and published evidence-based practice guidelines in 2006. The guidelines attempt to address the prevention and management of obesity at both the individual and population levels in both children and adults. The European Union published clinical practice guidelines in 2008 in an effort to address the rising rates of obesity in Europe. Australia came out with practice guidelines in 2004.

Research

Temporary, controllable gastric pseudo-bezoars (swallowable, swellable foreign bodies in the stomach meant to reduce gastric volume from inside the organ) are being tested. Treatment with naltrexone plus bupropion in a phase three trial resulted in a weight lose of 5–6% versus 1% for a placebo.

Breast Cancer Awareness

Breast cancer awareness is an effort to raise awareness and reduce the stigma of breast cancer through education on symptoms and treatment. Supporters hope that greater knowledge will lead to earlier detection of breast cancer, which is associated with higher long-term survival rates, and that money raised for breast cancer will produce a reliable, permanent cure.

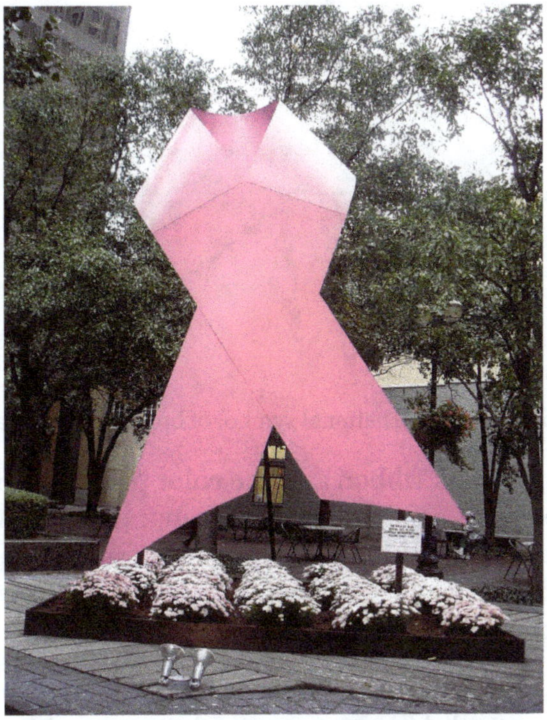

Breast Cancer Awareness, Louisville, Kentucky

Breast cancer advocacy and awareness efforts are a type of health advocacy. Breast cancer advocates raise funds and lobby for better care, more knowledge, and more patient empowerment. They may conduct educational campaigns or provide free or low-cost services. Breast cancer culture, sometimes called pink ribbon culture, is the cultural outgrowth of breast cancer advocacy, the social movement that supports it, and the larger women's health movement.

The pink ribbon is the most prominent symbol of breast cancer awareness, and in many countries the month of October is National Breast Cancer Awareness Month. Some national breast cancer organizations receive substantial financial support from corporate sponsorships.

Marketing Approaches

The goal of breast cancer awareness campaigns is to raise the public's "brand awareness" for breast cancer, its detection, its treatment, and the need for a reliable, permanent cure. Increased awareness has increased the number of women receiving mammograms, the number of breast cancers detected, and the number of women receiving biopsies. Overall, as a result of awareness, breast cancers are being detected at an earlier, more treatable stage. Awareness efforts have successfully utilized marketing approaches to reduce the stigma associated with the disease.

Generally speaking, breast cancer awareness campaigns have been highly effective in getting attention for the disease. Breast cancer receives significantly more media coverage than other prevalent cancers, such as prostate cancer.

Breast Cancer as a Brand

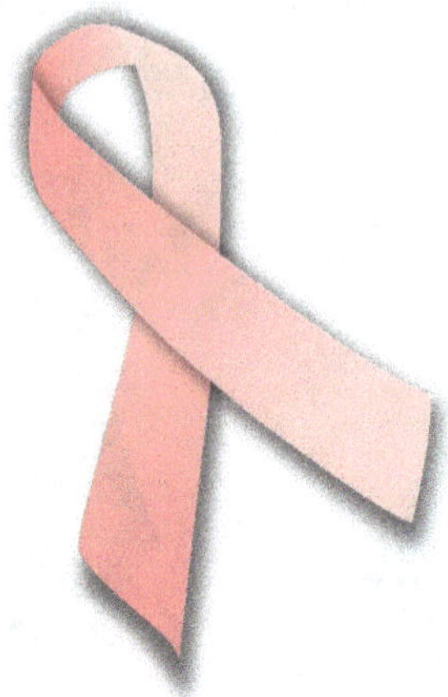

A pink ribbon, an international symbol of breast cancer awareness.

Breast cancer advocacy uses the pink ribbon and the color pink as a concept brand to raise money and increase screening. The breast cancer brand is strong: people who support the "pink brand" are members of the socially aware niche market, who are in favor of improved lives for women, believe in positive thinking, trust biomedical science to be able to solve any problem if given enough money, and prefer curative treatments to prevention.

The brand ties together fear of cancer, hope for early identification and successful treatment, and the moral goodness of women with breast cancer and anyone who visibly identifies themselves with breast cancer patients. This brand permits and even encourages people to substitute conscientious consumption and individual symbolic actions, like buying or wearing a pink ribbon, for concrete, practical results, such as collective political action aimed at discovering non-genetic causes of breast cancer.

The establishment of the brand and the entrenchment of the breast cancer movement has been uniquely successful, because no countermovement opposes the breast cancer movement or believes that breast cancer is desirable.

Pink Ribbon

A pink ribbon is a symbol of breast cancer awareness. It may be worn to honor those who have been diagnosed with breast cancer, or to identify products that a manufacturer would like to sell to consumers that are interested in breast cancer. Pink ribbons are sometimes sold as fundraisers, much like poppies on Remembrance Day.

The pink ribbon is associated with individual generosity, faith in scientific progress, and an optimistic "can-do" attitude. It encourages individuals to focus on the emotionally appealing ultimate vision of a cure for breast cancer, rather than the reality that there is no certain cure for breast cancer, and no guarantee there will ever be such a cure. The practice of blindly wearing or displaying a pink ribbon without making other, more concrete efforts to cure breast cancer has been described as a kind of slacktivism due to its lack of real effects, and has been compared to equally simple yet ineffective "awareness" practices like the drive for women to post the colors of their bras on Facebook. Critics say that the feel-good nature of pink ribbons and "pink consumption" distracts society from the lack of progress in curing breast cancer. It is also criticized for reinforcing gender stereotypes and objectifying women and their breasts.

Events

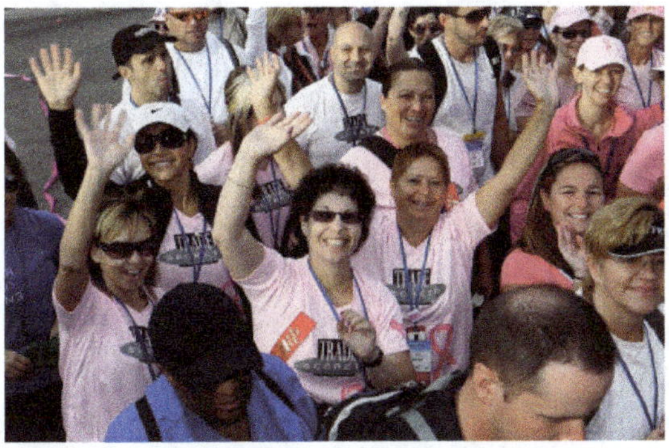

Large events, such as walkathons, promote breast cancer awareness.

Each year, the month of October is recognized as National Breast Cancer Awareness Month by many governments, the media, and cancer survivors. The month-long campaign has been called *Pinktober* because of the increased production of pink goods for sale, and *National Breast Cancer Industry Month* by critics like Breast Cancer Action. NBCAM was begun in 1985 by the American Cancer Society and pharmaceutical company AstraZeneca. The organization that runs the official NBCAM aims to promote mammography and other forms of early detection as the most effective means of fighting breast cancer.

Typical NBCAM events include fundraising-based foot races, walk-a-thons, and bicycle rides. Participants solicit donations to a breast cancer-related charity in return for running, walking, or riding in the event. Through mass-participation events, breast cancer survivors form a single, united group that speaks and acts consistently and shares a coherent set of beliefs. They also reinforce the cultural connection between each individual's physical fitness and moral fitness. Events organized by Avon or Komen are known to allocate around 25%-33% of donations to the funds needed to organize the event and advertise it.

A Breast Cancer Awareness programme is in progress in India among Muslim women by a NGO. December, 2013.

Various landmarks are illuminated in pink lights as a visible reminder of breast cancer, and public events, such as American football games, may use pink equipment or supplies. In 2010, all King Features Syndicate comic strips on one Sunday were printed in shades of red and pink, with a pink ribbon logo appearing prominently in one panel.

Private companies may arrange a "pink day", in which employees wear pink clothes in support of breast cancer patients, or pay for the privilege of a relaxed dress code, such as Lee National Denim Day. Some events are directed at people in specific communities, such as the Global Pink Hijab Day, which was started in America to encourage appropriate medical care and reduce the stigma of breast cancer among Muslim women, and *Male Breast Cancer Awareness Week*, which some organizations highlight during the third week of October. Most events are well-received, but some, like the unauthorized painting of the Pink Bridge in Huntington, West Virginia, are controversial.

Companies and Consumers

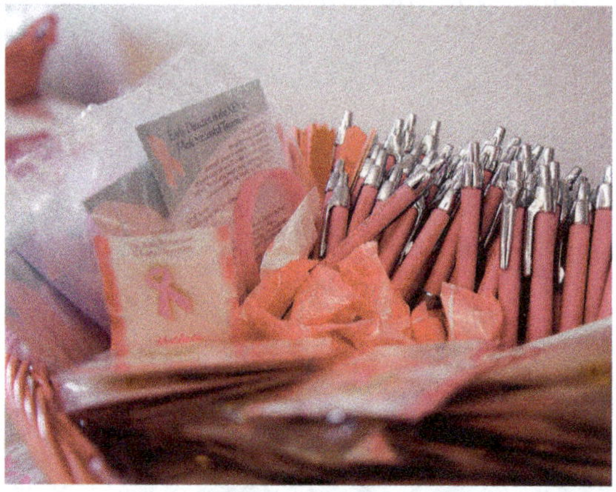

The basket contains an assortment of pink ribbon-branded promotional merchandise, including awareness bracelets, ink pens, candy, and emery boards.

Thousands of breast cancer-themed products are developed and sold each year. Some of these items are everyday products that have been repackaged or repositioned to take advantage of cause-related marketing, such as teddy bears, clothing, jewelry, candles, and coffee mugs. These blended value objects offer consumers an opportunity to simultaneously buy an object and make a donation to a breast cancer organization. Some of these products are produced and/or sold by breast cancer survivors or charities for fundraising purposes, while others are for profits in addition to fundraising. Manufacturers also produce products with pink labels or pink ribbon logos to donate a sum of money to support the cause. The donation is typically capped so that it is reached after a fixed level of sales, although in some cases the company is providing only free advertising for a selected charity. Although advertising costs are rarely disclosed, some companies have been found to spend far more money advertising "pink products" and tie-ins than they donate to charitable organizations supporting research or patients. For example, in 2005, 3M spent US $500,000 advertising post-it notes printed with a pink ribbon logo. Sales were nearly double what the company expected, but the campaign resulted in a $300,000 donation.

Advertisers and retail consultants have said that because of consumer cynicism, a company can benefit from marketing its support for a cause such as breast cancer awareness only when the company treats that support as "a commitment and not a marketing opportunity". Andrew Benett, an executive at Euro RSCG said that because consumers "have become more mindful, more thoughtful, about how they consume, where they consume, why they consume", companies cannot succeed by "just slapping a pink ribbon on a product and [expecting that] people will buy more". Pink products have also been condemned as promoting consumerism, materialism, and environmental degradation. Critics are also concerned that the ubiquity of pink products may mislead people into thinking that significant progress has been made, and that small, individual actions, like buying a breast cancer-themed product, are sufficient. Responding to criticism, Komen CEO Nancy G. Brinker said that corporate promotions enabled the organization to reach new audiences and that "America is built on consumerism. To say we shouldn't use it to solve the social ills that confront us doesn't make sense to me."

The first breast cancer awareness stamp in the U.S., featuring a pink ribbon, was issued in 1996. As it did not sell well, a semi-postal stamp without a pink ribbon, the breast cancer research stamp, was designed in 1998. Products like these emphasize the relationship between being a consumer and supporting women with breast cancer. In Canada, the Royal Canadian Mint produced 30 million 25-cent coins with pink ribbons during 2006 for normal circulation. Designed by the mint's director of engraving, Cosme Saffioti (reverse), and Susanna Blunt (obverse), this colored coin is the second in history to be put into regular circulation.

Business marketing campaigns, particularly sales promotions for products that increase pollution or have been linked to the development of breast cancer, such as alcohol, high-fat foods, some pesticides, or the parabens and phthalates used by most cosmetic companies, have been condemned as pinkwashing (a portmanteau of *pink ribbon* and *whitewash*). Such promotions generally result in a token donation to a breast cancer-related charity by taking advantage of the consumers' fear of cancer and grief for people who have died to drive sales. Critics say that these promotions, which net more than US $30 million each year just for fundraising powerhouse Susan G. Komen for the Cure, do little more than support the marketing machines that produce them. Komen says that corporate sponsorships are necessary to pay for the organization's efforts: in the 2010 fiscal year it spent $175 million on public health education and awareness campaigns, $75 million on medical research and about $67 million on treatment and screenings for patients.

Two significant campaigns against pink consumption are the National Breast Cancer Coalition's "Not Just Ribbons" campaign, and Breast Cancer Action's "Think Before You Pink" campaign. NBCC's "Not Just Ribbons" campaign sought to focus awareness efforts onto substantive issues such as genetic discrimination, access to cancer treatment, patient rights, and environmental breast cancer research. "Think Before You Pink" encouraged consumers to ask questions about pink products (e.g., to find out how much of a donation was being made).

Advertisements

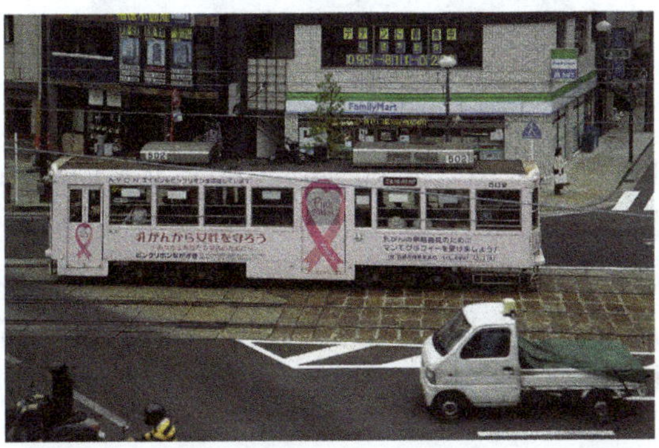

This trolley advertisement promotes cosmetics company Avon Products, Inc. and breast cancer awareness. Because of the pink ribbon brand's strength, the advertisement is easily recognized as a promotion for breast cancer awareness, even among people who cannot read the Japanese text.

Many corporate and charitable organizations run advertisements related to breast cancer, especially during National Breast Cancer Awareness Month, in the hope of increasing sales by aligning themselves with a positive, helpful message. In addition to selling pink products, corporate advertisements may promote the company's progressive policies, or may provide free advertising for a chosen charity. Medical institutions may run advertisements for mammogram or other breast-related services. Non-profit organizations often benefit from public service announcements, which are free advertisements provided by newspapers, radio and television stations, and other media.

Some marketing blurs the line between advertisements and events, such as flash mobs as a form of guerrilla marketing. The typical participant in the breast cancer movement, and therefore the advertisers' target audience, is a white, middle-aged, middle-class, well-educated woman.

Some corporate sponsors are criticized for having a conflict of interest. For example, some of the prominent sponsors of these advertisements include businesses that sell the expensive equipment needed to perform screening mammography; an increase in the number of women seeking mammograms means an increase in their sales, which has led critics to say that their sponsorship is not a voluntary act of charity, but an effort to increase sales. The regulated drug and medical device industry uses the color pink, positive images, and other themes of the pink ribbon culture in direct-to-consumer advertising to associate their breast cancer products with the fear, hope, and wholesome goodness of the breast cancer movement. This is particularly evident in advertisements designed to sell screening mammograms.

Social Role of the Woman with Breast Cancer

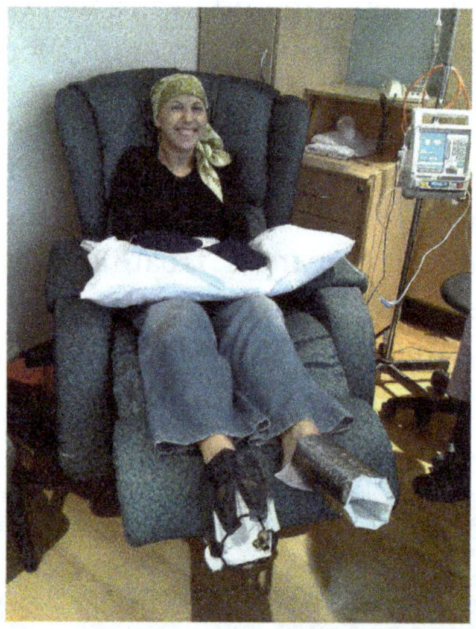

A woman being treated with docetaxel chemotherapy for breast cancer. Cold mittens and wine coolers are placed on her hands and feet to reduce harm to her nails.

The marketing of breast cancer awareness allows people to incorporate support for awareness into their personal identity or lifestyle. Socially aware, pro-woman individuals, businesses, politicians, and organizations use pink ribbons and other trappings of breast cancer awareness to signal their support for women, health, and mainstream medicine.

The She-ro

The term "she-ro", derived from hero, is used in discussions of breast cancer to refer to women who have been diagnosed with breast cancer, and sometimes to those who have survived breast cancer. The term describes an "idealized" patient who combines assertiveness, optimism, femininity and sexuality, despite the effects of treatment, and as a "paragon [who] uses a diagnosis of breast cancer as a catalyst for a personal transformation".

Sociologist Gayle Sulik analysis of the she-ro's social role ascribes it qualities that include being an educated medical consumer with a brave, pleasant and optimistic public appearance and demean-

or who aggressively fights breast cancer through compliance with screening guidelines and "disciplined practice of 'breast health'". In America the she-ro is diagnosed early due to adherence to early screening recommendations, and, by definition, survives her diagnosis. The role emphasizes the femininity and female gender role of the she-ro, offsetting the masculine characteristics of assertiveness, selfishness and "fighting" cancer by cultivating a feminine appearance and concern for others. After treatment, the she-ro regains her femininity by using breast reconstruction, prosthetic devices, wigs, cosmetics, and clothing to present an aesthetically appealing, upper-class, heterosexual feminine appearance and by maintaining relationships in which she can nurture other people. Ensuring the proper feeling rules of the breast cancer culture is encouraged, including remaining optimistic of a full cure, rationalizing the selfishness of treatment as a temporary measure and feeling guilty that it forces her to put her needs momentarily above the needs of others or due to her perceived inadequacy in caring for her family or other women with cancer. Also included in the role is a form of have-it-all superwoman, cultivating a normal appearance and activity level and minimizing the disruption that breast cancer causes to people around her.

Consequences

The effort of maintaining the role of a she-ro can be stressful. The role encourages women to care for others rather than themselves, which the patient may find comforting, but this may lead to the reluctance or inability to ask for help they need or want which can lead to bitterness that their friends and family did not offer these services unbidden. The success of the patient's normalization efforts may paradoxically increase their dissatisfaction, as their apparent ability to handle it all discourages people from offering help. The breast cancer culture celebrates women who display the attitude deemed correct, which implies that their continued survival is due to this positive attitude and fighting spirit. While cheerfulness, hope, and good social support can be advantageous to health outcomes, it cannot determine survival rates. Women who reject the she-ro model may find themselves socially isolated by the breast cancer support groups that are nominally supposed to help them. Support from "the sisterhood" favors the "passionately pink", and tends to overlook those whose response is incompatible with the pink ribbon culture because it is angry, unhappy, or afraid.

The breast cancer culture is ill-equipped to deal with women who are dying or who have died and their experiences may not be memorialized, validated or represented as part of the movement, instead being ignored or shunned as failures and as hope-destroying examples of reality. Similarly, the culture is also ill-equipped to deal with the news that a previously hyped treatment or screening procedure has been determined to be ineffective, with women advocating for the acceptance and promotion of inexpedient activities and inefficient or even sometimes harmful drugs.

Breast Cancer Culture

Breast cancer culture, or pink ribbon culture, is the set of activities, attitudes, and values that surround and shape breast cancer in public. The dominant values are selflessness, cheerfulness, unity, and optimism. It is pro-doctor, pro-medicine, and pro-mammogram. Health care professionals are sources of information, but the rightness of their advice is not to be seriously questioned by women with breast cancer. Patients are not encouraged to ask where research money is going or if the research industry is making progress in finding the "cure". The emphasis on cheerfulness allows society to blame women for developing breast cancer and limits their responses to certain culturally determined scripts. The requirement of cheerful optimism arose from the theory that cancer had a psychosomatic origin and that people who were diagnosed with cancer had a "cancer personality" that was depressed, repressed, and self-loathing. Psychotherapy was therefore considered an adjunct treatment used to produce a cheerful, self-affirming identity. This theory was predominant among psychiatrists through the 1970s, but has since been discredited. In a process called benefit finding, the she-ro uses the emotional trauma of being diagnosed with breast cancer and the suffering of extended treatment to transform herself into a stronger, happier and more sensitive person who is grateful for the opportunity to become a better person. In particular, she sees breast cancer as an opportunity to give herself permission for necessary personal growth that she felt she was prohibited from or unable to make before. Breast cancer thereby becomes a rite of passage rather than a disease, with pink ribbon culture honoring the suffering of its she-roes by selecting them based on the amount of misery they have experienced and leading women whose treatment is less painful or debilitating to feel excluded and devalued. The suffering, particularly the extended suffering of months of chemotherapy and radiation treatment, forms a metaphorical type of ordeal or rite of passage that initiates women into the inner circle of breast cancer culture. Barbara Ehrenreich describes it as:

Understood as a rite of passage, breast cancer resembles the initiation rites so exhaustively studied by Mircea Eliade: First there is the selection of the initiates—by age in the tribal situation, by mammogram or palpation here. Then come the requisite ordeals—scarification or circumcision within traditional cultures, surgery and chemotherapy for the cancer patient. Finally, the initiate emerges into a new and higher status—an adult and a warrior—or in the case of breast cancer, a "survivor."

Mainstream pink ribbon culture has aspects that are deemed trivializing, silencing, and infantilizing. Women with breast cancer are surrounded by childish kitsch such as pink teddy bears and crayons, but there is no equivalent gift of toy cars for men diagnosed with prostate cancer. Women who choose not to conform to the culture may feel excluded and isolated; those who cannot conform to the prescribed triumphant script report feeling unable to share their stories honestly. Anger, negativity and fatalism transgress the feeling rules, and women with breast cancer who express anger or negativity are corrected by other women with breast cancer and members of the breast cancer support organizations. Appearing unattractive—such as going out in public with a bare, bald head if treatment causes temporary hair loss—transgresses the approved, upper-class style of pink femininity and provokes shaming comments from strangers. Programs such as Reach to Recovery and Look Good, Feel Better inform breast cancer patients of this cultural standard and help them conform to it. This standard is not universally adhered to, with "the question of wigs versus baldness [defining] one of the few real disagreements in breast-cancer culture," and some women have used the effects of their breast cancer treatments as an opportunity to engage in *avant-garde* makeovers:

One decorates her scalp with temporary tattoos of peace signs, panthers, and frogs; another expresses herself with a shocking purple wig; a third reports that unadorned baldness makes her feel 'sensual, powerful, able to recreate myself with every new day' using temporary tattoos, colored wigs or open baldness to reinvent their appearances according to radical, natural or cosmetically enhanced tastes.

Since the beginning of the 21st century, breast cancer culture has become more sexualized, and many awareness campaigns now reflect the old advertising truism that sex sells. The "booby campaigns", such as "Save the Tatas" and the "I ♥ Boobies" gel bracelets, rely on a cultural obsession with breasts and a market that is already highly aware of breast cancer. This message trivializes women and reflects a belief that breast cancer is important because cancer and its treatment makes women feel less sexually desirable and interferes with men's sexual access to women's breasts. These campaigns tend to attract a younger audience than traditional campaigns.

At the same time, breast cancer culture tends to overlook men with breast cancer and women who do not fit the white, middle-class archetype. African-Americans involved with breast cancer organizations often feel like their role is to be the token minority.

Feminism and the Breast Cancer Wars

The breast cancer wars were a series of conflicts between advocates and others about the causes, treatments, and societal responses to breast cancer. Women in the late 1980s and 1990s followed the successful approach used by ACT-UP and other AIDS awareness groups, of staging media-friendly protests to increase political pressure. Prominent women who made the "wrong" choice were publicly excoriated, as when Nancy Reagan chose mastectomy over lumpectomy followed by six weeks of radiation therapy. The abortion–breast cancer hypothesis was formulated when an early study showed a connection between voluntary abortions and the development of breast cancer in premenopausal women, which pitted breast cancer advocates against abortion rights advocates.

Advocates for women's issues have said that breast cancer is special because of its status as a largely female disease, society's response to it is an ongoing indication of the status of women and the existence of sexism. Breast cancer activist Virginia Soffa wrote that "[a]s long as it is not a national priority, the breast cancer epidemic will remain a metaphor for how society treats women". Barbara Ehrenreich writes that, before the feminist movement "medicine was a solid patriarchy," and women with breast cancer were often treated as passive, dependent objects, incapable of making appropriate choices, whose role was to accept whatever treatment was decreed by the physicians and surgeons, who held all of the power. Because of sexism in education, female surgeons were far outnumbered by their male counterparts, and until the 1990s, when Susan Love of the University of California, Los Angeles Breast Center published *Dr. Susan Love's Breast Book*, the physicians who provided breast cancer treatments were generally men. Love said that some male physicians tended to impose their own values on women, such as recommending mastectomy to older women because, being past the age of child bearing and breastfeeding, they no longer "needed" their breasts. The women's health movement promoted mutual aid, self-help, networking, and an active, informed role in the patient's health care. Since the end of the breast cancer wars, feminists have again objected to the breast cancer culture's treatment of women with breast cancer as little girls who need to be obedient to authority figures, cooperative, pleasant and pretty.

Achievements of the Breast Cancer Movement

Social Progress

Breast cancer has been known to educated women and caregivers throughout history, but modesty and horror at the consequences of a largely untreatable disease made it a taboo subject. The breast cancer movement, which developed in the 1980s and 1990s out of 20th century feminist movements and the women's health movement, has mostly removed those taboos through its modern advocacy and awareness campaigns.

Educated, Empowered Patients

At the beginning and middle of the 20th century, breast cancer was usually discussed in hushed tones, as if it were shameful. As an example, the *New York Times* refused to publish an advertisement for a breast cancer support group in the early 1950s, stating that it would not print either the word "breast" or the word "cancer". Later, however, several celebrities publicly disclosed their own health challenges, and the resulting publicity reduced the stigma. One of the first was Shirley Temple Black, the former child star, who announced her diagnosis in 1972. In October 1974, Betty Ford, the wife of the then-President of the United States, openly discussed her breast cancer diagnosis and mastectomy. Two weeks later, the wife of the then-Vice President also had a mastectomy for breast cancer. The next year, journalist Rose Kushner published her book, *Breast Cancer: A Personal History and Investigative Report*, which she had written while recovering from a modified radical mastectomy. The media reported these women's health and their treatment choices, and even invited some to appear on talk shows to discuss breast cancer frankly.

The breast cancer movement has resulted in widespread acceptance of second opinions, the development of less invasive surgical procedures, the spread of support groups, and other advances in patient care. The movement successfully separated diagnostic biopsy from mastectomy surgery; before about 1980, it was common to perform the biopsy and, if a quick review of tissues indicated a probable need, a mastectomy in the same surgery. The one-step surgery prevented women from seeking different opinions about their treatment, and sent them into the surgery without knowing whether their breasts would be removed that day. In response to women's concerns over lymphedema after routine removal of lymph nodes during mastectomy, the more limited approach of sentinel node biopsy was developed. Advocacy efforts also led to the formal recommendation against the routine use of the Halsted radical mastectomy in favor of simple mastectomies and lumpectomies.

The breast cancer movement has supported practical, educational, emotional, and financial care for women with breast cancer. Support groups, individual counseling opportunities, and other resources are made available to patients.

Increased Resources for Treatment and Research

Supporting breast cancer was seen as a distinctively pro-woman stance popular among public official. This has resulted in better access to care. For example, in much of the United States, low-income women with breast cancer may qualify for taxpayer-funded health care benefits, such as screening mammography, biopsies, or treatment, while women with the same income, but another form of cancer or a medical condition other than cancer, do not.

Breast cancer advocates have successfully increased the amount of public money being spent on cancer research and shifted the research focus away from other diseases and towards breast cancer. Breast cancer advocates also raise millions of dollars for research into cures each year, although most of the funds they raise is spent on screening programs, education and treatment. Most breast cancer research is funded by government agencies.

The high level of awareness and organized political lobbying has resulted in a disproportionate level of funding and resources given to breast cancer research and care. Favoring breast cancer with disproportionate research may have the unintended consequence of costing lives elsewhere. In 2001 UK MP Ian Gibson said, "The treatment has been skewed by the lobbying, there is no doubt about that. Breast cancer sufferers get better treatment in terms of bed spaces, facilities and doctors and nurses".

Risks of Over-Awareness

Awareness has also led to increased anxiety for women. Early detection efforts result in overdiagnosis of precancerous and cancerous tumors that would never risk the woman's life (about one-third of breast cancers diagnosed through screening programs), and result in her being subjected to invasive and sometimes dangerous radiological and surgical procedures.

In recent years, the definition of breast cancer has expanded to include non-invasive, non-cancerous conditions like lobular carcinoma in situ (LCIS) and pre-cancerous or "stage 0" conditions like ductal carcinoma in situ (DCIS). Despite the now-regretted decision to use the word *carcinoma* in these relatively common conditions (almost a quarter of "breast cancer" diagnoses in the USA), they are not life-threatening cancers. Women with these conditions are promoted as breast cancer survivors due to the fear they experienced before they became educated about their condition, rather than in respect of any real threat to their lives. This effectively increases the market size for breast cancer organizations, medical establishments, pharmaceutical manufacturers, and the makers of mammography equipment.

Women fear dying from breast cancer more than dying from heart disease, even though women are eleven times more likely to die from heart disease or stroke than from breast cancer. According to cardiologist Lisa Rosenbaum, this may be because women "view heart disease as the consequence of having done something bad, whereas to get breast cancer is to have something bad happen to you".

An emphasis on educating women about lifestyle changes that may have a small impact on preventing breast cancer often makes women feel guilty if they do develop breast cancer. Some women decide that their own cancer resulted from poor diet, lack of exercise, or other modifiable lifestyle factor, even though most cases of breast cancer are due to non-controllable factors, like genetics or naturally occurring background radiation. Adopting such a belief may increase their sense of being in control of their fate. Increased awareness inadvertently increases victim blaming. Women who resist screening mammography or breast self-exams are subjected to social pressure, scare tactics, guilt, and threats from some physicians to terminate the relationship with the patient. Similarly, the emphasis on early detection results in many women wrongly blaming themselves if their cancer is not detected at an early stage.

The promotion of research to make screening programs find ever more cancers is also criticized. One-third of diagnosed breast cancers might recede on their own. In addition to efficiently finding most deadly cancers, screening programs also find most non-life-threatening, asymptomatic breast cancers and pre-cancers, and miss some fast growing, aggressive, dangerous cancers. According to H. Gilbert Welch of the Dartmouth Institute for Health Policy and Clinical Practice, "I'm certainly not asking anyone to stop getting mammograms. I am asking my profession to tell women the truth about overdiagnosis." Welch said that research on screening mammography has taken the "brain-dead approach that says the best test is the one that finds the most cancers" rather than the one that finds dangerous cancers.

Clinicians have responded that they are unwilling to consider the possibility of leaving potential deadly cancers alone because it is "far-riskier" than the alternative. Eric Winer, director of the breast cancer program at Dana-Farber Cancer Institute in Boston, says, "I don't know anyone who offers women the option of doing nothing." Further complicating the issue of early diagnosis is the fact that it is currently impossible to distinguish malicious cancers from benign ones. Otis Brawley, a top official for the American Cancer Society, says that "even if we overdiagnose 1 in 5, we have numerous studies showing that by treating all these women, we save a bunch of lives". For instance, a 2011 Cochrane review showed a sample of mammogram screening programs resulted in a 15% reduction in mortality rate despite over-diagnosis, indicating that mammography programs save lives regardless of over-diagnosis.

Independence of Breast Cancer Organizations

Some critics say that breast cancer awareness has transformed the disease into a market-driven industry of survivorship and corporate sales pitches. Corporate marketing machines promote early detection of breast cancer, while also opposing public health efforts, such as stricter environmental legislation, that might decrease the incidence rate of breast cancer. These critics believe that some of the breast cancer organizations, particularly the highly visible Susan G. Komen for the Cure, have become captive companies that support and provide social capital to the breast cancer industry, including pharmaceutical companies, mammography equipment manufacturers, and pollution-causing industries, as well as large corporations, creating or exacerbating other problems.

For example, Ford Motor Company ran a "Warriors in Pink" promotion on their Ford Mustang sports car, which critics say was intended to sell cars and counter the bad publicity the company received by reducing its workforce by tens of thousands of people, causing many of them to lose their health insurance, rather than to prevent or cure breast cancer. A Ford spokesperson acknowledged that the objective of the promotion was to "do good works throughout the community and derive some marketing exposure at the same time", but said that over the promotion's 15 years the company had donated $100 million and that the company continued the program during the automotive industry crisis of 2008–2010 because "It's part of our DNA now." Ford believes that the recipient of the funds, Susan G. Komen for the Cure, benefited because Ford helped it reach "people who might not have thought of this organization before or may be supporting other organizations."

However, the primary sponsors are part of the breast cancer industry, particularly cancer drug makers like AstraZeneca, Bristol-Myers Squibb, and Novartis. Because the national breast cancer organizations are dependent on corporate sponsorships for survival, this situation may represent a conflict of interest that prevents these organizations from representing the needs of current and future people with breast cancer when those needs conflict with the profit-making motives of the corporate sponsors.

The structure of the breast cancer movement may allow large organizations to claim to be the voice of women with breast cancer, while simultaneously ignoring their desires.

Some breast cancer organizations, such as Breast Cancer Action, refuse to accept funds from medical or other companies they disapprove of.

Environmental Breast Cancer Movement

Most of the money raised by advocates is spent on increasing awareness, cancer screening, and existing treatments. Only a small fraction of the funds is spent on research, and less than 7% of the total research funding provided by breast cancer organizations goes to prevention. Instead, most of the charities fund research into detection and treatment. Advocates like Breast Cancer Action and women's health issues scholar Samantha King, whose book inspired the 2011 documentary *Pink Ribbons, Inc.*, are unhappy that relatively little money or attention is devoted to identifying the non-genetic causes of breast cancer or to preventing breast cancer from occurring. The mainstream breast cancer culture has been criticized for focusing on detecting and curing existing breast cancer cases, rather than on preventing future cases.

As a result, screening mammography is promoted by the breast cancer culture as the sole possible approach to public health for breast cancer. Alternatives, such as pollution prevention, are largely ignored.

As the majority of women with breast cancer have no risk factors other than sex and age, the environmental breast cancer movement suspects pollution as a significant cause, possibly from pesticides, plastics, and industrial runoff in ground water. Large organizations, such as Susan G. Komen for the Cure and the American Cancer Society, are not part of the environmental breast cancer movement. These large organizations benefit the most from corporate sponsorships that critics deride as *pinkwashing*, e.g., polluting industries trying to buy public goodwill by publishing advertisements emblazoned with pink ribbons, rather than stopping their pollution under the precautionary principle.

The non-genetic factors with consistent evidence increasing breast cancer risk include "ionizing radiation, combination estrogen–progestin hormone therapy, and greater postmenopausal weight.... for many other factors, the evidence from human studies is more limited, contradictory, or absent" and called for additional research. Conducting research into whether a chemical causes cancer is difficult, because "suspect chemicals cannot ethically be given to people to see if they cause cancer. People exposed in the past can be studied, but information about the dose and timing may be sketchy. Animal studies can provide useful information, but do not always apply to humans. And people are often exposed to mixtures of chemicals that may interact in complex ways, with effects that may also vary depending on an individual's genetic makeup".

Samantha King says that prevention research is minimized by the breast cancer industry because there is no way to make money off of cases of breast cancer that do not happen, whereas a mammography imaging system that finds more possible cancers, or a "magic bullet" that kills confirmed cancers, would be highly profitable.

Breast Cancer Action

Breast Cancer Action is an American grassroots education and advocacy organization that promotes breast cancer awareness and public health issues relating to breast cancer, and advocates for system-wide change based on prevention. Breast Cancer Action is also known for its *Think Before You Pink* campaign, launched in 2002, which encourages consumers to ask critical questions before buying pink ribbon products.

Dissent Through Art

While the pink ribbon culture is dominant, there are alternatives. The environmental breast cancer movement is one type of dissent. Another is the rejection of compliant optimism, aesthetic normalization, and social pleasingness that the pink ribbon culture promotes.

In 1998, the Art.Rage.Us art collective published a book that collected some of the art work from their traveling collection. This included art that was shocking, painful and realistic rather than beautiful, such as several self-portraits that showed mastectomy scars.

Another art form has a wider range: the illness narrative has become a staple of breast cancer literature and is prominent in women's magazines. This may take the form of a restitution or cure narrative (the protagonist seeks a physical or spiritual return to a pre-diagnosis life), a quest narrative (the protagonist must meet a goal before dying), or a chaos narrative (the situation inexorably goes from bad to worse). The cure and quest narratives fit neatly with the breast cancer culture. Chaos narratives, which are rarer in stories about breast cancer, oppose it.

History

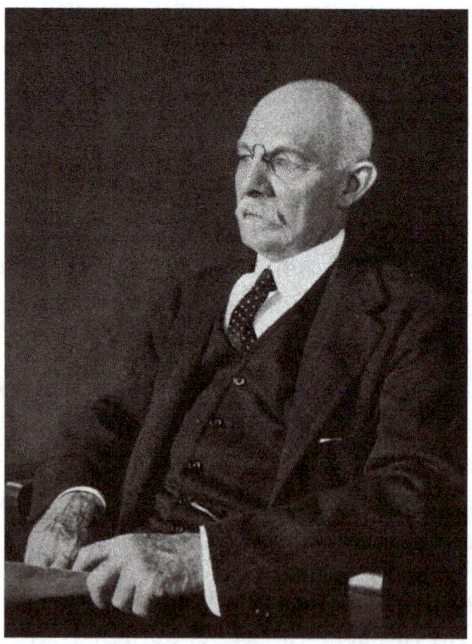

William Stewart Halsted, responsible for the radical mastectomy that dramatically reduced death rates due to breast cancer, but later proved to be controversial in its own right.

Breast cancer has been known since ancient times. With no reliable treatments, and with surgical outcomes often fatal, women tended to conceal the possibility of breast cancer as long as possible. With the dramatic improvement in survival rates at the end of the 19th century—the radical mastectomy promoted by William Stewart Halsted raised long-term survival rates from 10% to 50%—efforts to educate women about the importance of early detection and prompt action were begun.

Early campaigns included the "Women's Field Army", run by the American Society for the Control of Cancer (the forerunner of the American Cancer Society) during the 1930s and 1940s. Explicitly using a military metaphor, they promoted early detection and prompt medical intervention as every woman's duty in the war on cancer. In 1952, the first peer-to-peer support group, called Reach to Recovery, was formed. Later taken over by the American Cancer Society, it provided post-mastectomy, in-hospital visits from women who had survived breast cancer, who shared their own experiences, practical advice, and emotional support, but never medical information. This was the first program designed to promote restoration of a feminine appearance, e.g., through providing breast prostheses, as a goal.

Organizations

A wide variety of charitable organizations are involved in breast cancer awareness and support. These organizations do everything from providing practical support, to educating the public, to dispensing millions of dollars for research and treatment. Thousands of small breast cancer organizations exist. The largest and most prominent are:

- Susan G. Komen for the Cure: Komen is the largest and best funded organization, with highly visible fundraisers.
- National Breast Cancer Coalition: This large umbrella organization played key roles in several prominent pieces of American legislation, such as the creation of the United States Department of Defense's Breast Cancer Research Program, genetic non-discrimination laws, and the patients' bill of rights. They are committed to evidence-based medicine.
- Breast Cancer Action: Famous for its "Think Before You Pink" campaign against pinkwashing, BCA emphasizes the need for research into pollution as a cause of breast cancer. Like the National Women's Health Network, they refuse funding from any group that may have a conflict of interest, such as pharmaceutical companies, medical imaging companies, or pollution-causing industries.
- National Breast Cancer Organization: Closed in 2004. A dissenter to the notion of mandatory public unity, it provided case management and other services.

Alcohol Education

Alcohol education is the planned provision of information and skills relevant to living in a world where alcohol is commonly misused. The World Health Organisations (WHO) Global Status Report on Alcohol and Health, highlights the fact that alcohol will be a larger problem in later years, with estimates suggesting it will be the leading cause of disability and death. Informing people on alcohol and harmful drinking should become a priority.

History in the United States

Teaching about alcohol consumption has been a controversial topic for schools in the United States due to the differing viewpoints of Americans on the subject. A variety of educational methods that reflect these viewpoints have been developed and tried over the last century, but have yielded little behavioural change. These methods have included:

- an abstinence model — simply "don't do it"
- a social-economic model — which employs statistics demonstrating the likely effects of irresponsible drinking
- an alcoholism approach — which treats consumption of alcohol as a disease.
- an alternative approach — which seeks to offer alternatives to drinking

Kindergarten to 12th Grade

Alcohol education standards in K–12 public schools vary from state to state. In rare cases, some states such as Alaska do not require a statewide alcohol education program in their public schools. In other states, such as Delaware, the requirements are much more stringent. Delaware's students must complete 10 hours of drug and alcohol training per year in grades K-4 and 15 hours in grades 5–12.

Many studies such as Project SAFE have shown that targeting people as young as 6–8 is crucial in order to prevent them from abusing alcohol later on in life. People who begin drinking before the age of 15 are five times more likely to abuse alcohol later on in life. SAMSHA (Substance Abuse and Mental Health Services Administration) claims that "approximately 10 percent of 12-year-olds say they have used alcohol at least once. By age 13 that number doubles."

In past alcohol education programs in American schools, scare tactics were used in an attempt to persuade adolescents not to drink. According to a non-profit organization known as Prevention First, the use of scare tactics in alcohol awareness programs can actually be counterproductive. This is due to the fact that students learn better from someone who is honest and does not present them with fallacies.

Once programs that used scare tactics were disproved, evidence-based programs became the new norm. Evidence-based programs are programs that are backed by studies proving their effectiveness. One evidence-based alcohol prevention program that has proven very effective in reducing alcohol use is the LST (Life Skills Training Program). The LST program is designed for students grade 3-10. If administered every year, it would consist of 64 classroom sessions focused specifically on substance abuse. The officials with the LST claim that there has been up to a 60 percent reduction in alcohol use among students who completed the program. Although it may seem hard to believe that one program could cause such a significant reduction in alcohol use, the LST program's effectiveness has been proven by many studies published in scholarly journals such as The Journal of Behavioral Medicine, The Journal of Studies on Alcohol, and The Journal of the American Medical Association.

College

Alcohol programs and courses as a requirement of college students is a current, widespread movement to educate underage students about alcohol consumption in efforts to make binge drinking decrease, and safer students.

Currently 747 schools in the United States require some sort of alcohol education. Students must complete a program which educates them on the consequences of binge drinking. MADD states in a recent publication that 4 out of 5 college students drink and 100% of students surveyed said that drinking alcohol while in college has social benefits. Most colleges have alcohol policies which restrict underage drinking and have consequences. Many schools also require an entrance program to be attended by all transfer students as well as freshman that make the dangers and the policies regarding alcohol clear. A documentary about the late 18-year-old Gordie Bailey, is shown at many colleges.

Online courses are used in many schools. A course commonly used by institutions is AlcoholEdu, a population-level prevention program typically administered to all high school or college freshmen. AlcoholEdu's purpose is to change or influence how college students feel about drinking, as well as educate students on the harmful and negative risks associated with heavy consumption of alcohol by presenting students with realistic case studies to influence students not to over consume.

In the United States, Collegedrinkingprevention.gov is a government funded website based through the National Institute on Alcohol Abuse and Alcoholism which aims to change the drinking culture of college. Their report *A Call to Action: Changing the Culture of Drinking at U.S. Colleges* details how colleges and universities conduct alcohol programs. Publicly funded universities must comply with their standards as stated in their report.

Cost and Benefit

People often wonder if alcohol education programs are worth the money. According to the article "What We Can—and Cannot—Expect from School-Based Drug Prevention," out of The Journal of Drug and Alcohol Review, an average substance abuse program costing $150 can save $840 in social costs per participant. Granted this study focused on more than just alcohol, but at 28 percent alcohol was responsible for the second highest amount of social savings. Social savings can be seen in the form of healthcare expenditures, incarcerations, impaired productivity, premature death, and so on. The authors of this article also claim that a reduction in premature childbirth and other drug usage, along with better school performance and higher graduation rates are extra benefits of using a substance abuse program.

Effective Education

Protecting youth and keeping them safe from harm has to be a goal of any alcohol education program. Such programs need to:

1. Provide accurate, truthful and unbiased information about alcohol and its consumption.
2. Distinguish between abuse and use of alcohol.
3. Teach the possible consequences of underage purchase, possession and/or consumption of alcoholic beverages under the legal age.
4. Teach effective ways to reduce the potential threat/harm that can be a result from the abuse of alcohol.

History in Australia

In Australia teenage alcohol use is a growing problem, in 2011 74% of Australian students aged between 12 and 17 had tried alcohol in the past year, and in 2010 a study showed that 31% of 16- to 17-year-old students had consumed more than 20 standard drinks in one session. Every year, 5,500 people in Australia die, and around 157,000 are hospitalised from directly drinking alcohol. 400 more lives are lost from alcohol-related assaults. It is costing the country around $36 billion annually. The Australian Government has set up various organisations and campaigns to try and tackle the rise in teenage drinking, reduce the amount deaths and injuries that occur, as well as informing people of the adverse effects that can result from binge drinking.

Government Organizations

DrinkWise Australia

DrinkWise Australia is the most prominent organization in Australia aimed at educating the public on alcohol use, mainly focused on teenagers. Their recent campaign urging school leavers to drink responsibly (titled "How to Drink Properly") is believed to have been successful. One in three 18- to 24-year-olds who saw the campaign said they reduced their drinking on a night out, and just over half of young adults said the campaign helped them discuss their drinking habits. The campaign won a Silver Spike award at the 2014 Spike Asia awards.

Current methods in schools for educating about alcohol include:

- Using an approach relating to social influence
- Involve parental participation and work on building connections in the community
- Focus on interacting highly with students for a hands on delivery

There are four main types of alcohol education programs used in Australia

- School-based (classroom or whole school)
- Family-based
- Community-based
- Combination (of school- and community-based programs)

Alcohol.gov.au

This website from the Australian Government Department of Health gives relative information regarding alcohol related health issues, and also provides the policies from the government. The resource is helpful to Australians of all ages, and is extremely accessible.

Information available from the main site include:

- National Alcohol Strategy 2006-2011
- Australian Alcohol Guidelines
- Alcohol resources and publications

- National binge drinking strategies
- Women want to know (information regarding alcohol and pregnancy)

Foundation for Alcohol Research and Education (FARE)

FARE is an, "independent, non-profit organisation working to stop the harm caused by alcohol." It too is trying to prevent the growing alcohol problem in Australian communities.

FARE Goals

The FARE Strategic Plan lists the 5 goals for 2014 to 2017, with the aim to reduce harms to individuals and the costs to communities.

1. World-leading research: to undertake and communicate strategic research.
2. Strategic policy and advocacy: develop and advocate for policies and programs that work.
3. Working together: mobilise communities and organisations to work collectively.
4. Defending the public interest: promote open decision making and hold the alcohol industry to account.
5. Leading change: build an enduring world-class organisation that effects health and social change.

The Funding Structure

The Foundation for Alcohol Research and Education (FARE), has set up a Capital Fund to support their own work in assisting communities and their strategic policy priorities.

School-based Programs in Australia

Australian States each have different programs set up by their state governments aimed at high school students as well as multiple studies to research the effect that school-based education had on drinking habits.

Western Australia's Commissioner for Children and Young People (CCYP) sought out how teenagers aged 14–17 view alcohol and the negative consequences that could result from consuming it as well as knowledge about standard drinks and the national alcoholic guidelines in 2011. The CCYP also promoted two programs - SDERA (School Drug Education and Road Awareness) and SHAHRP (School Health and Alcohol Harm Reduction Project) - to educate the high school students about prevention and reduction of alcohol induced harm. SDERA targeted prevention and was taught as part of the health and physical education curriculum in WA, whereas SHAHRP targeted the reducing possible harm and was conducted by the National Drug Research Institute at Curtin University.

Victorian Department of Education and Training implemented the 'Get Ready' program in 2012. The program was aimed at students in years 7-9 and taught students about drug and alcohol risks.

Similarly, Queensland's Department of Education, Training and Employment worked with their Curriculum and Assessment Authority to create their education program 'Alcohol and other drugs education program.' The program addresses alcohol and drugs through the health and physical education curriculum and is aimed at high school student in years 7-12. The program works alongside the 'safe night out strategy' which is about violence caused by drugs and alcohol.

Similar to The foundation for alcohol research and Education, Alcohol Education Trust (AET), have a main goal of helping adolescents enter adulthood with a responsible relationship to alcohol, using an evidence based highly evaluated programme talk about alcohol.

Patient Education

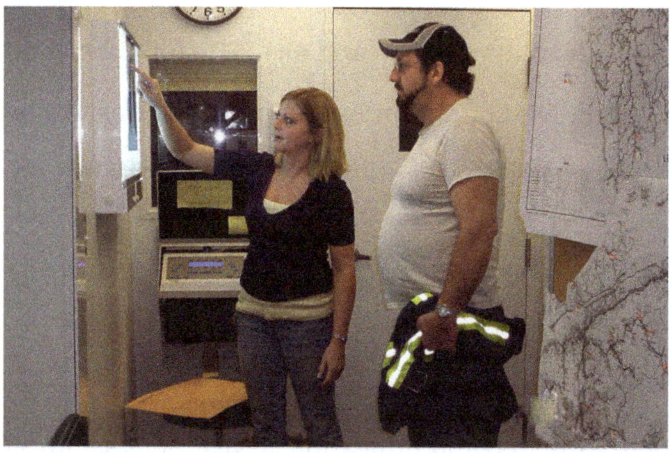

A Radiographer explains an x-ray to a coal miner participating in screening. Patient education can include explaining the results of diagnostic tests.

Patient education is the process by which health professionals and others impart information to patients and their caregivers that will alter their health behaviors or improve their health status.

Overview

Education may be provided by any healthcare professional who has undertaken appropriate training education, education on patient communication and education is usually included in the healthcare professional's training.

Health education is also a tool used by managed care plans, and may include both general preventive education or health promotion and disease or condition specific education.

Important elements of patient education are skill building and responsibility: patients need to know when, how, and why they need to make a lifestyle change. Group effort is equally important: each member of the patient's health care team needs to be involved.

The value of patient education can be summarized as follows:

- Improved understanding of medical condition, diagnosis, disease, or disability.

- Improved understanding of methods and means to manage multiple aspects of medical condition.
- Improved self-advocacy in deciding to act both independently from medical providers and in interdependence with them.
- Increased Compliance – Effective communication and patient education increases patient motivation to comply.
- Patient Outcomes – Patients more likely to respond well to their treatment plan – fewer complications.
- Informed Consent – Patients feel you've provided the information they need.
- Utilization – More effective use of medical services – fewer unnecessary phone calls and visits.
- Satisfaction and referrals – Patients more likely to stay with your practice and refer other patients.
- Risk Management – Lower risk of malpractice when patients have realistic expectations.
- Enhance patients' safety - Prevent fatality at home, specially a patient with lifelong tracheostomy.

The competencies of a health educator include the following:

- Incorporate a personal ethic in regards to social responsibilities and services towards others.
- Provide accurate, competent, and evidence-based care.
- Practice preventative health care.
- Focus on relationship-centered care with individuals and their families.
- Incorporate the multiple determinants of health when providing care.
- Be culturally sensitive and be open to a diverse society.
- Use technology appropriately and effectively.
- Be current in the field and continue to advance education.

There are many areas where patient education can improve the outcomes of treatment.

- For example, in patients with amputations, patient education has been shown to be effective when approached from all angles by the healthcare team (nurse, primary care physician, prosthetist, physical therapist, occupational therapist etc.). Support groups have been shown to be a helpful method for dealing with depression in this population. Preoperative patient education helped patients with their decision making process by informing them of factors related to pain, limb loss, and functional restriction faced after amputation.

- In the case of arthritis, patient education was found to be administered through three methods, including individual face to face meetings with healthcare professionals, patient groups, online support programs. Category I evidence was found for individual, face to face counseling. Meeting with rheumatologists, occupational therapists, physical therapists, nurses, and other healthcare providers was found to be effective in creating adherence to treatment, medication, and for improving overall patient health.
- In the case of rheumatoid arthritis, patient education has been shown as an effective non-pharmacological treatment.

Chronic Care Management

Chronic care management encompasses the oversight and education activities conducted by health care professionals to help patients with chronic diseases and health conditions such as diabetes, high blood pressure, lupus, multiple sclerosis and sleep apnea learn to understand their condition and live successfully with it. This term is equivalent to disease management for chronic conditions. The work involves motivating patients to persist in necessary therapies and interventions and helping them to achieve an ongoing, reasonable quality of life.

Chronic Care and the Medical System

Historically, there has been little coordination across the multiple settings, providers and treatments of chronic illness care. In addition, the treatments for chronic diseases are often complicated, making it difficult for patients to comply with treatment protocols.

Effective medical care usually requires longer visits to the doctor's office than is common in acute care. Moreover, in treating chronic illnesses, the same intervention, whether medical or behavioral, may differ in effectiveness depending on when in the course of the illness the intervention is suggested. Fragmentation of care is a risk for patients with chronic diseases, because frequently multiple chronic diseases coexist. Necessary interventions can require input from multiple specialists that may not usually work together, and to be effective, they require close, careful coordination.

As a consequence, patients with chronic conditions can fare poorly in the current acute-care model of care delivery.

Historically, reimbursement has been challenging for care coordination services. Medicare recently started paying for services related to chronic care management. Medicare pays a monthly fee for patients who consent to treatment for a minimum of 20 minutes of telehealth services.

Personal Chronic Care Management

Patients with chronic conditions have an important role in the management of their conditions, as they are often the ones administering the treatments in everyday life. They also play an important role in monitoring their health and changes in their health by means of Observations of Daily Living (ODLs). Resulting information may inform both self care and clinical care.A Care management solution can play an important role in making the participation of patients in his own healthcare, easier and more effective.

Importance

Certain problems related to chronic illness are not specifically medical, but involve patients' interactions with families and workplaces. Interventions often require patients and families to make difficult lifestyle changes. Patients need to be educated on the benefits of treatment and the risks of not properly following their treatment regimen. They need to be motivated to comply because treatment usually produces an improved state, rather than the results that most patients desire—a cure. Chronic care management helps patients systematically monitor their progress and coordinate with experts to identify and solve any problems they encounter in their treatment.

It would appear from the above, that chronically ill persons are better cared for by primary care physicians. Considering the diverse nature of chronic health problems and the roles that psychosocial environments play in their course, a purely biological model of care is usually inadequate. The biopsychosocial model of care is the ideal alternative.

History

Although acute care has characterized all medical care until recently, several varieties of managed care have emerged in the past decades in an effort to improve care, reduce unnecessary service utilization and control spiraling costs. Despite its initial promise, however, managed care has not achieved truly coordinated care. In actual operation it appears to emphasize its fiscal goals. Moreover, managed care does not address the complexity of chronic conditions, and in the interests of cost-cutting, tends to reduce time with patients rather than increase it.

Chronic Care Models

In the latter part of the 20th century, researchers began to develop care models for the assessment and treatment of the chronically ill.

Nurse researchers, such as S. Wellard, C. S. Burckhardt, C. Baker and P. N. Stern, and I. M. Lubkin and P. D. Larson, were often on the front lines of actual care for patients with ongoing treatments for conditions such as diabetes or renal failure. They stated that their patients experienced a series of "phases", and that during some of these phases the patients responded to the same interventions quite differently.

Individuals who suffered from chronic illnesses, such as C. Register and S. Wells, have given detailed accounts of their experiences and made recommendations about how to manage chronic conditions. Associations proliferated for those with specific conditions (Sjögren's syndrome, chronic fatigue syndrome, peripheral neuropathy, etc.), and these groups have engaged in advocacy work, acted as clearinghouses for information, and began funding research.

Edward H. Wagner, M.D., Director of The MacColl Institute for Healthcare Innovation, Director of The Robert Wood Johnson Foundation national program "Improving Chronic Illness Care", and Senior Investigator at Group Health Research Institute in Seattle, WA developed the Chronic Care Model, or CCM. The CCM summarizes the basic elements for improving care in health systems on different levels. These elements are the community, the health system, self-management support, delivery system design, decision support and clinical information systems. Evidence-based change concepts under each element, in combination, foster productive interactions between informed patients who take an active part in their care and providers with resources and expertise. The Chronic Care Model can be applied to a variety of chronic illnesses, health care settings and target populations. The bottom line is healthier patients, more satisfied providers, and cost savings.

The Stanford Self-Management Program is a community-based self-management program that helps people with chronic illness gain self-confidence in their ability to control their symptoms and manage how their health problems will affect their lives.

Partnership for Solutions, a Johns Hopkins/Robert Wood Johnson collaborative, conducts research to improve the care and quality of life for individuals with chronic health conditions.

J. O. Prochaska and his colleagues, investigating issues associated with the treatment of addictions, have described a transtheoretical model of behavior change as a process rather than an event. They have advocated assessment and treatment based on the patient's stage in the process.

Patricia Fennell, working on the experiences of imposed change (such as illness, grief, or trauma), has developed the Fennell Four Phase Model of chronic illness. Fennell says people commonly experience four phases as they learn to incorporate their changed physical abilities or psychological outlook into their personality and lifestyle: Crisis, Stabilization, Integration, and Resolution.

Established by the investment banking firm Wyatt Matas, the term Care Cycle Management is a chronic care business model that integrates interventional disease management with care delivery to manage the care of high-cost patients.

The Flinders Human Behaviour & Health Research Unit (based in Adelaide, South Australia) has developed the Flinders ProgramTM, a generic set of tools and processes that allows for assessment of chronic condition management behaviours, collaborative identification of problems and goal setting leading to the development of individualised care plans with the goal of raising the quality of life for people living with chronic disease. The Flinders ProgramTM has been adapted to specific contexts to meet the needs of Indigenous Australians and veterans.

References

- Joint Committee on Terminology (2001). "Report of the 2000 Joint Committee on Health Education and Promotion Terminology". American Journal of Health Education. 32 (2): 89–103
- Sullivan, S. (2015). "Endoscopic Treatment of Obesity". In Jonnalagadda, S.S. Gastrointestinal Endoscopy: New Technologies and Changing Paradigms. Springer. pp. 61–82. ISBN 9781493920327. Retrieved 18 March 2016
- World Health Organization. (1998). List of Basic Terms. Health Promotion Glossary. (pp. 4). Retrieved May 1, 2009
- Sulik, Gayle (2010). Pink Ribbon Blues: How Breast Cancer Culture Undermines Women's Health. New York: Oxford University Press. ISBN 0-19-974045-3. OCLC 535493589
- Kann L.; Brener N.D.; Allensworth D.D. (2001). "Health education: Results from the School Health Policies and Programs Study 2000". Journal of School Health. 71 (7): 266–278. doi:10.1111/j.1746-1561.2001.tb03504.x
- Institute of Medicine (2012). Breast Cancer and the Environment: A Life Course Approach (Institute of Medicine). Washington, D.C: National Academies Press. ISBN 0-309-22069-6
- Coalition of National Health Education Organizations. Introduction. Health Education Code of Ethics. November 8, 1999, Chicago, IL. Retrieved May 1, 2009

- Rosenbaum, Lisa (February 2014). ""Misfearing"—Culture, Identity, and Our Perceptions of Health Risks". New England Journal of Medicine. 370 (7): 595–7. doi:10.1056/NEJMp1314638. PMID 24521105
- King, Samantha (2006). Pink Ribbons, Inc.: Breast Cancer and the Politics of Philanthropy. Minneapolis: University of Minnesota Press. ISBN 0-8166-4898-0
- "FDA Briefing Document NDA 21-888 Zimulti (rimonabant) Tablets, 20 mg Sanofi Aventis Advisory Committee" (PDF). Food and Drug Administration. June 13, 2007. Retrieved 2008-09-19
- Mukherjee, Siddhartha (2010). The Emperor of All Maladies: A Biography of Cancer (1st Scribner hardcover ed.). New York: Scribner. ISBN 1439181713

4

Preventive Healthcare: An Overview

The measures taken to prevent diseases and generate proper awareness related to hygiene is known as preventive healthcare. Health promotions can be of various sorts like workplace health promotion, health literacy, peer education and breastfeeding promotion. The major components of preventive healthcare are discussed in this chapter.

Preventive Healthcare

Preventive healthcare (alternately preventive medicine or prophylaxis) consists of measures taken for disease prevention, as opposed to disease treatment. Just as health encompasses a variety of physical and mental states, so do disease and disability, which are affected by environmental factors, genetic predisposition, disease agents, and lifestyle choices. Health, disease, and disability are dynamic processes which begin before individuals realize they are affected. Disease prevention relies on anticipatory actions that can be categorized as primal, primary, secondary, and tertiary prevention.

Each year, millions of people die of preventable deaths. A 2004 study showed that about half of all deaths in the United States in 2000 were due to preventable behaviors and exposures. Leading causes included cardiovascular disease, chronic respiratory disease, unintentional injuries, diabetes, and certain infectious diseases. This same study estimates that 400,000 people die each year in the United States due to poor diet and a sedentary lifestyle. According to estimates made by the World Health Organization (WHO), about 55 million people died worldwide in 2011, two thirds of this group from non-communicable diseases, including cancer, diabetes, and chronic cardiovascular and lung diseases. This is an increase from the year 2000, during which 60% of deaths were attributed to these diseases. Preventive healthcare is especially important given the worldwide rise in prevalence of chronic diseases and deaths from these diseases.

There are many methods for prevention of disease. It is recommended that adults and children aim to visit their doctor for regular check-ups, even if they feel healthy, to perform disease screening, identify risk factors for disease, discuss tips for a healthy and balanced lifestyle, stay up to date with immunizations and boosters, and maintain a good relationship with a healthcare provider. Some common disease screenings include checking for hypertension (high blood pressure), hyperglycemia (high blood sugar, a risk factor for diabetes mellitus), hypercholesterolemia (high blood cholesterol), screening for colon cancer, depression, HIV and other common types of sexually transmitted disease such as chlamydia, syphilis, and gonorrhea, mammography (to screen for breast cancer), colorectal cancer screening, a pap test (to check for cervical cancer), and screening for osteoporosis. Genetic testing can also be performed to screen for mutations that cause genetic disorders or predisposition to certain diseases such as breast or ovarian cancer. However, these measures are not affordable for every individual and the cost effectiveness of preventive healthcare is still a topic of debate.

Levels of Prevention

Preventive healthcare strategies are described as taking place at the primal, primary, secondary, and tertiary prevention levels. In the 1940s, Hugh R. Leavell and E. Gurney Clark coined the term primary prevention. They worked at the Harvard and Columbia University Schools of Public Health, respectively, and later expanded the levels to include secondary and tertiary prevention. Goldston (1987) notes that these levels might be better described as "prevention, treatment, and rehabilitation", though the terms primary, secondary, and tertiary prevention are still in use today. The concept of primal prevention has been created much more recently, in relation to the new developments in molecular biology over the last fifty years, more particularly in epigenetics, which point to the paramount importance of environmental conditions - both physical and affective - on the organism during its fetal and newborn life (or so-called primal life).

Level	Definition
Primal and primordial prevention	Any measure aimed at helping future parents provide their upcoming child with adequate attention, as well as secure physical and affective environments from conception to first birthday (i.e., over the child's *primal period* of life). Primordial prevention refers to measures designed to avoid the development of risk factors in the first place, early in life.
Primary prevention	Methods to avoid occurrence of disease either through eliminating disease agents or increasing resistance to disease. Examples include immunization against disease, maintaining a healthy diet and exercise regimen, and avoiding smoking.
Secondary prevention	Methods to detect and address an existing disease prior to the appearance of symptoms. Examples include treatment of hypertension (a risk factor for many cardiovascular diseases), cancer screenings
Tertiary prevention	Methods to reduce the harm of symptomatic disease, such as disability or death, through rehabilitation and treatment. Examples include surgical procedures that halt the spread or progression of disease
Quaternary prevention	Methods to mitigate or avoid results of unnecessary or excessive interventions in the health system

Primal and Primordial Prevention

A separate category of "health promotion" has recently been propounded. This health promotion *par excellence* is based on the 'new knowledge' in molecular biology, in particular on epigenetic knowledge, which points to how much affective - as well as physical - environment during fetal and newborn life may determine each and every aspect of adult health. This new way of promoting health is now commonly called primal prevention. It consists mainly in providing future parents with pertinent, unbiased information on *primal health* and supporting them during their child's *primal period of life* (i.e., "from conception to first anniversary" according to definition by the Primal Health Research Centre, London). This includes adequate parental leave - ideally for both parents - with kin caregiving and financial help where needed.

Another related concept is primordial prevention which to refers to all measures designed to prevent the development of risk factors in the first place, early in life.

Primary Prevention

Primary prevention consists of traditional "health promotion" and "specific protection." Health promotion activities are current, non-clinical life choices. For example, eating nutritious meals and exercising daily, that both prevent disease and create a sense of overall well-being. Preventing disease and creating overall well-being, prolongs our life expectancy. Health-promotional activities do not target a specific disease or condition but rather promote health and well-being on a very general level. On the other hand, specific protection targets a type or group of diseases and complements the goals of health promotion. In the case of a sexually transmitted disease such as syphilis health promotion activities would include avoiding microorganisms by maintaining personal hygiene, routine check-up appointments with the doctor, general sex education, etc. whereas specific protective measures would be using prophylactics (such as condoms) during sex and avoiding sexual promiscuity.

Food is very much the most basic tool in preventive health care. The 2011 National Health Interview Survey performed by the Centers for Disease Control was the first national survey to include questions about ability to pay for food. Difficulty with paying for food, medicine, or both is a problem facing 1 out of 3 Americans. If better food options were available through food banks, soup kitchens, and other resources for low-income people, obesity and the chronic conditions that come along with it would be better controlled A "food desert" is an area with restricted access to healthy foods due to a lack of supermarkets within a reasonable distance. These are often low-income neighborhoods with the majority of residents lacking transportation . There have been several grassroots movements in the past 20 years to encourage urban gardening, such as the GreenThumb organization in New York City. Urban gardening uses vacant lots to grow food for a neighborhood and is cultivated by the local residents. Mobile fresh markets are another resource for residents in a "food desert", which are specially outfitted buses bringing affordable fresh fruits and vegetables to low-income neighborhoods. These programs often hold educational events as well such as cooking and nutrition guidance. Programs such as these are helping to provide healthy, affordable foods to the people who need them the most.

Scientific advancements in genetics have significantly contributed to the knowledge of hereditary diseases and have facilitated great progress in specific protective measures in individuals who are carriers of a disease gene or have an increased predisposition to a specific disease. Genetic testing has allowed physicians to make quicker and more accurate diagnoses and has allowed for tailored treatments or personalized medicine. Similarly, specific protective measures such as water purification, sewage treatment, and the development of personal hygienic routines (such as regular hand-washing) became mainstream upon the discovery of infectious disease agents such as bacteria. These discoveries have been instrumental in decreasing the rates of communicable diseases that are often spread in unsanitary conditions.

Secondary Prevention

Secondary prevention deals with latent diseases and attempts to prevent an asymptomatic disease from progressing to symptomatic disease. Certain diseases can be classified as primary or secondary. This depends on definitions of what constitutes a disease, though, in general, primary prevention addresses the root cause of a disease or injury whereas secondary prevention aims to detect and treat a disease early on. Secondary prevention consists of "early diagnosis and prompt treatment" to contain the disease and prevent its spread to other individuals, and "disability limitation" to prevent potential future complications and disabilities from the disease. For example, early diagnosis and prompt treatment for a syphilis patient would include a course of antibiotics to destroy the pathogen and screening and treatment of any infants born to syphilitic mothers. Disability limitation for syphilitic patients includes continued check-ups on the heart, cerebrospinal fluid, and central nervous system of patients to curb any damaging effects such as blindness or paralysis.

Tertiary Prevention

Finally, tertiary prevention attempts to reduce the damage caused by symptomatic disease by focusing on mental, physical, and social rehabilitation. Unlike secondary prevention, which aims to prevent disability, the objective of tertiary prevention is to maximize the remaining capabilities and functions of an already disabled patient. Goals of tertiary prevention include: preventing pain and damage, halting progression and complications from disease, and restoring the health and functions of the individuals affected by disease. For syphilitic patients, rehabilitation includes measures to prevent complete disability from the disease, such as implementing work-place adjustments for the blind and paralyzed or providing counseling to restore normal daily functions to the greatest extent possible.

Leading Causes of Preventable Death

United States

The leading cause of death in the United States was tobacco. However, poor diet and lack of exercise may soon surpass tobacco as a leading cause of death. These behaviors are modifiable and public health and prevention efforts could make a difference to reduce these deaths.

Leading causes of preventable deaths in the United States in the year 2000		
Cause	**Deaths caused**	**% of all deaths**
Tobacco smoking	435,000	18.1
Poor diet and physical inactivity	400,000	16.6
Alcohol consumption	85,000	3.5
Infectious diseases	75,000	3.1
Toxicants	55,000	2.3
Traffic collisions	43,000	1.8
Firearm incidents	29,000	1.2
Sexually transmitted infections	20,000	0.8
Drug abuse	17,000	0.7

Worldwide

The leading causes of preventable death worldwide share similar trends to the United States. There are a few differences between the two, such as malnutrition, pollution, and unsafe sanitation, that reflect health disparities between the developing and developed world.

Leading causes of preventable death worldwide as of the year 2001	
Cause	**Deaths caused (millions per year)**
Hypertension	7.8
Smoking	5.0
High cholesterol	3.9
Malnutrition	3.8
Sexually transmitted infections	3.0
Poor diet	2.8
Overweight and obesity	2.5
Physical inactivity	2.0
Alcohol	1.9
Indoor air pollution from solid fuels	1.8
Unsafe water and poor sanitation	1.6

Infant and Child Mortality

In 2010, 7.6 million children died before reaching the age of 5. While this is a decrease from 9.6 million in the year 2000, it is still far from the fourth Millennium Development Goal to decrease child mortality by two-thirds by the year 2015. Of these deaths, about 64% were due to infection (including diarrhea, pneumonia, and malaria). About 40% of these deaths occurred in neonates (children ages 1–28 days) due to pre-term birth complications. The highest number of child deaths occurred in Africa and Southeast Asia. In Africa, almost no progress has been made in reducing neonatal death since 1990. India, Nigeria, Democratic Republic of the Congo, Pakistan, and China contributed to almost 50% of global child deaths in 2010. Targeting efforts in these countries is essential to reducing the global child death rate.

Child mortality is caused by a variety of factors including poverty, environmental hazards, and lack of maternal education. The World Health Organization created a list of interventions in the following table that were judged economically and operationally "feasible," based on the healthcare resources and infrastructure in 42 nations that contribute to 90% of all infant and child deaths. The table indicates how many infant and child deaths could have been prevented in the year 2000, assuming universal healthcare coverage.

Leading preventive interventions that reduce deaths in children 0–5 years old worldwide	
Intervention	**Percent of all child deaths preventable**
Breastfeeding	13
Insecticide-treated materials	7
Complementary feeding	6
Zinc	4
Clean delivery	4
Hib vaccine	4
Water, sanitation, hygiene	3
Antenatal steroids	3

Newborn temperature management	2
Vitamin A	2
Tetanus toxoid	2
Nevirapine and replacement feeding	2
Antibiotics for premature rupture of membranes	1
Measles vaccine	1
Antimalarial intermittent preventive treatment in pregnancy	<1%

Preventive Methods for Different Diseases

Obesity

Obesity is a major risk factor for a wide variety of conditions including cardiovascular diseases, hypertension, certain cancers, and type 2 diabetes. In order to prevent obesity, it is recommended that individuals adhere to a consistent exercise regimen as well as a nutritious and balanced diet. A healthy individual should aim for acquiring 10% of their energy from proteins, 15-20% from fat, and over 50% from complex carbohydrates, while avoiding alcohol as well as foods high in fat, salt, and sugar. Sedentary adults should aim for at least half an hour of moderate-level daily physical activity and eventually increase to include at least 20 minutes of intense exercise, three times a week. Preventive health care offers many benefits to those that chose to participate in taking an active role in the culture. The medical system in our society is geared toward curing acute symptoms of disease after the fact that they have brought us into the emergency room. An ongoing epidemic within American culture is the prevalence of obesity. Eating healthier and routinely exercising plays a huge role in reducing an individuals risk for type 2 diabetes. About 23.6 million people in the United States have diabetes. Of those, 17.9 million are diagnosed and 5.7 million are undiagnosed. Ninety to 95 percent of people with diabetes have type 2 diabetes. Diabetes is the main cause of kidney failure, limb amputation, and new-onset blindness in American adults.

Sexually Transmitted Infections

STIs are common both in history and in today's society. STIs can be asymptomatic or cause a range of symptoms. Condom and other barrier use reduces the risk of acquiring some STIs. STI prophylaxis includes: condom use, abstinence, testing and screening a partner, regular health check-ups, and certain medications such as Truvada.

Thrombosis

Thrombosis is a serious circulatory disease affecting thousands, usually older persons undergoing surgical procedures, women taking oral contraceptives and travelers. Consequences of thrombosis can be heart attacks and strokes. Prevention can include: exercise, anti-embolisim stockings, pneumatic devices, and pharmacological treatments.

Cancer

In recent years, cancer has become a global problem. Low and middle income countries share a majority of the cancer burden largely due to exposure to carcinogens resulting from industrialization and globalization. However, primary prevention of cancer and knowledge of cancer risk factors can reduce over one third of all cancer cases. Primary prevention of cancer can also prevent other diseases, both communicable and non-communicable, that share common risk factors with cancer.

Lung Cancer

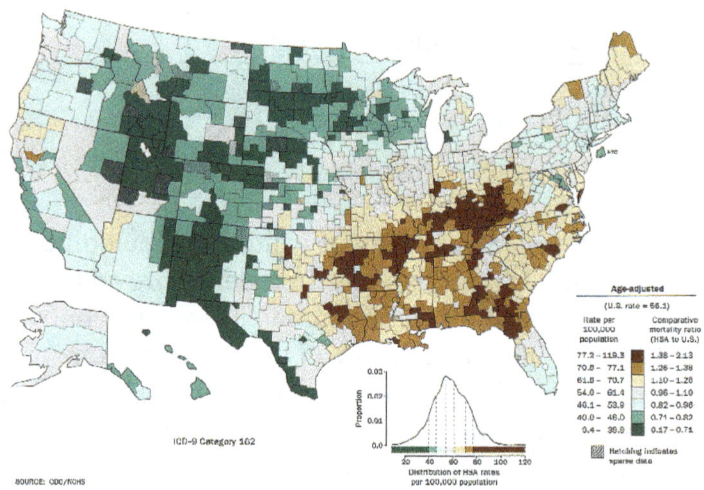

Distribution of lung cancer in the United States

Lung cancer is the leading cause of cancer-related deaths in the United States and Europe and is a major cause of death in other countries. Tobacco is an environmental carcinogen and the major underlying cause of lung cancer. Between 25% and 40% of all cancer deaths and about 90% of lung cancer cases are associated with tobacco use. Other carcinogens include asbestos and radioactive materials. Both smoking and second-hand exposure from other smokers can lead to lung cancer and eventually death. Therefore, prevention of tobacco use is paramount to prevention of lung cancer.

Individual, community, and statewide interventions can prevent or cease tobacco use. 90% of adults in the US who have ever smoked did so prior to the age of 20. In-school prevention/educational programs, as well as counseling resources, can help prevent and cease adolescent smoking. Other cessation techniques include group support programs, nicotine replacement therapy (NRT), hypnosis, and self-motivated behavioral change. Studies have shown long term success rates (>1 year) of 20% for hypnosis and 10%-20% for group therapy.

Cancer screening programs serve as effective sources of secondary prevention. The Mayo Clinic, Johns Hopkins, and Memorial Sloan-Kettering hospitals conducted annual x-ray screenings and sputum cytology tests and found that lung cancer was detected at higher rates, earlier stages, and had more favorable treatment outcomes, which supports widespread investment in such programs.

Legislation can also affect smoking prevention and cessation. In 1992, Massachusetts (United States) voters passed a bill adding an extra 25 cent tax to each pack of cigarettes, despite intense lobbying and a $7.3 million spent by the tobacco industry to oppose this bill. Tax revenue goes toward tobacco education and control programs and has led to a decline of tobacco use in the state.

Lung cancer and tobacco smoking are increasing worldwide, especially in China. China is responsible for about one-third of the global consumption and production of tobacco products. Tobacco control policies have been ineffective as China is home to 350 million regular smokers and 750 million passive smokers and the annual death toll is over 1 million. Recommended actions to reduce tobacco use include: decreasing tobacco supply, increasing tobacco taxes, widespread educational campaigns, decreasing advertising from the tobacco industry, and increasing tobacco cessation support resources. In Wuhan, China, a 1998 school-based program, implemented an anti-tobacco curriculum for adolescents and reduced the number of regular smokers, though it did not significantly decrease the number of adolescents who initiated smoking. This program was therefore effective in secondary but not primary prevention and shows that school-based programs have the potential to reduce tobacco use.

Skin Cancer

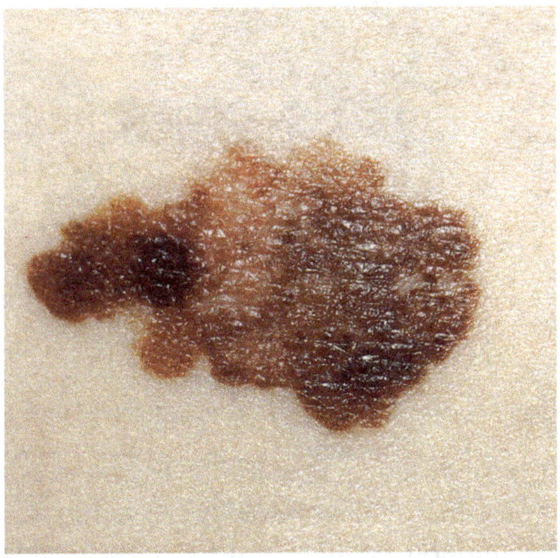

An image of melanoma, one of the deadliest forms of skin cancer

Skin cancer is the most common cancer in the United States. The most lethal form of skin cancer, melanoma, leads to over 50,000 annual deaths in the United States. Childhood prevention is particularly important because a significant portion of ultraviolet radiation exposure from the sun occurs during childhood and adolescence and can subsequently lead to skin cancer in adulthood. Furthermore, childhood prevention can lead to the development of healthy habits that continue to prevent cancer for a lifetime.

The Centers for Disease Control and Prevention (CDC) recommends several primary prevention methods including: limiting sun exposure between 10 AM and 4 PM, when the sun is strongest, wearing tighter-weave natural cotton clothing, wide-brim hats, and sunglasses as protective covers, using sunscreens that protect against both UV-A and UV-B rays, and avoiding tanning salons. Sunscreen should be reapplied after sweating, exposure to water (through swimming for example) or after several hours of sun exposure. Since skin cancer is very preventable, the CDC recommends school-level prevention programs including preventive curricula, family involvement, participation and support from the school's health services, and partnership with community, state, and national agencies and organizations to keep children away from excessive UV radiation exposure.

Most skin cancer and sun protection data comes from Australia and the United States. An international study reported that Australians tended to demonstrate higher knowledge of sun protection and skin cancer knowledge, compared to other countries. Of children, adolescents, and adults, sunscreen was the most commonly used skin protection. However, many adolescents purposely used sunscreen with a low sun protection factor (SPF)in order to get a tan. Various Australian studies have shown that many adults failed to use sunscreen correctly; many applied sunscreen well after their initial sun exposure and/or failed to reapply when necessary. A 2002 case-control study in Brazil showed that only 3% of case participants and 11% of control participants used sunscreen with SPF >15.

Cervical Cancer

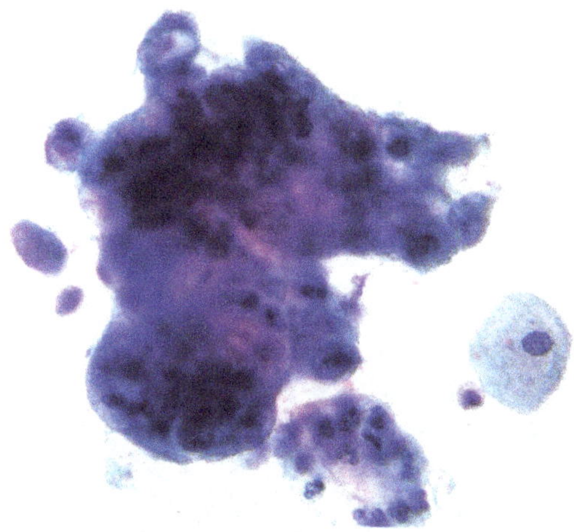

The presence of cancer (adenocarcinoma) detected on a pap test

Cervical cancer ranks among the top three most common cancers among women in Latin America, sub-Saharan Africa, and parts of Asia. Cervical cytology screening aims to detect abnormal lesions in the cervix so that women can undergo treatment prior to the development of cancer. Given that high quality screening and follow-up care has been shown to reduce cervical cancer rates by up to 80%, most developed countries now encourage sexually active women to undergo a pap test every 3–5 years. Finland and Iceland have developed effective organized programs with routine monitoring and have managed to significantly reduce cervical cancer mortality while using fewer resources than unorganized, opportunistic programs such as those in the United States or Canada.

In developing nations in Latin America, such as Chile, Colombia, Costa Rica, and Cuba, both public and privately organized programs have offered women routine cytological screening since the 1970s. However, these efforts have not resulted in a significant change in cervical cancer incidence or mortality in these nations. This is likely due to low quality, inefficient testing. However, Puerto Rico, which has offered early screening since the 1960s, has witnessed an almost a 50% decline in cervical cancer incidence and almost a four-fold decrease in mortality between 1950 and 1990. Brazil, Peru, India, and several high-risk nations in sub-Saharan Africa which lack organized screening programs, have a high incidence of cervical cancer.

Colorectal Cancer

Colorectal cancer (also called bowel cancer, colon cancer, or rectal cancer) is globally the second most common cancer in women and the third-most common in men, and the fourth most common cause of cancer death after lung, stomach, and liver cancer, having caused 715,000 deaths in 2010.

It is also highly preventable; about 80 percent of colorectal cancers begin as benign growths, commonly called polyps, which can be easily detected and removed during a colonoscopy. Other methods of screening for polyps and cancers include fecal occult blood testing. Lifestyle changes that may reduce the risk of colorectal cancer include increasing consumption of whole grains, fruits and vegetables, and reducing consumption of red meat.

Health Disparities and Barriers to Accessing Care

Access to healthcare and preventive health services is unequal, as is the quality of care received. A study conducted by the Agency for Healthcare Research and Quality (AHRQ)revealed health disparities in the United States. In the United States, elderly adults (>65 years old)received worse care and had less access to care than their younger counterparts. The same trends are seen when comparing all racial minorities (black, Hispanic, Asian) to white patients, and low-income people to high-income people. Common barriers to accessing and utilizing healthcare resources included lack of income and education, language barriers, and lack of health insurance. Minorities were less likely than whites to possess health insurance, as were individuals who completed less education. These disparities made it more difficult for the disadvantaged groups to have regular access to a primary care provider, receive immunizations, or receive other types of medical care. Additionally, uninsured people tend to not seek care until their diseases progress to chronic and serious states and they are also more likely to forgo necessary tests, treatments, and filling prescription medications.

These sorts of disparities and barriers exist worldwide as well. Oftentimes there are decades of gaps in life expectancy between developing and developed countries. For example, Japan has an average life expectancy that is 36 years greater than that in Malawi. Low-income countries also tend to have fewer physicians than high-income countries. In Nigeria and Myanmar, there are fewer than 4 physicians per 100,000 people while Norway and Switzerland have a ratio that is ten-fold higher. Common barriers worldwide include lack of availability of health services and healthcare providers in the region, great physical distance between the home and health service facilities, high transportation costs, high treatment costs, and social norms and stigma toward accessing certain health services.

Economics of Lifestyle-based Prevention

With lifestyle factors such as diet and exercise rising to the top of preventable death statistics, the economics of healthy lifestyle is a growing concern. There is little question that positive lifestyle choices provide an investment in health throughout life. To gauge success, traditional measures such as the quality years of life method (QALY), show great value. However, that method does not account for the cost of chronic conditions or future lost earnings because of poor health. Developing future economic models that would guide both private and public investments as well as drive future policy to evaluate the efficacy of positive lifestyle choices on health is a major topic for economists globally.

Americans spend over three trillion a year on health care but have a higher rate of infant mortality, shorter life expectancies, and a higher rate of diabetes than other high-income nations because of negative lifestyle choices. Despite these large costs, very little is spent on prevention for lifestyle-caused conditions in comparison. The Journal of American Medical Association estimates that $101 billion was spent in 2013 on the preventable disease of diabetes, and another $88 billion was spent on heart disease. In an effort to encourage healthy lifestyle choices, workplace wellness programs are on the rise; but the economics and effectiveness data are still continuing to evolve and develop.

Health insurance coverage impacts lifestyle choices. In a study by Sudano and Baker, even intermittent loss of coverage has negative effects on healthy choices. The potential repeal of the Affordable Care Act (ACA) could significantly impact coverage for many Americans, as well as "The Prevention and Public Health Fund" which is our nation's first and only mandatory funding stream dedicated to improving the public's health. Also covered in the ACA is counseling on lifestyle prevention issues, such as weight management, alcohol use, and treatment for depression. Policy makers can have substantial effects on the lifestyle choices made by Americans.

Because chronic illnesses predominate as a cause of death in the US and pathways for treating chronic illnesses are complex and multifaceted, prevention is a best practice approach to chronic disease when possible. In many cases, prevention requires mapping complex pathways to determine the ideal point for intervention. In addition to efficacy, prevention is considered a cost-saving measure. Cost-effectiveness analysis of prevention is achievable, but impacted by the length of time it takes to see effects/outcomes of intervention. This makes prevention efforts difficult to fund—particularly in strained financial contexts. Prevention potentially creates other costs as well, due to extending the lifespan and thereby increasing opportunities for illness. In order to establish reliable economics of prevention for illnesses that are complicated in origin, knowing how best to assess prevention efforts, i.e. developing useful measures and appropriate scope, is required.

Effectiveness

Overview

There is no general consensus as to whether or not preventive healthcare measures are cost-effective, but they increase the quality of life dramatically. There are varying views on what constitutes a "good investment." Some argue that preventive health measures should save more money than they cost, when factoring in treatment costs in the absence of such measures. Others argue in favor of "good value" or conferring significant health benefits even if the measures do not save money Furthermore, preventive health services are often described as one entity though they comprise a myriad of different services, each of which can individually lead to net costs, savings, or neither. Greater differentiation of these services is necessary to fully understand both the financial and health effects.

A 2010 study reported that in the United States, vaccinating children, cessation of smoking, daily prophylactic use of aspirin, and screening of breast and colorectal cancers had the most potential to prevent premature death. Preventive health measures that resulted in savings included vaccinating children and adults, smoking cessation, daily use of aspirin, and screening for issues with alcoholism, obesity, and vision failure. These authors estimated that if usage of these services in the United States increased to 90% of the population, there would be net savings of $3.7 billion, which comprised only about -0.2% of the total 2006 United States healthcare expenditure. Despite the potential for decreasing healthcare spending, utilization of healthcare resources in the United States still remains low, especially among Latinos and African-Americans. Overall, preventive services are difficult to implement because healthcare providers have limited time with patients and must integrate a variety of preventive health measures from different sources.

While these specific services bring about small net savings not every preventive health measure saves more than it costs. A 1970s study showed that preventing heart attacks by treating hypertension early on with drugs actually did not save money in the long run. The money saved by evading treatment from heart attack and stroke only amounted to about a quarter of the cost of the drugs. Similarly, it was found that the cost of drugs or dietary changes to decrease high blood cholesterol exceeded the cost of subsequent heart disease treatment. Due to these findings, some argue that rather than focusing healthcare reform efforts exclusively on preventive care, the interventions that bring about the highest level of health should be prioritized.

Cohen et al. (2008) outline a few arguments made by skeptics of preventive healthcare. Many argue that preventive measures only cost less than future treatment when the proportion of the population that would become ill in the absence of prevention is fairly large. The Diabetes Prevention Program Research Group conducted a 2012 study evaluating the costs and benefits (in quality-adjusted life-years or QALY's) of lifestyle changes versus taking the drug metformin. They found that neither method brought about financial savings, but were cost-effective nonetheless because they brought about an increase in QALY's. In addition to scrutinizing costs, preventive healthcare skeptics also examine efficiency of interventions. They argue that while many treatments of existing diseases involve use of advanced equipment and technology, in some cases, this is a more efficient use of resources than attempts to prevent the disease. Cohen et al. (2008) suggest that the preventive measures most worth exploring and investing in are those that could benefit a large portion of the population to bring about cumulative and widespread health benefits at a reasonable cost.

Cost-Effectiveness of Childhood Obesity Interventions

There are at least four nationally implemented childhood obesity interventions in the United States: the Sugar-Sweetened Beverage excise tax (SSB), the TV AD program, active physical education (Active PE) policies, and early care and education (ECE) policies. They each have similar goals of reducing childhood obesity. The effects of these interventions on BMI have been studied, and the cost-effectiveness analysis (CEA) has led to a better understanding of projected cost reductions and improved health outcomes. The Childhood Obesity Intervention Cost-Effectiveness Study (CHOICES) was conducted to evaluate and compare the CEA of these four interventions.

Gortmaker, S.L. et al. (2015) states: "The four initial interventions were selected by the investigators to represent a broad range of nationally scalable strategies to reduce childhood obesity using a mix of both policy and programmatic strategies... 1. an excise tax of $0.01 per ounce of sweetened beverages, applied nationally and administered at the state level (SSB), 2. elimination of the tax deductibility of advertising costs of TV advertisements for "nutritionally poor" foods and beverages seen by children and adolescents (TV AD), 3. state policy requiring all public elementary schools in which physical education (PE) is currently provided to devote ≥50% of PE class time to moderate and vigorous physical activity (Active PE), and 4. state policy to make early child educational settings healthier by increasing physical activity, improving nutrition, and reducing screen time (ECE)."

The CHOICES found that SSB, TV AD, and ECE led to net cost savings. Both SSB and TV AD increased quality adjusted life years and produced yearly tax revenue of 12.5 billion US dollars and 80 million US dollars, respectively.

Some challenges with evaluating the effectiveness of child obesity interventions include:

1. The economic consequences of childhood obesity are both short and long term. In the short term, obesity impairs cognitive achievement and academic performance. Some believe this is secondary to negative effects on mood or energy, but others suggest there may be physiological factors involved. Furthermore, obese children have increased health care expenses (e.g. medications, acute care visits). In the long term, obese children tend to become obese adults with associated increased risk for a chronic condition such as diabetes or hypertension. Any effect on their cognitive development may also affect their contributions to society and socioeconomic status.

2. In the CHOICES, it was noted that translating the effects of these interventions may in fact differ among communities throughout the nation. In addition it was suggested that limited outcomes are studied and these interventions may have an additional effect that is not fully appreciated.

3. Modeling outcomes in such interventions in children over the long term is challenging because advances in medicine and medical technology are unpredictable. The projections from cost-effective analysis may need to be reassessed more frequently.

The Economics of Preventive Care in the US

The cost-effectiveness of preventive care is a highly debated topic. While some economists argue that preventive care is valuable and potentially cost saving, others believe it is an inefficient waste of resources. Preventive care is composed of a variety of clinical services and programs including annual doctor's check-ups, annual immunizations, and wellness programs.

Clinical Preventive Services & Programs

Research on preventive care addresses the question of whether it is cost saving or cost effective and whether there is an economics evidence base for health promotion and disease prevention. The need for and interest in preventive care is driven by the imperative to reduce health care costs while improving quality of care and the patient experience. Preventive care can lead to improved health outcomes and cost savings potential. Services such as health assessments/screenings, prenatal care, and telehealth and telemedicine can reduce morbidity or mortality with low cost or cost savings. Specifically, health assessments/screenings have cost savings potential, with varied cost-effectiveness based on screening and assessment type. Inadequate prenatal care can lead to an increased risk of prematurity, stillbirth, and infant death. Time is the ultimate resource and preventive care can help mitigate the time costs. Telehealth and telemedicine is one option that has gained consumer interest, acceptance and confidence and can improve quality of care and patient satisfaction.

Understanding the Economics for Investment

There are benefits and trade-offs when considering investment in preventive care versus other types of clinical services. Preventive care can be a good investment as supported by the evidence base and can drive population health management objectives. The concepts of cost saving and cost-effectiveness are different and both are relevant to preventive care. For example, preventive care that may not save money may still provide health benefits. Thus, there is a need to compare interventions relative to impact on health and cost.

Preventive care transcends demographics and is applicable to people of every age. The Health Capital Theory underpins the importance of preventive care across the lifecycle and provides a framework for understanding the variances in health and health care that are experienced. It treats health as a stock that provides direct utility. Health depreciates with age and the aging process can be countered through health investments. The theory further supports that individuals demand good health, that the demand for health investment is a derived demand (i.e. investment is health is due to the underlying demand for good health), and the efficiency of the health investment process increases with knowledge (i.e. it is assumed that the more educated are more efficient consumers and producers of health).

The prevalence elasticity of demand for prevention can also provide insights into the economics. Demand for preventive care can alter the prevalence rate of a given disease and further reduce or even reverse any further growth of prevalence. Reduction in prevalence subsequently leads to reduction in costs.

Economics for Policy Action

There are a number of organizations and policy actions that are relevant when discussing wthe economics of preventive care services. The evidence base, viewpoints, and policy briefs from the Robert Wood Johnson Foundation, the Organisation for Economic Co-operation and Development (OECD), and efforts by the U.S. Preventive Services Task Force (USPSTF) all provide examples that improve the health and well-being of populations (e.g. preventive health assessments/ screenings, prenatal care, and telehealth/telemedicine). The Patient Protection and Affordable Care Act (PPACA, ACA) has major influence on the provision of preventive care services, although it is currently under heavy scrutiny and review by the new administration. According to the Centers for Disease Control and Prevention (CDC), the ACA makes preventive care affordable and accessible through mandatory coverage of preventive services without a deductible, copayment, coinsurance, or other cost sharing.

The U.S. Preventive Services Task Force (USPSTF), a panel of national experts in prevention and evidence-based medicine, works to improve health of Americans by making evidence-based recommendations about clinical preventive services. They do not consider the cost of a preventive service when determining a recommendation. Each year, the organization delivers a report to Congress that identifies critical evidence gaps in research and recommends priority areas for further review.

The National Network of Perinatal Quality Collaboratives (NNPQC), sponsored by the CDC, supports state-based perinatal quality collaboratives (PQCs) in measuring and improving upon health care and health outcomes for mothers and babies. These PQCs have contributed to improvements such as reduction in deliveries before 39 weeks, reductions in healthcare associated blood stream infections, and improvements in the utilization of antenatal corticosteroids.

Telehealth and telemedicine has realized significant growth and development recently. The Center for Connected Health Policy (The National Telehealth Policy Resource Center) has produced multiple reports and policy briefs on the topic of Telehealth and Telemedicine and how they contribute to preventive services.

Policy actions and provision of preventive services do not guarantee utilization. Reimbursement has remained a significant barrier to adoption due to variances in payer and state level reimbursement policies and guidelines through government and commercial payers. Americans use preventive services at about half the recommended rate and cost-sharing, such as deductibles, co-insurance, or copayments, also reduce the likelihood that preventive services will be used. Further, despite the ACA's enhancement of Medicare benefits and preventive services, there were no effects on preventive service utilization, calling out the fact that other fundamental barriers exist.

The Affordable Care Act and Preventive Healthcare

The Patient Protection and Affordable Care Act also known as just the Affordable Care Act or Obamacare was passed and became law in the United States on March 23, 2010. The finalized and newly ratified law was to address my issues in the U.S. healthcare system, which included expansion of coverage, insurance market reforms, better quality, and the forecast of efficiency and costs. Under the insurance market reforms the act required that insurance companies no longer exclude people with pre-existing conditions, allow for children to be covered on their parents plan until the age of 26, expand appeals that dealt with reimbursement denials. The Affordable Care Act also banned the limited coverage imposed by health insurances and insurance companies were to include coverage for preventive health care services. The U.S. Preventive Services Task Force has categorized and rated preventive health services as either '"A" or "B", as to which insurance companies must comply and present full coverage. Not only has the U.S. Preventive Services Task Force provided graded preventive health services that are appropriate for coverage they have also provided many recommendations to clinicians and insurers to promote better preventive care to ultimately provide better quality of care and lower the burden of costs.

Health insurance and Preventive Care

Healthcare insurance companies are willing to pay for preventive care despite the fact that patients are not acutely sick in hope that it will prevent them from developing a chronic disease later on in life. Today, health insurance plans offered through the Marketplace, mandated by the Affordable Care Act are required to provide certain preventive care services free of charge to patients. Section 2713 of the Affordable Care Act, specifies that all private Marketplace and all employer-sponsored private plans (except those grandfathered in) are required to cover preventive care services that are ranked A or B by the US Preventive Services Task Force free of charge to patients. For example, UnitedHealthcare insurance company has published patient guidelines at the beginning of the year explaining their preventive care coverage.

Evaluating Incremental Benefits of Preventive Care

Evaluating the incremental benefits of preventive care requires longer period of time when compared to acute ill patients. Inputs into the model such as, discounting rate and time horizon can have significant effects of the results. One controversial subject is use of 10-year time frame to assess cost effectiveness of diabetes preventive services by the Congressional Budget Office.

The preventive care services mainly focuses on chronic disease, the Congressional Budget Office has provided guidance that further research in the area of the economic impacts of obesity in the US before the CBO can estimate budgetary consequences. A bipartisan report published in May 2015, recognizes that the potential of the preventive care to improve patients health at individual and population levels while decreasing the healthcare expenditure.

Health Promotion

Health promotion is "the process of enabling people to increase control over their health and its determinants, and thereby improve their health", according to the World Health Organization's (WHO) 2005 Bangkok Charter for Health Promotion in a Globalized World.

Health promotion involves public policy that addresses health determinants such as income, housing, food security, employment, and quality working conditions. More recent work has used the term Health in All Policies to refer to the actions to incorporate health into all public policies. Health promotion is aligned with health equity and can be a focus of NGOs dedicated to social justice or human rights. Health literacy can be developed in schools, while aspects of health promotion such as breastfeeding promotion can depend on laws and rules of public spaces. Health promotion is focused on preventative healthcare rather than a medical model of curative care.

There is a tendency among public health officials and governments—and this is especially the case in neoliberal nations such as Canada and the USA—to reduce health promotion to health education and social marketing focused on changing behavioral risk factors.

History

The "first and best known" definition of health promotion, promulgated by the *American Journal of Health Promotion* since at least year 1986, is "the science and art of helping people change their lifestyle to move toward a state of optimal health". This definition was derived from the 1974 Lalonde report from the Government of Canada,<refcap name=Minkler1989/> which contained a health promotion strategy "aimed at informing, influencing and assisting both individuals and organizations so that they will accept more responsibility and be more active in matters affecting mental and physical health". Another predecessor of the definition was the 1979 *Healthy People* report of the Surgeon General of the United States, which noted that health promotion "seeks the development of community and individual measures which can help... [people] to develop lifestyles that can maintain and enhance the state of well-being".

At least two publications led to a "broad empowerment/environmental" definition of health promotion in the mid-1980s:

- In year 1984 the World Health Organization (WHO) Regional Office for Europe defined health promotion as "the process of enabling people to increase control over, and to improve, their health". In addition to methods to change lifestyles, the WHO Regional Office advocated "legislation, fiscal measures, organisational change, community development and spontaneous local activities against health hazards" as health promotion methods.

- In 1986, Jake Epp, Canadian Minister of National Health and Welfare, released *Achieving health for all: a framework for health promotion* which also came to be known as the "Epp report". This report defined the three "mechanisms" of health promotion as "self-care"; "mutual aid, or the actions people take to help each other cope"; and "healthy environments".

The WHO, in collaboration with other organizations, has subsequently co-sponsored international conferences on health promotion as follows:

- 1st International Conference on Health Promotion, Ottawa, 1986, which resulted in the "Ottawa Charter for Health Promotion". According to the Ottawa Charter, health promotion:
    - "is not just the responsibility of the health sector, but goes beyond healthy lifestyles to well-being"
    - "aims at making... [political, economic, social, cultural, environmental, behavioural and biological factors] favourable through advocacy for health"
    - "focuses on achieving equity in health"
    - "demands coordinated action by all concerned: by governments, by health and other social organizations.

Workplace

Work site health focus on the prevention and the intervention that reduce the health risks of the employee. The U.S. Public Health Service recently issued a report titled "Physical Activity and Health: A Report of the Surgeon General" which provides a comprehensive review of the available scientific evidence about the relationship between physical activity and an individual's health status. The report shows that over 60% of Americans are not regularly active and that 25% are not active at all. There is very strong evidence linking physical activity to numerous health improvements. Health promotion can be performed in various locations. Among the settings that have received special attention are the community, health care facilities, schools, and worksites. Worksite health promotion, also known by terms such as "workplace health promotion," has been defined as "the combined efforts of employers, employees and society to improve the health and well-being of people at work". WHO states that the workplace "has been established as one of the priority settings for health promotion into the 21st century" because it influences "physical, mental, economic and social well-being" and "offers an ideal setting and infrastructure to support the promotion of health of a large audience".

Worksite health promotion programs (also called "workplace health promotion programs," "worksite wellness programs," or "workplace wellness programs") include exercise, nutrition, smoking cessation and stress management.

According to the Centers for Disease Control and Prevention (CDC), "Regular physical activity is one of the most effective disease prevention behaviors." Physical activity programs reduce feelings of anxiety and depression, reduce obesity (especially when combined with an improved diet), reduce risk of chronic diseases including cardiovascular disease, high blood pressure, and type 2 diabetes; and finally improve stamina, strength, and energy.

Reviews and meta-analyses published between 2005 and 2008 that examined the scientific literature on worksite health promotion programs include the following:

- A review of 13 studies published through January 2004 showed "strong evidence... for an effect on dietary intake, inconclusive evidence for an effect on physical activity, and no evidence for an effect on health risk indicators".
- In the most recent of a series of updates to a review of "comprehensive health promotion and disease management programs at the worksite," Pelletier (2005) noted "positive clinical and cost outcomes" but also found declines in the number of relevant studies and their quality.
- A "meta-evaluation" of 56 studies published 1982–2005 found that worksite health promotion produced on average a decrease of 26.8% in sick leave absenteeism, a decrease of 26.1% in health costs, a decrease of 32% in workers' compensation costs and disability management claims costs, and a cost-benefit ratio of 5.81.
- A meta-analysis of 46 studies published in 1970–2005 found moderate, statistically significant effects of work health promotion, especially exercise, on "work ability" and "overall well-being"; furthermore, "sickness absences seem to be reduced by activities promoting healthy lifestyle".
- A meta-analysis of 22 studies published 1997–2007 determined that workplace health promotion interventions led to "small" reductions in depression and anxiety.
- A review of 119 studies suggested that successful work site health-promotion programs have attributes such as: assessing employees' health needs and tailoring programs to meet those needs; attaining high participation rates; promoting self care; targeting several health issues simultaneously; and offering different types of activities (e.g., group sessions as well as print materials).

Entities and Projects by Country

Worldwide, government agencies (such as health departments) and non-governmental organizations have substantial efforts in the area of health promotion. Some of these entities and projects are:

International and Multinational

The WHO and its Regional Offices such as the Pan American Health Organization are influential in health promotion around the world. The main eight health promotion campaigns marked by WHO are World Health Day, World Tuberculosis Day, World Blood Donor Day, World Immunization Week, World Malaria Day, World No Tobacco Day, World Hepatitis Day and World AIDS Day.

The International Union for Health Promotion and Education, based in France, holds international, regional, and national conferences.

The European Union is co-funding a Joint Action on Chronic Diseases and Healthy Ageing across the Life Cycle (JA-CHRODIS) with a strong focus on health promotion.

Australia

The Australian Health Promotion Association, a professional body, was incorporated in year 1988. In November 2008, the National Health and Hospitals Reform Commission released a paper recommending a national health promotion agency. ACT Health of the Australian Capital Territory supports health promotion with funding and information dissemination. The Victorian Health Promotion Foundation (VicHealth) from the state of Victoria is "the world's first health promotion foundation to be funded by a tax on tobacco. ". The Australian Government has come up with some initiatives to help Australians achieve a healthy lifestyle. These initiatives are:

- Get Set 4 Life - Habits for Healthy Kid
- The Stephanie Alexander Kitchen Garden National Program
- Healthy Spaces and Place
- Learning from Successful Community Obesity Initiative
- Healthy Weight information and resources.

Health Promotion is strong and well-established in Australia. Since 2008 there has been a number of graduate courses people can take to be involved within Health Promotion in Australia. The government since 2008 has included an initiative that involves the Aboriginal and Torres Strait Island citizens in the preventive health sector.

Health Promotion In Australian Schools

School programs are based on curriculum documents from state and territory councils. Schools mainly focus on health issues that are being supported by funding and special events. Funding for many health issues are the main basis for school curriculum's health subject.

Health Promotion for Aboriginal and Torres Strait Islander Citizens

Aboriginal and Torres Strait Island citizens in Australia in the last couple of centuries have had poor health. The reason behind the poor health conditions is due to major events in the history of Australia, There is an increasing advancement in the promotion of health for Torres Strait Islander and Aboriginal citizens, but this cannot be achieved without the co-operation of non-indigenous Australians. For this Health promotion to be a success the citizens of Australia need to put the history between non-indigenous and indigenous citizens behind them and co-operate as equals.

Canada

The province of Ontario appointed a health promotion minister to lead its Ministry of Health Promotion in year 2005.

The Ministry's vision is to enable Ontarians to lead healthy, active lives and make the province a healthy, prosperous place to live, work, play, learn and visit. Ministry of Health Promotion sees that its fundamental goals are to promote and encourage Ontarians to make healthier choices at all ages and stages of life, to create healthy and supportive environments, lead the development of healthy public policy, and assist with embedding behaviours that promote health.

The Canadian Health Network was a "reliable, non-commercial source of online information about how to stay healthy and prevent disease" that was discontinued in 2007.

The BC Coalition for Health Promotion is "a grassroots, voluntary non-profit society dedicated to the advancement of health promotion in British Columbia".

Ireland

Health Promotion Research in Ireland

The Health Promotion Research Centre (HPRC) at the National University of Ireland Galway was established in 1990 with support from the Department of Health to conduct health promotion related research on issues relevant to health promotion in an Irish context. The Centre is unique in that it is the only designated research centre in Ireland dedicated to health promotion. It produces high quality research of national and international significance that supports the development of best practice and policy in the promotion of health. The Centre is a World Health Organisation (WHO) Collaborating Centre for Health Promotion Research, has an active multidisciplinary research programme, and collaborates with regional, national and international agencies on the development and evaluation of health promotion interventions and strategies.

Objectives of the HPRC include:

- The generation and dissemination of health promotion research that is of national and international relevance.
- The translation of research that will lead to the development of healthy public policy and evidence-informed practice.

New Zealand

The Health Promotion Forum (HPF) of New Zealand is the national umbrella organization of over 150 organisations committed to improving health. HPF has worked with The Cancer Society in order to produce a personal development plan for health promoters, which may be helpful to inform personal development reviews, to identify the competencies of individuals and to provide ideas for future development.

The Health Promotion Agency (HPA), formed July 1, 2012, is a Crown institution that has been established under the New Zealand Public Health and Disability Amendment Act 2012. Its board has been appointed by the Minister of Health. The work of HPA is divided into three main areas:

- Promoting the wellbeing and health of the community

- Enabling health promoting initiatives and environments
- Informing the public on health promoting policies and practices

HPA has a variety of programs based around many areas of work, including alcohol, immunisation, mental health, and skin cancer prevention. The agency aims to promote the wellbeing of individuals and encourage healthy lifestyles, prevent disease, illness and injury, enable environments that support health and wellbeing, and to reduce personal, economic and social harm.

Health Workforce New Zealand (HWNZ) is an organisation that is part of the National Health Board which provides national leadership on the development of the health workforce. Some health promotional programs supported by HWNZ include education and training initiatives, and the Voluntary Bonding Scheme, which rewards medical, midwifery and nursing graduates who agree to work in hard-to-staff communities, and sonography, medical physicist and radiation therapy graduates who stay in New Zealand.

Health promotion in New Zealand has become an established approach in addressing public problems since the 1980s, through increasing use of intersectoral action, the use of public policy and mass media as promotional strategies, and the increasing control Maori have taken over the provision and purchase of health promotion services. An example of health promotional initiatives is the action put in place to reduce childhood obesity in primary schools. Research was completed to identify the barriers to improving school food environments and promoting healthy nutrition in primary schools in New Zealand.

Considerable progress has also been made in the health impact assessment (HIA) research on the impact of policies on health in New Zealand. The approach has an important contribution to make in the strengthening of health and wellbeing in policymaking in New Zealand.

Sri Lanka

In 2015, the life expectancy of Sri Lankan people was 72 for male and 78 for female. The disease burden has started to shift towards non-communicable diseases related to lifestyle and environmental factors. The 2012 estimated "healthy life expectancy" at birth of all Sri Lanka population is 68 for females, 63 for males, and 65 overall.

The development of the Sri Lankan National Health Promotion Policy is related to the State Policy and Strategy for Health and the Health Master Plan 2007–2016. It emphasises advocacy and empowerment to enable individuals and communities to take control of their own health, as well as improving the management of health promotion interventions across sectors.

United Kingdom

The Royal Society for Public Health was formed in October 2008 by the merger of the Royal Society for the Promotion of Health (also known as the Royal Society of Health or RSH) and the Royal Institute of Public Health (RIPH). Earlier, July 2005 saw the publication by the Department of Health and Welsh Assembly Government of Shaping the Future of Public Health: Promoting Health in the NHS. Following discussions with the Department of Health and Welsh Assembly Government officials, the Royal Society for Public Health and three national public health bodies agreed, in 2006, to work together to take forward the report's recommendations, working in partnership with other organisations. Accordingly:

1. the Royal Society for Public Health (RSPH) leads and hosts the collaboration, and focuses on advocacy for health promotion and its workforce;
2. The Institute of Health Promotion and Education (IHPE) works with the RSPH Royal Society for Public Health to give a voice to the workforce;
3. the Faculty of Public Health (FPH) focuses on professional standards, education and training; and
4. (4) the UK Public Health Register (UKPHR) is responsible for regulation of the workforce.

In Northern Ireland, the government's Health Promotion Agency for Northern Ireland which was set up to "provide leadership, strategic direction and support, where possible, to all those involved in promoting health in Northern Ireland". The Health Promotion Agency for Northern Ireland was incorporated into the Public Health Agency for Northern Ireland in April 2009.

Recent work in the UK *(Delphi consultation exercise due to be published late 2009 by Royal Society of Public Health and the National Social Marketing Centre)* on relationship between health promotion and social marketing has highlighted and reinforce the potential integrative nature of the approaches. While an independent review (NCC 'It's Our Health!' 2006) identified that some social marketing has in past adopted a narrow or limited approach, the UK has increasingly taken a lead in the discussion and developed a much more integrative and strategic approach which adopts a holistic approach, integrating the learning from effective health promotion approaches with relevant learning from social marketing and other disciplines. A key finding from the Delphi consultation was the need to avoid unnecessary and arbitrary 'methods wars' and instead focus on the issue of 'utility' and harnessing the potential of learning from multiple disciplines and sources. Such an approach is arguably how health promotion has developed over the years pulling in learning from different sectors and disciplines to enhance and develop.

United States

Government agencies in the U.S. concerned with health promotion include the following:

- The Centers for Disease Control and Prevention has a Coordinating Center for Health Promotion who mission is "Prevent disease, improve health, and enhance human potential through evidence based interventions and research in maternal and child health, chronic disease, disabilities, genomics, and hereditary disorders".
- The National Institute for Occupational Safety and Health has developed Total Worker Health, a strategy incorporating elements of occupational safety and health and health promotion, to advance the health and well-being of employees.
- The United States Army Center for Health Promotion and Preventive Medicine "provide[s] worldwide technical support for implementing preventive medicine, public health, and health promotion/wellness services into all aspects of America's Army and the Army Community".

Nongovernmental organizations in the U.S. concerned with health promotion include:

- The Public Health Education and Health Promotion Section is an active component of the American Public Health Association.
- The National Commission for Health Education Credentialing offers the NCHEC, a competency-based tool used to measure possession, application and interpretation of knowledge in the Seven Areas of Responsibility for Health Education Specialists. The exam reflects the entry-level Sub-competencies of these Areas of Responsibility.
- The Wellness Council of America is an industry trade group that supports workplace health promotion programs.
- URAC accredits comprehensive wellness programs "that focus on health promotion, chronic disease prevention and health risk reduction".

Breastfeeding Promotion

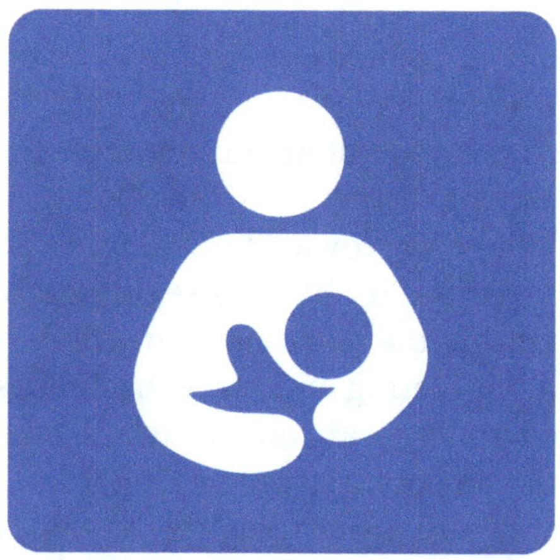

International Breastfeeding Symbol

Breastfeeding promotion refers to coordinated activities and policies to promote health among women, newborns and infants through breastfeeding.

The World Health Organization (WHO) recommends infants should be exclusively breastfed for the first six months of life to achieve optimal health and development, followed by complementary foods while continuing breastfeeding for up to two years or beyond. However, currently fewer than 40% of infants under six months of age are exclusively breastfed worldwide.

Public health awareness events such as World Breastfeeding Week, as well as training of health professionals and planning, aim to increase this number.

Significance of Breastfeeding Promotion in the United States

Breastfeeding promotion is a movement that came about in the twentieth century in response to high rates of bottle-feeding among mothers, and in recognition of the many health benefits to both mothers and children that breastfeeding offers. While infant formula had been introduced in developed countries in the 1920s as a healthy way to feed one's children, the emergence of research on health benefits of breastfeeding precipitated the beginning of the breastfeeding promotion movement in the United States. In the 1950s, La Leche League meetings began. The United States began incorporating benefits specific to breastfeeding promotion into its Women, Infants, and Children program in 1972. In 1989, WIC state agencies began being required to spend funds targeted at breastfeeding support and promotion, including the provision of education materials in different languages and the purchase of breast pumps and other supplies. In 1998, WIC state agencies were authorized to use funds earmarked for food to purchase breast pumps.

Each year, the Centers for Disease Control and Prevention release a Breastfeeding Report Card, detailing breastfeeding rates and promotion programs nationally and in all fifty states. In 2013, 76.5% of US women had ever breastfed their children; 16.4% exclusively breastfed up to six months of age. The Healthy People 2020 target for exclusive breastfeeding at six months is 25.5%. The proportion of infants who were breastfed exclusively or non-exclusively at six months was 35% in 2000 and increased to 49% by 2010.

Promotion Techniques

Prenatal Care

The discussion of breastfeeding during early prenatal care can positively effect a woman's likelihood to breastfeed her child. During regular checkups, a woman's physician, midwife or other healthcare provider can initiate a conversation about the benefits of breastfeeding, which can influence a woman to breastfeed her child for a longer period of time than she might have otherwise. In addition, the involvement of lactation consultants in the prenatal visits of low-income women increases the likelihood that they will breastfeed.

Peer Support and Counseling

Peer support techniques can be used before, during, and after pregnancy to encourage exclusive breastfeeding, particularly among groups with low breastfeeding rates. Breastfeeding peer counselors, who are ideally women who have breastfed who can provide information, support, and troubleshooting to mothers, have had a positive effect on the breastfeeding rate in American Indian populations. Peer counseling has also been effective at increasing breastfeeding initiation rates and breastfeeding rates up to three months after birth in Hispanic populations in the United States. In addition, peer counseling can be effective in encouraging not only exclusive breastfeeding, but also breastfeeding rates in combination with formula, or "any breastfeeding".

Peer counseling has had a strong effect on breastfeeding initiation and duration in developing countries such as Bangladesh and in areas where home births are more prevalent than hospital births. When combined with nutrition support, particularly the WIC program in the United States, the presence of peer counselors can have a significant effect on incidence of breastfeeding among low-income women.

Support during and immediately after childbirth can also help women initiate and continue breastfeeding while working through common concerns related to breastfeeding. This support can be non-medical, as doula care is. Culturally sensitive care (for example, care from a peer of a similar ethnic background) may be most effective at encouraging high-risk women to breastfeed.

Lactation Consultants

Lactation consultants are health care professionals whose primary goal is to promote breastfeeding and assist mothers with breastfeeding on an individualized or group basis. They work in a variety of health care settings, including hospitals, private doctor's offices, and public health clinics. Lactation consultants are board-certified by the International Board of Lactation Consultant Examiners. The majority of lactation consultants hold a certification in another healthcare profession, often as a nurse, midwife, dietician or physician. However, there is no specific post-secondary education required to become a lactation consultant.

In low-income contexts, interventions by breastfeeding consultants can be effective in promoting breastfeeding among high-risk populations. In one study, while exclusive breastfeeding rates were low in both control and intervention groups, black and Latina low-income women who had prenatal and postnatal support from a lactation consultant were more likely to breastfeed at 20 weeks than women who had not accessed this support. In general, lactation consultants give a greater proportion of positive feedback to mothers regarding breastfeeding than either physicians or nurses do; the amount of positive advice that a first-time mother receives regarding breastfeeding from any health care provider can influence her likelihood to continue breastfeeding for a longer period of time.

Social Marketing and Media

Social marketing has been shown to influence women's decision to breastfeed their children. One study found that in years when Parents magazine ran formula advertisements at a higher frequency, the proportion of women who breastfed often decreased in the following year. Conversely, women who are exposed to marketing that promotes breastfeeding are likely to breastfeed at higher rates.

The growth of the Internet's influence has also influenced women's choices in infant feeding. The Internet has served as both a vector for formula advertisement and a means by which women can connect with other mothers to gain support and share experiences from breastfeeding. In addition, social media is a category of advertising that did not exist when the International Code of Marketing of Breast-milk Substitutes was published; thus, while some advertising practices undertaken by formula companies on the Internet violated the Code, they did so in ways that could not have been anticipated.

One social medium used to promote breastfeeding is video. These videos are often independently filmed and produced by lactation consultants who seek a new way to reach clients. While the efficacy of these videos has not been formally studied, they are a relatively new medium of conveying messages about breastfeeding to women.

Cultural and Social Factors

Ethnicity and Breastfeeding Promotion

Breastfeeding initiation and duration varies significantly by race and ethnicity. The National Immunization Survey in the United States found that while 73.4% of all women in the United States initiated breastfeeding upon the birth of their child, only 54.4% of black, non-Hispanic women and

69.8% of American Indian and Alaska Native women did. White non-Hispanic women initiated breastfeeding 74.3% of the time and Hispanic women had an initiation rate of 80.4%. However, one study found that in a low-income environment, foreign-born black women had a similar breastfeeding rate to Hispanic women; both of these rates were higher than that of non-Hispanic white women. In addition, native-born black women had a somewhat higher rate of breastfeeding than white women.

Immigrant status in the United States is a predictor for breastfeeding adherence. In particular, the Hispanic paradox plays a role in the high breastfeeding rates observed among Hispanic/Latina women in the United States. Breastfeeding initiation rates among this population are higher for less acculturated immigrants; Hispanic women who have been in the United States for longer are less likely to breastfeed. This disparity does not depend on age, income level, or education level; more acculturated Hispanics are likely to cite the same reasons for bottle-feeding as native-born white women do. In many cases, the connection that Hispanic women feel to their culture and its values can strongly influence their decision regarding breastfeeding.

Access to prenatal care, socioeconomic status, cultural influence, and postpartum breastfeeding support all influence the differing rates of breastfeeding in different ethnic groups. In the United States, black women are more likely than white women to report that they "prefer bottle-feeding" to breastfeeding, and they are also more likely to be low-income and unmarried and to have lower levels of education. The decision to bottle-feed rather than breastfeed is of similar importance to low birth weight in predicting infant mortality, particularly in regards to the black-white infant mortality gap. Thus, breastfeeding promotion initiatives focused on black women should emphasize education and encourage black women to prefer breastfeeding to bottle-feeding.

Experts attribute high mortality rates and under nutrition amongst infants to the decreasing number of woman who breastfeed. This delay in breastfeeding initiation increases the risk of neonatal mortality. Experts suggest breastfeeding within the first day of birth until the infant is 6-months old. Promotion of breastfeeding during this period could potentially reduce the mortality rates by 16% if infant was breast fed since day one and 22% if the infant was breastfed within the first hour. Rates of breastfeeding initiation vary with ethnicity and socioeconomic situations. Studies suggest that college educated women over their 30 are more likely to initiate breastfeeding in comparison to other women who have different levels of educational attainment. Ethnicity, age, education, employment, marital status, and location are reported factors of delayed breastfeeding and infant under nutrition. Low- income mothers are specifically at risk for under nutrition and high mortality rates amongst their infants because they replace breast milk with formula. They do so because they lack a supportive environment, embarrassment of nursing, or the need to return to school or work. About 16.5% of low-income mothers breastfed for the recommended time. Studies suggest that scarce financial and social resources are consistent with the high mortality rates amongst the infants of low-income mothers.

An example of neonatal and infant mortality that is directly correlated with delayed initiation of breastfeeding is seen is sub-Saharan, Africa. Mortality rates are highest in this region of the world and have had the slowest progress to achieving reductions to the overall child mortality. Even if low-income mothers exclusively breast fed their infants for the 6 month – 1-year period, their infant is still at risk because most women commonly delay first day initiation of breast-feeding. Most women aren't aware that absence in breast milk put their infant at risk for serious health problems in the future. The Centers for Disease Control and Prevention (CDC) implements programs that promote and support breastfeeding and the benefits for infants and children. They compile many types of data so states can monitor progress and to educate expecting parents on the subject . But for other countries these programs aren't so common.

Socioeconomic Influence

Socioeconomic status of mothers likely has a larger influence on breastfeeding adherence than race or ethnicity, as many women who are members of groups with low breastfeeding rates also have a low socioeconomic status. Among women born in the United States, women who are wealthier are more likely to breastfeed. In addition, employment can influence the decision to breastfeed. When either parent was unemployed or held a lower-status occupation (such as labor or sales), their children were more likely to never have been breastfed. In addition, women with public insurance or with no health insurance are more likely to never have breastfed their children, as are women who receive WIC.

The time commitment of exclusive breastfeeding is also an economic constraint. The time required per week to breastfeed rather than bottle-feed or feed solids to children can be a significant burden for women without other childcare or who need to spend this time doing paid work. However, some evidence suggests that the long-term benefits of exclusive breastfeeding outweigh the short-term costs. In the United States, workplace policy surrounding breastfeeding and parental leave often does not reflect these benefits. In addition, women are often unable to risk the loss of their jobs or loss of income due to breastfeeding adherence, so bottle-feeding is the best solution for the short-term.

Supporting Adolescent Mothers Breastfeed

In recent times adolescent mothers have become a target population for breastfeeding education. In industrialized regions of the world including Canada, the United Kingdom, Australia and the United States, single, young mothers, under age 20, are less likely to initiate breastfeeding and more likely to have lower rates of breastfeeding duration. Studies have found that social barriers to continuing breastfeeding are insufficiently recognized and addressed by healthcare professionals. Studies suggest that one of the greatest barriers to improving breastfeeding rates among adolescent mothers are the expectations made by health care providers who assume young mother are too immature to breastfeed successfully. Therefore, these young mothers receive even less education and support than adult mothers even though they need it most. Participants of the various studies reported that medical staff directed them towards the hospital's vast supply of formula milk instead of receiving lactation consultations even when they wished to breastfeed.

Adolescent mothers have particular needs due to levels of education, employment, exposure (or lack thereof) to breastfeeding, self-esteem, support from others, of cognitive and psychological immaturity. These factors contribute to a young mother's likelihood to experience distress during their breastfeeding experiences and may even lead first time adolescent mothers to have different concerns and anxieties regarding breastfeeding from those of adult first time mothers.

Studies suggest that even when young mothers are informed about the health benefits of breast-feeding other social norms take precedence. The potential social embarrassment was present in the minds of expecting adolescent mothers and a major factor that influenced their choice of feeding method. Adolescent mothers have also described conflicts between their wish to resume activities outside of the home in the post-natal period and the baby's need to be fed. Public breastfeeding was seen as risking social disapproval, thus, discouraged from breastfeeding. Some of the adolescent participants of these studies described how their fears become a reality when they were asked to stop breastfeeding in public areas.

The breastfeeding promotion and support of adolescent mothers must take into account the context of the individual and their cultural norms. Few teenagers can withstand the cultural pressure which categorizes bottle feeding as a norm. Therefore, new teenage mothers need more concerted prenatal anticipatory guidance, specialized lactation education and an increase of face-to-face postpartum support. To succeed with the task at hand, inpatient nursing care will have to be tailor to the unique needs of this population. Positive perception of inpatient postpartum nursing care have been found to be an incredible influence in a young mother's success with breastfeeding. In a study conducted in the United States, young mothers reported positive postpartum experiences, especially in respect to breastfeeding initiation and mother-infant bonding, when their nursing care was targeted for adolescent mothers. The mothers reported that they felt better cared for and more motivated to initiate and sustain breastfeeding when nurses where friendly, patient, respectful and understanding of their individual needs. Maternal self-confidence is a contributing factor that influences positive breastfeeding outcomes especially among adolescent mothers. Empowerment, compassion, understanding and patience are key when caring for young moms.

Support outside of clinical settings is also important. Changes to policies have been introduced in the California (U.S.) legislature that identify schools as key institution of support for adolescent mothers. On February 12, 2015, State Assembly Member Cristina Garcia from Los Angeles, introduced and amendment to AB 302. AB 302 is a law which requires an employer to provide break time to accommodate employees to express breast milk for the employee's infant child, breast-feed an infant child or address other needs related to breast-feeding. This amendment requires public schools to provide similar accommodations to lactating students. These accommodations include but are not limited to access to a private or secure room, other than a restroom, permission to bring into a school campus any equipment used to express breast milk, access to a power source for said equipment, and access to store expressed breast milk. The bill does not mandate the construction of new space to make these accommodations possible. The policy hopes to validate young mothers' wishes to continue breastfeeding their infant children without shame.

On a global scale, recommendations have been made to educate school age children using curriculum that promotes healthy nutrition which includes breastfeeding. The World Health Organization's Global Strategy for Infant and Young Child Feeding recommend education authorities help form positive attitudes through the promotion of evidence-based science regarding the benefits of breastfeeding and other nutrition programs.

Worldwide Efforts

La Leche League

La Leche League International was founded in 1956 after breastfeeding rates in the United States dropped to about 20%. Today, La Leche League has groups in all 50 states and many countries worldwide. Its goals include promoting understanding of breastfeeding as a part of child development and providing support and education for breastfeeding mothers. La Leche League utilizes peer support groups in breastfeeding promotion in addition to supporting World Breastfeeding Week and other breastfeeding promotion initiatives. All La Leche League support group leaders have been specially trained and accredited in breastfeeding support. La Leche League also operates an online help form, online discussion forums, and podcasts to enable remote access to breastfeeding support resources.

Baby Friendly Hospital Initiative

The Baby Friendly Hospital Initiative (BFHI) is an initiative of the World Health Organization and UNICEF that seeks to encourage initiation of breastfeeding among mothers who give birth to their children in hospitals. Facilities that achieve its "Ten Steps to Successful Breastfeeding" and implement the International code of Marketing Breast-milk Substitutes can be recognized as a Baby-Friendly facility by the BFHI. In the United States, accreditation by the BFHI allows facilities to approach the Healthy People 2020 breastfeeding initiation goals. Worldwide, facilities that fulfill the requirements of the BFHI have been able to greatly increase their breastfeeding initiation rates among patients. The guidelines of the BFHI have also been effective in increasing breastfeeding initiation rates among populations that typically have lower incidences of breastfeeding, such as black women. In one study, the rate of infants exclusively breastfeeding more than quintupled over a four-year period upon the implementation of the BFHI.

World Breastfeeding Week

World Breastfeeding Week is an international initiative of the World Alliance for Breastfeeding Action that seeks to promote exclusive breastfeeding. Since 1992, it has been held each year from August 1 through August 7. In 2013, the theme of World Breastfeeding Week was "Breastfeeding Support: Close to Mothers"; past themes include early initiation of breastfeeding, the role of communication in breastfeeding, and breastfeeding policy. World Breastfeeding Week provides informational materials about breastfeeding to healthcare providers and breastfeeding specialists via download or purchase. In addition, groups or individuals worldwide are able to "pledge" that they will undergo promotion activities related to World Breastfeeding Week in order to show their support for the initiative.

WHO and UNICEF Initiatives

In addition to overseeing the Baby-Friendly Hospital Initiative, the WHO and UNICEF have promoted breastfeeding on an international level. In 1990, the Innocenti Declaration On the Protection, Promotion, and Support of Breastfeeding was published after a joint meeting of WHO and UNICEF policymakers. The Innocenti Declaration set forth goals of exclusive breastfeeding up to 4–6 months, helping women be confident in their ability to breastfeed, and national policies regarding breastfeeding to be determined by individual countries, among other benchmarks. In addition, UNICEF has published "Ten Steps to Successful Breastfeeding" which has been implemented in the Baby-Friendly Hospital Initiative.

The WHO and UNICEF also undertake independent research and reviews of recent research on breastfeeding in order to inform their future recommendations. UNICEF, alongside its recommendations for nutrition for children and adults, advocates exclusive breastfeeding up to six months of age and complementary feeding up to two years of age for young children. With these guidelines in mind, UNICEF believes that with optimal breastfeeding practices, up to 1.4 million deaths of children under 5 in the developing world can be prevented.

International Code of Marketing of Breast-Milk Substitutes

The International Code of Marketing of Breast-milk Substitutes was adopted in May 1981 by the Health Assembly of WHO and UNICEF. It sets forth standards for health care systems, health care workers, and formula distributors regarding the promotion of formula in comparison to breastfeeding. It also delineates the responsibilities of formula manufacturers to monitor the safety of breast-milk substitutes and governments to monitor the implementation of policies that promote breastfeeding. Although the Code has been successful in some settings, it has faced some opposition and non-compliance from the pharmaceutical industry. This has caused hospitals in different regions of the world to face unsolicited advertising from breast-milk substitute manufacturers, which inhibits their ability to make unbiased, evidence-based recommendations to patients.

Africa

Uganda

In Uganda, campaigns to promote breastfeeding have been conducted in the mass media, including public service announcements via radio, television, posters, newspapers and magazines, leading to improved knowledge of the benefits of breastfeeding for infants and mothers among individuals and communities.

Asia

Bangladesh

In Bangladesh, prelacteal feeding is a common custom; this is the practice of feeding other foods to infants before breast milk during the first three days of life. A study found that in a region of rural Bangladesh, 89.3% of infants were fed prelacteally, and only 18.8% of these infants were exclusively breastfed between three days and three months postpartum. 70.6% of infants who were not fed prelacteally were exclusively breastfed up to three months. Peer counseling and support programs have been shown to have a positive effect on exclusive breastfeeding rates in rural Bangladesh.

Australia

Australia implemented its first national breastfeeding policy in 2010, aimed at protecting, promoting, supporting and monitoring breastfeeding through each level of government and in non-government organisation.

Europe

Russia

In Russia, the Association of Natural Feeding Consultants (AKEV) promotes breastfeeding. AKEV provides mother-to-mother support, educates breastfeeding consultants as well as participates in public outreach about breastfeeding importance. AKEV is a regional group of the International Baby Food Action Network in Russia.

North America

Canada

In Canada, the provinces of Quebec and New Brunswick have mandated the implementation of the Baby Friendly Hospital Initiative, known as the Baby-Friendly Initiative (BFI) in Canada, which is designed to support best practices in hospitals and communities to ensure informed feeding decisions and enable families to sustain breastfeeding. Other provinces and territories are implementing strategies around the BFI at regional and local levels. The Canadian adaptation of the Baby-Friendly Hospital Initiative is designed to promote breastfeeding through a variety of facilities and settings; thus, the word "Hospital" is omitted from its title.

Cuba

The Cuban constitution contains a provision that allows one hour per day to breastfeed for women who return to their jobs after giving birth. Cuba also operates regional maternity homes for women who are undergoing high-risk pregnancies; after giving birth, 80% of women in these facilities will breastfeed.

United States

In the United States, breastfeeding promotion often relates to activities required to be carried out by state and local agencies using federal funds provided for nutrition education and administrative services under the Special Supplemental Nutrition Program for Women, Infants and Children (WIC program). States are required to use a portion of funds they receive to promote breastfeeding by postpartum mothers participating in the program.

Controversies

Breastfeeding and HIV

It has been argued that, in hindsight, the campaign for the universal promotion of breastfeeding prior to the acknowledgement of HIV contraction via mother-to-child transmission (MTCT) fails to consider affected mothers in developing countries who have limited or no access to procedures that would minify the chance of spreading the virus to their young ones. Initiatives for a decreased percentage of infants contracting HIV include administering Antiretroviral therapy (ART) to their mothers and providing milk formula in hand with proper water sterilization techniques to prevent disease from contamination. The majority of opposition comes from local and global policy makers who argue about the non-feasibility of these projects. However others argue that there is limited say of the women directly affected, resulting in further segregation of women in developing nations from preventive aid and health care systems.

Infant Formula Marketing in Hospitals

In many hospitals, women who are being discharged after giving birth are given discharge packs branded by a formula company that include formula samples. Many breastfeeding experts argue that these commercial discharge packs decrease the likelihood that a woman will breastfeed and, if she does breastfeed, the length of time she will do so. Studies have found that marketing of infant formula in hospitals makes it likelier that a woman will breastfeed for a shorter amount of time due to the perceived convenience of bottle-feeding. Formula companies often offer these discharge packs, as well as a general supply of formula, to hospitals at no cost, which can place some facilities at an economic disadvantage if they choose to give up these benefits. However, not accepting free formula is one of the criteria that determine whether a facility can be certified as Baby-Friendly; thus, the economic burden of giving up access to formula for free can be a significant barrier for disadvantaged facilities that wish to achieve Baby-Friendly status.

Workplace Health Promotion

Workplace health promotion is the combined efforts of employers, employees, and society to improve the mental and physical health and well-being of people at work. The term workplace health promotion denotes a comprehensive analysis and design of human and organizational work levels with the strategic aim of developing and improving health resources in an enterprise.

The World Health Organization has prioritized the workplace as a setting for health promotion because of the large potential audience and influence on all spheres of a person's life. The Luxembourg Declaration provides that health and well-being of employees at work can be achieved through a combination of:

- Improving the organization and the working environment
- Promoting active participation
- Encouraging personal development.

Workplace health promotion combines alleviation of health risk factors with enhancement of health strengthening factors and seeks to further develop protection factors and health potentials. Workplace health promotion is complementary to the discipline of occupational safety and health, which consists of protecting workers from hazards.

Successful workplace health promotion strategies include the principles of participation, project management, integration, and comprehensiveness:

- Participation: all staff must be included in all program stages
- Project management: programs must be oriented toward the problem-solving cycle
- Integration: programs must be incorporated into company management practices and workplace health-promotion strategies should influence corporate planning
- Comprehensiveness: programs must incorporate interdisciplinary individual-directed and environment-directed health strategies.

A report by the European Agency for Safety and Health at Work notes growing evidence that significant cost savings can be made by implementing workplace health promotion strategies, and over 90% of United States workplaces with greater than 50 employees have health promotion programs in place.

Strategies to Promote Health in the Workplace

Strategies for workplace health promotion need to be inclusive to account for diversity in the workforce, and behavioral economics is a key tool for implementing workplace health programs. The United States Department of Health and Human Services includes five strategic guidelines for workplace health promotion in its Healthy People 2010 initiative. These include:

- Health education, focused on skill development and lifestyle behavior change along with information dissemination and awareness building.
- Supportive social and physical environments, reflecting the organization's expectations regarding health behaviors and implementing policies promoting healthy behaviors.
- Integration of the worksite program into the organization's benefits, human resources infrastructure, and environmental health and safety initiatives.
- Links between health promotion and related programs like employee assistance.
- Screenings followed by counseling and education on how to best use medical services for necessary follow-up.

More generally, workplace health promotion efforts are implemented at three functional levels, including:

- Level I: awareness programs such as newsletters, health fairs, and educational classes that may or may not directly improve individual health or influence behavioral change.
- Level II: lifestyle modification programs of 8 to 12 weeks duration that are available to employees on an ongoing basis and directly influence health outcomes.
- Level III: the creation of a work environment that assists employees in sustaining healthy lifestyles and behaviors, such as workplace cafeterias offering healthy food choices or the provision of workplace exercise facilities.

In most instances physical activity interventions conform to Level II of this framework and may also include elements from Level III. Incentive-based Fitness Rewards Programs (FRPs) aim to influence employee behaviors and thereby conform to Level I.

Physical Activity Interventions

Approximately half of all current workplace health promotion programs are based on physical activity interventions given the relative ease by which employers can advocate such efforts to employees. Employer-sponsored activity interventions in the form of team sports originated as early as the 17th century in the United Kingdom, however, most 21st century interventions rely on employer sponsorship of employee access to health and fitness facilities. Employee convenience to sponsored fitness facilities strongly influences program participation, and facilities located near employee locations of residence hold lower time costs, receive increased use, and yield better program and health outcomes. Women frequently demonstrate lower participation in workplace exercise programs than men, and young, single individuals are often more predisposed to pursue employer-sponsored physical activity initiatives. In many cases, exercise-based workplace health promotion programs struggle to attract those who would benefit the most from such fitness efforts, including aging, sedentary, blue-collar, female, or less-educated employees.

The sedentary nature of many modern workplaces increases negative metabolic risk factors such as high body mass index (BMI), waist circumference, and blood pressure and elevated fasting glucose and triglyceride levels. Breaking up long periods of sedentary time is shown to improve these risks. Specifically, utilization of portable pedal exercise machines in office environments has been shown to improve employee health, and use was demonstrated feasible during working hours. Interventions using pedometers to influence employee behavior, decrease the duration of sedentary periods, and increase total movement during the work day have also proven successful. Smartphone applications and workplace signs promoting stair use are known to improve employee health, and many employers are now investing in wearable technologies to encourage employees to monitor physical activity. Workplace Tai Chi programs have also proven effective as a health intervention and means of reducing absenteeism, particularly in older workers. Despite these efforts, many health promotion programs struggle with poor participation, and the introduction of incentives is shown to improve employee involvement.

Incentive Based Programs

To encourage physical activity among the workforce, many employers offer financial incentives to employees through Fitness Rewards Programs (FRPs). Seeing that exercise and dieting produce immediate discomfort, the benefits of weight loss are often not noticeable in the short-term, and many people seek long-term health but succumb to near-term temptations of unhealthy eating and inactivity (hyperbolic discounting), maintaining employee involvement in wellness programs is difficult. To solve these problems of immediacy, salience, and hyperbolic discounting FRPs offer financial incentives to employees for healthy behaviors. Though lack of participation remains a problem even among well crafted FRPs, attrition is not random and greater weight loss success is associated with a reduction in later program dropout probability.

Effects of Workplace Health Promotion

The positive impact of workplace health promotion programs on productivity is widely discussed. The impact of workplace health promotion on absenteeism is substantial since productivity is impossible if an employee is absent. However, the effects of presenteeism are also significant, and working while sick is estimated to cost the United States economy more than $150 billion per year. Absenteeism is estimated to cost the average employer $660 annually per employee. Based on productivity costs, employees experiencing negative health conditions or at risk of developing impaired health cost employers up to $1601 more than healthy employees per year. Improvements in productivity and absenteeism following implementation of workplace health promotion programs can annually save employers $15.6 for every one dollar spent on health initiatives. More generally, employee health care costs and absentee day costs decrease by $3.27 and $2.73, respectively, for every dollar spent on workplace health promotion. In some cases, employer-based health programs have been shown to yield no reduction in health care spending or employer insurance outlay.

Relevant to health outcomes, workplace health promotion programs have demonstrated numerous short and long term benefits. Significantly, workplace physical activity interventions are shown to improve employee fitness, activity behavior, unhealthy lipid levels, work attendance, and job stress, and workplace exercise programs are known to reduce supervisor stress and abusive supervision of subordinates, increasing productivity. Additional improvements have been noted following workplace health programs in injury incidence, blood pressure, cholesterol levels, body mass index, cardiovascular disease risk, dynamic muscle performance, and maximal oxygen consumption. Some improvements vary by gender, with men often experiencing more consequential improvements in body mass index than women. Workplace health promotion is also known to improve the "perceived health status" of employees, enhancing productivity and improving health program participation.

Summarily, the expected outcomes of an ideal workplace health promotion program include:

- "Make workers aware of their health and how being in good health improves quality of life."
- "Workers should take 'ownership' of their behaviors and be accountable for health and cost outcomes."
- "High participation and active involvement in these programs. People should take advantage of the many programs offered."
- "Employees should lose weight, stop smoking, exercise more often, eat a healthy diet, better manage their stress levels, and generally adopt healthy habits."
- "Medical claims costs should go down. The company should experience a lower incidence of certain diseases linked to behaviors like diabetes, heart disease, cancer, chronic obstructive pulmonary disease (COPD), musculoskeletal disorders, and stroke."
- "Workers will be absent less often, disability costs will be controlled, accidents will be avoided, and injury rates should drop sharply."
- "These programs will attract the best talent—and turnover rates will be reduced because we are the employer of choice in the community."
- "Workers will perform at higher levels—they will be happier, have more energy, and produce better results for our company."
- "Establish a culture of health and well-being, where every worker feels valued and important to the enterprise—this will inspire greater loyalty and a high level of engagement."
- "The program will produce a positive return-on-investment (ROI) for the company—for every dollar spent, two or three will be saved."

Health Literacy

Health literacy is the ability to obtain, read, understand and use healthcare information to make appropriate health decisions and follow instructions for treatment. There are multiple definitions of health literacy, in part, because health literacy involves both the context (or setting) in which health literacy demands are made (e.g., health care, media, internet or fitness facility) and the skills that people bring to that situation (Rudd, Moeykens, & Colton, 1999). Studies reveal that only 12 percent of the adults in the U.S. have proficient health literacy. This means 77 million adults have basic or below basic health literacy. These individuals have difficulty with common health tasks including reading the label of a prescribed drug. Low health literacy reduces the success of treatment and increases the risk of medical error. Health literacy is essential to promote healthy individuals and communities.

Various interventions, such as simplified information and illustrations, avoiding jargon, "teach-back" methods and encouraging patients' questions, have improved health behaviors in persons with low health literacy. Health literacy is of continued and increasing concern for health professionals, as it is a primary factor behind health disparities. The proportion of adults aged 18 and over in the U.S., in the year 2010, who reported that their health care providers always explained things so they could understand them was about 60.6%. This number increased 1% from 2007 to 2010. The Healthy People 2020 initiative of the United States Department of Health and Human Services has included it as a pressing new topic, with objectives for addressing it in the decade to come.

Society as a whole is responsible for improving health literacy, but most importantly the healthcare, public health professionals, and the public health systems.

Characteristics

Plain Language

In order to have a population that understands health terms and can make proper health decisions, the language used by health professionals has to be a level that others who are not in the medical field can understand. Health professionals must know their audience in order to better serve their patient. The language used by these professionals should be plain language. Plain language is a strategy for making written and oral information easier to understand; it is communication that users can understand the first time they read or hear it.

Some key elements of plain language include:

- Organizing information so most important points come first
- Breaking complex information into understandable chunks
- Using simple language and defining technical terms
- Using active voice
- Using lists and tables to make complex material easier to understand

If health practitioners use plain language and ask their patients to teach back what they were told, individuals will be better able to take action, protect their health and wellness, and the health system will have better health outcomes.

Factors

Many factors determine the health literacy level of health education materials or other health interventions: reading level, numeracy level, current state of health, language barriers, cultural appropriateness, format and style, sentence structure, use of illustrations, interactiveness of intervention, and numerous other factors will affect how easily health information is understood and followed.

A study of 2,600 patients conducted in 1995 by two US hospitals found that between 26% and 60% of patients could not understand medication directions, a standard informed consent or basic health care materials.

History

The young and multidisciplinary field of health literacy emerged from two expert groups; physicians, other health providers, and health educators, and Adult Basic Education (ABE) and English as a Second Language (ESL) practitioners. Physicians are a source of groundbreaking patient comprehension and compliance studies. Adult Basic Education / English for Speakers of Languages Other Than English (ABE/ESOL) specialists study and design interventions to help people develop reading, writing, and conversation skills and increasingly infuse curricula with health information to promote better health literacy. A range of approaches to adult education brings health literacy skills to people in traditional classroom settings, as well as where they work and live.

Biomedical Approach

The biomedical approach to health literacy that became dominant (in the U.S.) during the 1980s and 1990s often depicted individuals as lacking, or "suffering" from, low health literacy, assumed that recipients are passive in their possession and reception of health literacy, and believed that models of literacy and health literacy are politically neutral and universally applicable. This approach is found lacking when placed in the context of broader ecological, critical, and cultural approaches to health. This approach has produced, and continues to reproduce, numerous correlational studies.

Where there are adequate levels of health literacy, that is where the population has sufficient knowledge and skills and where members of a community have the confidence to guide their own health, people are able to stay healthy, recover from illness and live with disease or disability.

McMurray states that health literacy is important in a community as it addresses health inequities, as those at the lower levels of health literacy are often the ones who live in lower socio-economic communities. Being aware of information relevant to improving their health, or how to access health resources creates higher levels of disadvantage. For some people, a lack of education and health literacy that would flow from education prevents them from becoming empowered at any time in their lives.

A more robust view of health literacy includes the ability to understand scientific concepts, content, and health research; skills in spoken, written, and online communication; critical interpretation of mass media messages; navigating complex systems of health care and governance; and knowledge and use of community capital and resources, as well as using cultural and indigenous knowledge in health decision making (Nutbeam, 2000; Ratzan, 2001; Zarcadoolas, Pleasant, & Greer, 2002).

This view sees health literacy as a social determinant of health that offers a powerful opportunity to reduce inequities in health.

This perspective defines health literacy as the wide range of skills, and competencies that people develop over their lifetimes to seek out, comprehend, evaluate, and use health information and concepts to make informed choices, reduce health risks, and increase quality of life (Zarcadoolas, Pleasant, & Greer, 2006). While definitions vary in wording, they all fall within the conceptual framework offered in this definition.

Defining health literacy in that manner builds the foundation for a multi-dimensional model of health literacy built around four central domains:

- fundamental literacy,
- scientific literacy,
- civic literacy, and
- cultural literacy.

There are several tests, which have verified reliability in the academic literature that can be administered in order to test one's health literacy. Some of these tests include the Medical Term Recognition Test (METER), which was developed in the United States (2 minute administration time) for the clinical setting. The METER includes many words from the Rapid Estimate of Adult Literacy in Medicine (REALM) test. The Short Assessment of Health Literacy in Spanish and English populations (SAHL-S&E) uses word recognition and multiple choice questions to test a person's comprehension. The CHC-Test is a test used to measure critical health competencies, which consists of 72 items and is designed to test a person's understanding of medical concepts, literature searching, basic statistics and design of experiments and samples.

Patient Safety and Outcomes

According to an Institute of Medicine (2004) report, low health literacy negatively affects the treatment outcome and safety of care delivery. The lack of health literacy affects all segments of the population. Although it is disproportionate in certain demographic groups, such as the elderly, ethnic minorities, recent immigrants and persons with low general literacy, it does not only affect the; it is an issue for all racial and ethnic groups. Anyone can face health literacy challenges including people with strong literacy skills. Nevertheless, elderlies, ethnic minorities, recent immigrants and people with low general literacy, have a higher risk of hospitalization and longer hospital stays, are less likely to comply with treatment, are more likely to make errors with medication, and are more ill when they seek medical care.

The mismatch between a clinician's level of communication and a patient's ability to understand can lead to medication errors and adverse medical outcomes. Health literacy skills are not only a problem in the public. Health care professionals (doctors, nurses, public health workers) can also have poor health literacy skills, such as a reduced ability to clearly explain health issues to patients and the public. A well arranged layout, pertinent illustrations, and intuitive format can improve the usability of health care literature. This in turn can help in effective communication between health care providers and patients and their families.

Risk Identification

Identifying patients at risk due to low health literacy is productive. Health behaviors such as correct medication use, taking advantage of health screening and effective preventive measures such as exercise and smoking cessation improved when low literacy patients were given visual aids, easy readability brochures or videotapes. Several tests of health literacy have been developed to validate research studies, but a practical, three-minute assessment can be completed in a doctor's office. A recent review on health literacy in the Journal of the American Medical Association's "Rational Clinical Examination Series" showed that single-item questions can be useful. The simple inquiry, "How confident are you in filling out medical forms by yourself?" gives a likelihood ratio (LR) for limited literacy of 5.0 (95% confidence interval [CI], 3.8-6.4) for an answer of "a little confident" or "not at all confident"; an LR of 2.2 (95% CI, 1.5-3.3) for "somewhat confident"; and an LR of 0.44 (95% CI, 0.24-0.82) for "quite a bit" or "extremely confident."

Intervention

Once identified, low health literacy patients benefit from providing limited but clear information at each visit, avoidance of medical jargon, using illustrations of important concepts and confirming information by a "teach back" method. A program called "Ask Me 3" is designed to bring public and physician attention to this issue, by letting patients know that they should ask three questions each time they talk to a doctor, nurse, or pharmacist:

- What is my main problem?
- What do I need to do?
- Why is it important for me to do this?

A public information program by the US Department of Health and Human Services encourages patients to improve healthcare quality and avoid errors by asking questions about health conditions and treatment.

The book *Decoding Medical Gobbleddygook - Health Literacy Puts Patients First* offers many resources on improving health literacy and is available free online.

The IROHLA (Intervention Research on Health Literacy of the Ageing population) project, funded by the EU, seeks to develop evidence based guidelines for policy and practice for approaches to improve health literacy of the ageing population in EU member states. The project has developed a framework, identified and validated interventions which together constitute a comprehensive approach of addressing health literacy needs of the older people. In November 2015 the IROHLA project will present its findings in an interactive web-portal informing professionals and local, regional and national policy makers.

Health Illiterate-related Diabetes Prevalence in Vietnamese-American Populations

Diabetes is a rapidly growing health problem among immigrants—affecting approximately 10 percent of Asian-Americans. It is the fifth-leading cause of death in Asian-Americans between the ages of 45 and 64. In addition, type 2 diabetes is the most common form of the disease. Those who are diagnosed with type 2 diabetes have high levels of blood glucose because the body does not effectively respond to insulin. It is a lifelong disease with no known cure. Diabetes is a chronic, debilitating, and costly social burden—costing healthcare systems about $100 billion annually.

Diabetes disproportionately affects underserved and ethnically diverse populations, such as Vietnamese-American communities. The relationship between the disease and health literacy level is in part because of an individual's ability to read English, evaluate blood glucose levels, and communicate with medical professionals. Other studies also suggest lack in knowledge of diabetes symptoms and complications. According to an observational cross-sectional study conducted, many Vietnamese-American diabetic patients show signs of poor blood glucose control and adherence due to inadequate self-management knowledge and experience. Diabetes health literacy research is needed to fully understand the burden of the chronic disease in Vietnamese-American communities, with respect to language and culture, health literacy, and immigrant status. Ethnic minority groups and immigrant communities have less knowledge of health promoting behavior, face considerable obstacles to health services, and experience poor communication with medical professionals. According to a recent review, studies has supported an independent relationship between literacy and knowledge of diabetes management and glucose control, but its impact on patients has not been sufficiently described. With the demand of chronic disease self-management (e.g., diabetic diet, glucose monitoring, etc.), a call for cultural-specific patient education is needed to achieve the control of diabetes and its adverse health outcomes in low- to middle-income Vietnamese-American immigrant communities.

eHealth Literacy

eHealth literacy is a term that describes the relatively modern concept of an individual's ability to search for, successfully access, comprehend, and appraise desired health information from electronic sources and to then use such information to attempt to address a particular health problem. Due to the increasing influence of the internet for information-seeking and health information distribution purposes, eHealth literacy has become an important topic of research in recent years. Stellefson (2011) states, "8 out of 10 Internet users report that they have at least once looked online for health information, making it the third most popular Web activity next to checking email and using search engines in terms of activities that almost everybody has done." Though in recent years, individuals may have gained access to a multitude of health information via the Internet, access alone does not ensure that proper search skills and techniques are being used to find the most relevant online and electronic resources. The lines between a reputable medical source and an amateur opinion from a so-called expert can often be blurred; however the ability to differentiate between the two is becoming increasing important.

Health literacy requires a combination of several different literacy skills in order to facilitate eHealth promotion and care. Six core skills are delineated by an eHealth literacy model referred to as the Lily model. The Lily Model's six literacies are organized into two central types: analytic and context-specific. Analytic type literacies are those skills that can be applied to a broad range of sources, regardless of topic or content (i.e., skills that can also be applied to shopping or researching a term paper in addition to health) whereas context-specific skills are those that are contextualized within a specific problem domain (can solely be applied to health). The six literacies are listed below, the first three of the analytic type and the latter three of the context-specific:

- Traditional literacy
- Media literacy
- Information literacy
- Computer literacy
- Scientific literacy
- Health literacy

According to Norman (2006), both analytical and context-specific literacy skills are "required to fully engage with electronic health resources." As the World Wide Web and technological innovations are more and more becoming a part of the health care environment, it is important for information technology to be properly utilized to promote health and deliver health care effectively.

It has been suggested that the move towards patient-centred care and the greater use of technology for self-care and self-management requires higher health literacy on the part of the patient.

Improvement

Incorporate Information Through the University Level

The United States Department of Health and Human Services created a National Action Plan to Improve Health Literacy. One of its goals is to incorporate health and science information in child-care and education through the university level. The target is to educate people at an early stage; that way individuals are raised with health literacy and will have a better quality of life. The earlier an individual is exposed to health literacy skills the better for the person and the community.

Programs such as Head Start and Women, Infants, and Children (WIC) have impacted our society and the low income population. Head Start provides low-income children and their families early childhood education, nutrition, and health. Health literacy is integrated in the program for both children and parents through the education they give the individuals. WIC serves low-income pregnant and after pregnancy mothers by supplementing them food, health care referrals, and nutrition education. Programs like these help both, the parent and the child with health literacy creating a more knowledgeable community with health education.

Although programs like Head Start and WIC have been working with the health literacy of a specific population, much more can be done with the education of children and young adults. Now, more and more adolescents are getting involved with their health care. Due to this, it is crucial to educate these individuals in order for them to make informed decisions.

Many schools in the country incorporate a health class in their curriculum. These classes provided an excellent opportunity to facilitate and develop health literacy in today's children and adolescents. The skills of how to read food labels, the meaning of common medical terms, the structure of the human body, and education on the most prevalent disease in the United States should be taught in both private and public schools. This way new generations will grow with health literacy and would hopefully make knowledgeable health decisions.

Framework and Potential Intervention Points

The National Library of Medicine defines health literacy as:

"The degree to which individuals have the capacity to obtain, process, and understand basic health literacy

information and services needed to make appropriate health decisions."

Based on this clinical definition, health literacy gives individuals the skills that they need to both understand and effectively communicate information and concerns. Bridging that gap between literacy skills and the ability of the individual in health contexts, the *Health Literacy Framework* highlights the health outcomes and costs associated with health contexts including cognitive abilities, social skills, emotional state, and physical conditions such as visual and auditory contributions.

Potential Intervention Points are illustrated in reflection of the *Health Literacy Framework*. Outlining interactions such as those of individuals and the education systems that they are engaged with, their health systems, and societal factors as they relate to health literacy, these potential intervention points are not however, components of a casual model. The three potential intervention points are culture and society, the health system, and the education system. Health outcomes and costs are the products of the health literacy developed during diversity of exposure to these three potential intervention points.

Referring to shared ideas, meanings, and values that influence an individual's beliefs and attitudes, cultural and societal influences are a significant intervention point for health literacy development. As interactions with healthcare systems often first occur at the family level, deeply rooted beliefs and values can shape the significance of the experience. Included components that reflect the development of health literacy both culturally and societally are native language, socioeconomic status, gender, race, and ethnicity, as well as mass media exposure. These are pathways to understanding American life paralleling conquests for a health literate America.

The health system is an intervention point in the *Health Literary Framework*. For the purposes of this framework, health literacy refers to an individual's interaction with people performing health-related activities in settings such as hospitals, clinics, physician's offices, home health care, public health agencies, and insurers.

In the United States, the education system consists of K-12 curricula. In addition to this standard educational setting, adult education programs are also environments in which individuals can develop traditional literacy skills founded in comprehension and real-world application of knowledge via reading and writing. Tools for educational development provided by these systems impact an individual's capacity to obtain specific knowledge regarding health. Reflecting components of traditional literacy such as cultural and conceptual knowledge, oral literacy (listening and speaking,) print literacy (reading and writing,) and numeracy, education systems are also potential intervention points for health literacy development.

Skills Needed for Development

Health Related Goals

- Promoting and protect health and prevent disease
- Understand, interpret, and analyze health information
- Apply health information over a variety of life events and situations
- Navigate the health-care system
- Actively participate in encounters with health-care professionals and workers
- Understand and give consent
- Understand and advocate for rights

Libraries

Libraries have increasingly recognised that they can play a role in health literacy since the 2000s, influenced by the Medical Library Association. Library initiatives have included running education programs, fostering partnerships with health organisations, and using outreach efforts.

Clinical Health Promotion

Clinical Health Promotion is Prevention, which includes elements of health promotion and rehabilitation, which takes place in the health care system together with patients.

The intention is to focus on and integrate prevention into patient pathway to reduce decease progression, prevent complications and relapse as well as maximize coping and quality of life. Clinical health promotion emanates from the health care system where the patient is the active/activated part and hence the efforts also include elements of health promotion and rehabilitation.

Emphasis is placed on keeping choice and accountability with the patient, as well as empathy, feedback and positive expectations for the patient. The target audience is patients and the arena may be primary or secondary care where professionals in interaction with patients are engaged in clinical health promotion.

Examples

Examples of clinical health promotion are:

- Smoking cessation for pregnant women
- Alcohol cessation before surgery
- Physical activity program for mentally ill
- Diabetes education
- Control of asthma patients.

Peer Education

Peer education is an approach to health promotion, in which community members are supported to promote health-enhancing change among their peers. Peer education is the teaching or sharing of health information, values and behavior in educating others who may share similar social backgrounds or life experiences.

Rather than health professionals educating members of the public, the idea behind peer education is that ordinary lay people are in the best position to encourage healthy behaviour to each other.

Areas of Application

Peer education has become very popular in the broad field of HIV prevention. It is a mainstay of HIV prevention in many developing countries, among groups including young people, sex workers, men who have unprotected sex with men, or people who use intravenous drugs.

Peer education is also associated with efforts to prevent tobacco, alcohol and other drug use among young people. Peer educators can be effective role models for young adolescents by promoting healthy behavior, helping to create and reinforce social norms that support safer behaviors, and also serve as an accessible and approachable health education resource both inside and outside the classroom.

Peer education is also useful in promoting healthy eating, food safety and physical activity amongst marginalized populations.

The Process

A peer education programme is usually initiated by health or community professionals, who recruit members of the *target* community to serve as peer educators. The recruited peer educators are trained in relevant health information and communication skills. Armed with these skills, the peer educators then engage their peers in conversations about the issue of concern, seeking to promote health-enhancing knowledge and skills. The intention is that familiar people, giving locally-relevant and meaningful suggestions, in appropriate local language and taking account of the local context, will be most likely to be able to promote health-enhancing behaviour change.

There is a great variety in the support provided to peer educators. Sometimes they are unpaid volunteers, sometimes they are given a small honorarium, sometimes they receive a reasonable salary. The peer educators may be supported by regular meetings and training, or expected to continue their work without formal supports.

Theories

A variety of theories are offered regarding the question of how peer education is supposed to achieve positive results.

Positive results of a Peer Educator are achieved through educating individuals to enhance their understanding about diseases, alcohol and drug abuse etc. and effectively communicate what they've learned to other at-risk peers in their community. The goal is to educate and reach as many people to limit the spread of disease and to learn how to overcome drug and alcohol abuse etc.

Kelly's Popular Opinion Leader Theory

The popular opinion leader theory suggests a parallel between peer education and the marketing of commercial products. Peer educators are seen as *opinion leaders*—respected and admired by other members of the community. These opinion leaders espouse a certain lifestyle (such as safer sex, or not smoking, etc.)—and their peers wish to emulate them.

Critical Consciousness

Campbell argues that what peer education ought to do is to promote the kind of critical consciousness theorised by Paulo Freire This means that peers use the peer education process to critically discuss their circumstances, especially the social factors impacting upon their health. Becoming critically aware of these forces is the first step to tackling them. So, for instance, if local norms regarding sexuality and gender put people's health at risk, this approach argues that peers should critically discuss those norms, so that they can then collectively seek to establish new more health-enhancing norms.

Social Learning Theory

Based on the work of Bandura and colleagues, social learning theory claims that modelling is an important component of the learning process. In the most basic sense, people observe behaviour taking place and then go on to adopt similar behaviour. Participants require the opportunity to practice modelled behavior and positive reinforcement if it is to be adopted successfully.

Differential Association Theory

Based on the work of Sutherland and Cressy, differential association theory has been applied to the study of crime. Rather than the result of biological or psychological disorders, crime is a learned behaviour. This learning happens in social situations by associating with those who can teach the necessary skills and techniques needed. Through this theory it can be understood that peers can be very influential for both positive and negative behaviours. Young people can learn both good and bad habits from each other. In differential association theory the mere association with others provides a learning opportunity. If social learning theory is essentially psychological, differential association theory is essentially sociological.

Role Theory

Sarbin argues that peer educators will adapt to the role expectations of a tutor and behave appropriately. Furthermore, through adopting a role, individuals develop a deeper understanding and commitment to it. The potential is that Peer educators can develop a stronger commitment and a greater appreciation of the relevance of the health topic. Role theory is also based on the premise that communication can be blocked by differences in culture between the teacher and learner. Peer educators who have a similar set of experiences and culture are therefore likely to be more effective in promoting learning.

Communication of Innovations Theory

Developed by Rogers and Shoemaker, the communication of innovations theory explains how innovations come to be adopted by communities and what factors influence the rate of adoption. These factors include the characteristics of those who adopt the innovation, the nature of the social system, the characteristics of the innovation and the characteristics of change agents. Rogers and Shoemaker argue that all innovations follow a similar pattern of adoption, with one group of people—the *innovators*—taking it up immediately. Then there are *early adopters*, the *early majority*, the *late majority* and finally the *laggards*, including some who never adopt the innovation. In this theory key people influence the opinion leaders within a community. Change agents can be viewed as health professionals while opinion leaders correlate with peer educators. Rogers and Shoemaker argue that effective communication occurs when the source and receiver are *homophilous*, that is, are similar in certain attributes. These include beliefs, values, education and social status. This would suggest that peers communicate better than those who are unequal or different.

Support

Peer educators are seen as credible sources of information. This has been shown to be particularly effective amongst the youth population. Peers and peer education are an important influence and approach in changing health behaviours.

One of the beliefs of peer education is that it is cost effective. Peer education has been identified as a more economical way to deliver health training.

A team of peer educators can extend health promotion outreach and be more accessible than paid health professionals. Peer educators help to bridge many of the gaps in service that occur through fear and suspicion of official health care providers, and to facilitate effective communication with community members and professional provider. Engaging youth peer educators helps professionals to extend their outreach of programs and services to ensure their efforts are impactful.

Peer education is empowering from both the standpoint of the peer educator and the individual receiving service. Peer education has been operative in encouraging knowledge, attitudes and intention to change behavior in AIDS prevention. Furthermore, nondirective peer support has been identified as the best way to motivate individuals in the preparation, action, or maintenance stages of readiness to change. Researchers have acknowledged that trained peer tutors were more effective than the untrained peers in influencing positive health outcomes. Peer education offers the educators the opportunity to benefit from taking on meaningful roles. Peer educators can act as enthusiastic advocates for the program and have a sense of purpose in their community outreach efforts.

Peer education is sustainable. This has been found to be an important issue for community-based health promotion interventions to make a difference over time. A grassroots initiative involving volunteers means that the health issue is reaching the target audience continuously with less of a threat of financial cutbacks impacting on their work. Research findings support the use of volunteer peer educators as a feasible and effective healthcare delivery strategy and as having promising indicators of sustainability over time. Sustainability through the engagement of peer educators can strengthen the social environment so that it is supportive of healthy behaviors.

Debates

Despite its popularity, the evidence about peer education is mixed, and there is no consensus on whether it works or how it works. Researchers have questioned the validity of the assumption that peer education influences behavior.

One important line of inquiry suggests that peer education may work in some contexts but not in others. A study comparing peer education among sex workers in India and South Africa found that the more successful Indian group benefited from a supportive social and political context, and a more effective community development ethos, rather than the biomedical focus of the South African intervention.

A key issue concerns what a peer is and who defines this. In some instances age is a central factor but in other contexts, commonalities such as status may be more relevant. Caution has been noted regarding selection of peer educators. Some argue that there can be a stigma held against peer educators who have faced adversities in their own lives, particularly by mainstream health service organizations and professionals. Alternatively, peers educators would need to have high status within their social group to be effective. Researchers have argued that peer educators sometimes receive inadequate training, which limits their ability to educate their peers effectively and further state that peer selection and training is very important.

An important analysis on the development of many peer education projects is that it is led by adult constructions of adolescence and adolescent health behaviour. A central question should therefore be whose agenda is being served by using peer education projects which manipulate and exploit the social worlds of young people?

Family Planning

Family planning is the practice of controlling the number of children in a family and the intervals between their births, particularly by means of artificial contraception or voluntary sterilization. Because "family" is included in the concept's name, consideration of a couple's desire to bear children, in the context of a family unit, is often considered primarily. Contemporary notions of family planning, however, tend to place a woman and her childbearing decisions at the center of the discussion, as notions of women's empowerment and reproductive autonomy have gained traction in many parts of the world. Family planning may involve consideration of the number of children a woman wishes to have, including the choice to have no children, as well as the age at which she wishes to have them. These matters are obviously influenced by external factors such as marital situation, career considerations, financial position, any disabilities that may affect their ability to have children and raise them, besides many other considerations. If sexually active, family planning may involve the use of contraception and other techniques to control the timing of reproduction. Other techniques commonly used include sexuality education, prevention and management of sexually transmitted infections, pre-conception counseling and management, and infertility management.

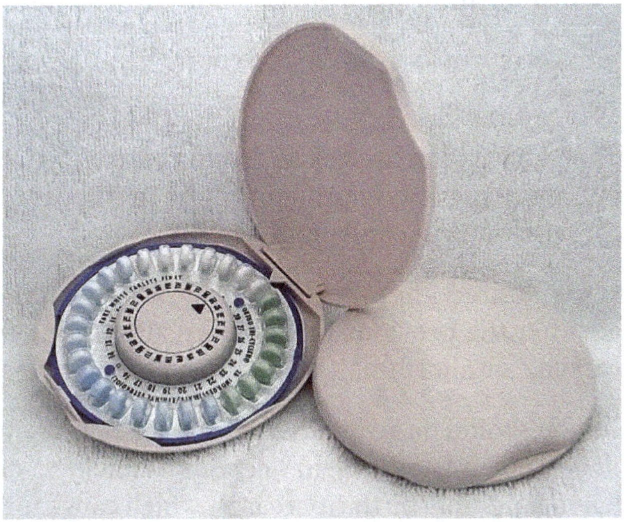

Combined oral contraceptives. Introduced in 1960, "the Pill" has played an instrumental role in family planning for decades.

Family planning is sometimes used as a synonym or euphemism for access to and the use of contraception. However, it often involves methods and practices in addition to contraception. Additionally, there are many who might wish to use contraception but are not, necessarily, planning a family (e.g., unmarried adolescents, young married couples delaying childbearing while building a career); family planning has become a catch-all phrase for much of the work undertaken in this realm. It is most usually applied to a female-male couple who wish to limit the number of children they have and/or to control the timing of pregnancy (also known as *spacing children*). Family planning may encompass sterilization, as well as abortion.

Family planning services are defined as "educational, comprehensive medical or social activities which enable individuals, including minors, to determine freely the number and spacing of their children and to select the means by which this may be achieved".

Purposes

"Raising" a child requires significant amounts of resources: time, social, financial, and environmental. Planning can help assure that resources are available. The purpose of family planning is to make sure that any couple, man, or woman who has the desire to have a child has the resources that are needed in order to complete this goal. With these resources a couple, man or women can explore the options of natural birth, surrogacy, artificial insemination, or adoption. In the other case, if the person does not wish to have a child at the specific time, they can investigate the resources that are needed to prevent pregnancy, such as birth control, contraceptives, or physical protection and prevention.

Health

The WHO states about maternal health that:

> "Maternal health refers to the health of women during pregnancy, childbirth and the post-partum period. While motherhood is often a positive and fulfilling experience, for too many women it is associated with suffering, ill-health and even death."

About 99% of maternal deaths occur in less developed countries; > ½ occur in sub-Saharan Africa and almost ⅓ in South Asia.

Both early and late motherhood have increased risks. Young teenagers face a higher risk of complications and death as a result of pregnancy. Waiting until the mother is at least 18 years old before trying to have children improves maternal and child health.

Also, if additional children are desired after a child is born, it is healthier for the mother and the child to wait at least 2 years after the previous birth before attempting to conceive (but not more than 5 years). After a miscarriage or abortion, it is healthier to wait at least 6 months.

When planning a family, women should be aware that reproductive risks increase with the age of the woman. Like older men, older women have a higher chance of having a child with autism or Down syndrome, the chances of having multiple births increases, which cause further late-pregnancy risks, they have an increased chance of developing gestational diabetes, the need for a Caesarian section is greater, older women's bodies are not as well-suited for delivering a baby. The risk of prolonged labor is higher. Older mothers have a higher risk of a long labor, putting the baby in distress.

"Family planning benefits the health and well-being of women and families throughout the world. Using contraception can help to avoid unwanted pregnancies and space births; protect against STDs, including HIV/AIDS; and provide other health benefits."

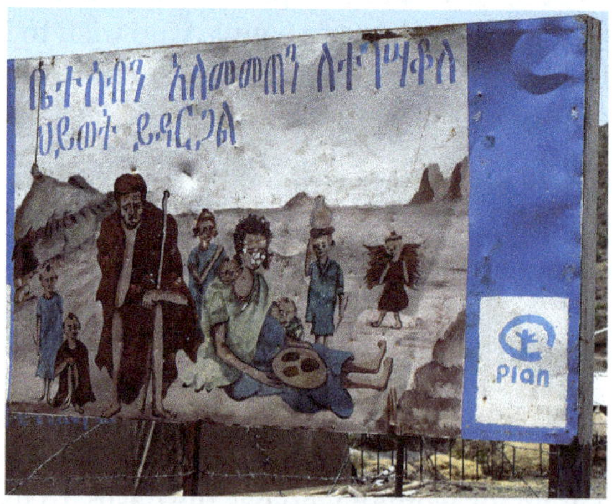

Placard showing negative effects of lack of family planning and having too many children and infants (Ethiopia)

Modern Methods

Modern methods of family planning include birth control, assisted reproductive technology and family planning programs.

The use of modern methods of contraception is an important basis for improving the long-term health of adolescent girls. The United Nations Population Fund (UNFPA) says that, "Contraceptives prevent unintended pregnancies, reduce the number of abortions, and lower the incidence of death and disability related to complications of pregnancy and childbirth." UNFPA states that, "If all women with an unmet need for contraceptives were able to use modern methods, an additional 24 million abortions (14 million of which would be unsafe), 6 million miscarriages, 70,000 maternal deaths and 500,000 infant deaths would be prevented."

In cases where couples may not want to have children just yet, family planning programs help a lot. Federal family planning programs reduced childbearing among poor women by as much as 29 percent, according to a University of Michigan study.

Adoption is sometimes used to build a family. There are seven steps that one must make towards adoption. You must decide to pursue an adoption, apply to adopt, complete an adoption home study, get approved to adopt, be matched with a child, receive an adoptive placement, and then legalize the adoption.

Contraception

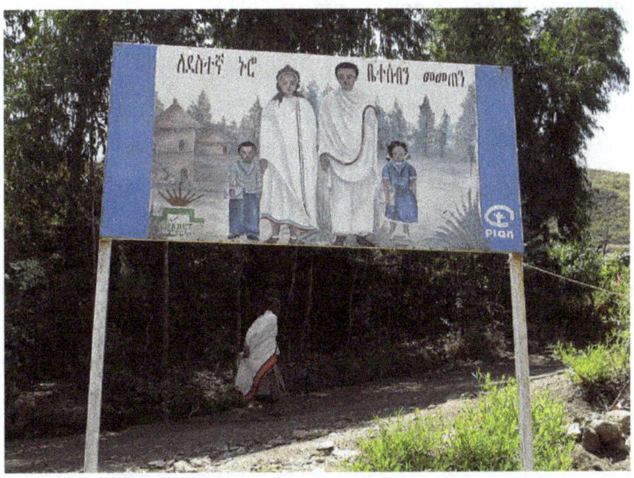

Placard showing positive effects of family planning (Ethiopia)

A number of contraceptive methods are available to prevent unwanted pregnancy. There are a range of contraceptive methods, each with particular advantages and disadvantages. Behavioral methods to avoid pregnancy that involve vaginal intercourse include the withdrawal and calendar-based methods, which have little up front cost and are readily available, but are much less effective in typical use than most other methods. Long-acting reversible contraceptive methods, such as intrauterine device (IUD) and implant are highly effective and convenient, requiring little user action. When cost of failure is included, IUDs and vasectomy are much less costly than other methods. In addition to providing birth control, male and/or female condoms protect against sexually transmitted diseases (STD). Condoms may be used alone, or in addition to other methods, as backup or to prevent STD. Surgical methods (tubal ligation, vasectomy) provide long-term contraception for those who have completed their families.

Assisted Reproductive Technology

When, for any reason, a woman is unable to conceive by natural means, she may seek assisted conception. For example, some families or women seek assistance through surrogacy, in which a woman agrees to become pregnant and deliver a child for another couple or person.

There are two types of surrogacy: traditional and gestational. In traditional surrogacy, the surrogate uses her own eggs *and* carries the child for her intended parents. This procedure is done in a doctor's office through IUI. This type of surrogacy obviously includes a genetic connection between the surrogate and the child. Legally, the surrogate will have to disclaim any interest in the child to complete the transfer to the intended parents. A gestational surrogacy occurs when the intended mother's or a donor egg is fertilized outside the body and then the embryos are transferred into the uterus. The woman who carries the child is often referred to as a gestational carrier. The legal steps to confirm parentage with the intended parents are generally easier than in a traditional because there is no genetic connection between child and carrier.

Sperm donation is another form of assisted conception. It involves donated sperm being used to fertilise a woman's ova by artificial insemination (either by intracervical insemination or intrauterine insemination) and less commonly by invitro fertilization (IVF), but insemination may also be achieved by a donor having sexual intercourse with a woman for the purpose of achieving conception. This method is known as natural insemination (NI).

Mapping of a woman's ovarian reserve, follicular dynamics and associated biomarkers can give an individual prognosis about future chances of pregnancy, facilitating an informed choice of when to have children.

Finances

Family planning is among the most cost-effective of all health interventions. "The cost savings stem from a reduction in unintended pregnancy, as well as a reduction in transmission of sexually transmitted infections, including HIV".

Childbirth and prenatal health care cost averaged $7,090 for normal delivery in the United States in 1996. U.S. Department of Agriculture estimates that for a child born in 2007, a U.S. family will spend an average of $11,000 to $23,000 per year for the first 17 years of child's life. (Total inflation-adjusted estimated expenditure: $196,000 to $393,000, depending on household income.) Breaks down cost by age, type of expense, region of country. Adjustments for number of children (one child — spend 24% more, 3 or more spend less on each child.)

Investing in family planning has clear economic benefits and can also help countries to achieve their "demographic dividend," which means that countries productivity is able to increase when there are more people in the workforce and less dependents. UNFPA says that, "For every dollar invested in contraception, the cost of pregnancy-related care is reduced by $1.47."

UNFPA states that,

"The lifetime opportunity cost related to adolescent pregnancy – a measure of the annual income a young mother misses out on over her lifetime – ranges from 1 per cent of annual gross domestic product in a large country such as China to 30 per cent of annual GDP in a small economy such as Uganda. If adolescent girls in Brazil and India were able to wait until their early twenties to have children, the increased economic productivity would equal more than $3.5 billion and $7.7 billion, respectively."

International Oversight

The world's largest international source of funding for population and reproductive health programs is the United Nations Population Fund (UNFPA). In 1994, the International Conference on Population and Development set the main goals of its Program of Action as:

- Universal access to reproductive health services by 2015
- Universal primary education and ending the gender gap in education by 2015
- Reducing maternal mortality by 75% by 2015
- Reducing infant mortality
- Increasing life expectancy at birth
- Reducing HIV infection rates in persons aged 15–24 years by 25% in the most-affected countries by 2005, and by 25% globally by 2010

The World Health Organization (WHO) and World Bank estimate that $3 per person per year would provide basic family planning, maternal and neonatal health care to women in developing countries. This would include contraception, prenatal, delivery, and post-natal care in addition to postpartum family planning and the promotion of condoms to prevent sexually transmitted infections.

Coercive Interfering with Family Planning

Forced Sterilization

Compulsory or forced sterilization programs or government policy attempt to force people to undergo surgical sterilization without their freely given consent. People from marginalized communities are at most risk of forced sterilization. Forced sterilization has occurred in recent years in Eastern Europe (against Roma women), and in Peru (during the 1990s against indigenous women). China's one-child policy was intended to limit the rise in population numbers, but in some situations involved forced sterilisation.

Sexual Violence

Rape can result in a pregnancy. Rape can occur in a variety of situations, including war rape, forced prostitution and marital rape, and those that result in pregnancy add to the long-term psychological and economic anguish of the victim, besides other things, disturbing her plans for creating a family of her choosing.

In Rwanda, the National Population Office has estimated that between 2,000 and 5,000 children were born as a result of sexual violence perpetrated during the genocide, but victims' groups gave a higher estimated number of over 10,000 children.

Family Planning, Human Rights & Development

Access to safe, voluntary family planning is a human right and is central to gender equality, women's empowerment and poverty reduction. The United Nations Population Fund (UNFPA) says that, "Some 225 million women who want to avoid pregnancy are not using safe and effective family planning methods, for reasons ranging from lack access to information or services to lack of support from their partners or communities." UNFPA says that, "Most of these women with an unmet need for contraceptives live in 69 of the poorest countries on earth."

Over the past 50 years, right-based family planning has enabled the cycle of poverty to be broken resulting in millions of women and children's lives being saved.

UNFPA says that, "Global consensus that family planning is a human right was secured at the 1994 International Conference on Population and Development, in Principle 8 of the Programme of Action: All couples and individuals have the basic right to decide freely and responsibly the number and spacing of their children and to have the information, education and means to do so."

As part of the United Nations Millennium Development Goals (MDGs) universal access to family planning is one of the key factors contributing to development and reducing poverty. Family planning creates benefits in areas such as, gender quality and women's health, access to sexual education and higher education, and improvements in maternal and child health.

UNFPA and the Guttmacher Institute say that,

"Serving all women in developing countries that currently have an unmet need for modern contraceptives would prevent an additional 54 million unintended pregnancies, including 21 million unplanned births, 26 million abortions (of which 16 million would have been unsafe) and seven million miscarriages; this would also prevent 79,000 maternal deaths and 1.1 million infant deaths."

Regional Variations

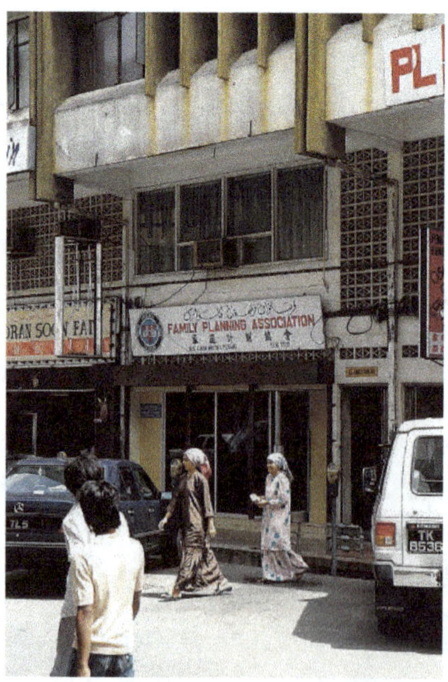

A family planning facility in Kuala Terengganu, Malaysia

Africa

Most of the countries with lowest rates of contraceptive use, highest maternal, infant, and child mortality rates, and highest fertility rates are in Africa. Only about 30% of all women use birth control, although over half of all African women would like to use birth control if it was available to them. The main problems that preventing access to and use of birth control are unavailability, poor health care services, spousal disapproval, religious concerns, and misinformation about the effects of birth control. The most available type of birth control is condoms. A rapidly growing population coupled with an increase in preventable diseases means countries in Sub-Saharan Africa face an increasingly younger population.

China

China's *Family planning policy* forced couples to have no more than one child. Beginning in 1979 and being officially phased out in 2015, the policy was instated to control the rapid population growth that was occurring in the nation at that time. With the rapid change in population, China was facing many impacts, including poverty and homelessness. As a developing nation, the Chinese government was concerned that a continuation of the rapid population growth that had been occurring would hinder their development as a nation. The process of family planning varied throughout China, as people differed in their responsiveness to the one-child policy, based on location and socioeconomic status. For example, many families in the cities accepted the policy more readily based on the lack of space, money, and resources that often occurs in the cities. Another example can be found in the enforcement of this rule; people living in rural areas of China were, in some cases, permitted to have more than one child, but had to wait several years after the birth of the first one. However, the people in rural areas of China were more hesitant in accepting this policy. China's population policy has been credited with a very significant slowing of China's population growth which had been higher before the policy was implemented. However, the policy has come under criticism that it has resulted in the abuse of women. Often implementation of the policy has involved forced abortions, forced sterilization, and infanticides. That families desired a male child had a part to play in the number of infanticides. The number of girls that die within their first year of birth is twice that of boys. Another drawback of the policy is that China's elderly population is now increasing rapidly. However, while the punishment of "unplanned" pregnancy is a large fine, both forced abortion and forced sterilization can be charged with intentional assault, which is punished with up to ten years' imprisonment. Another issue that is raised in the one-child policy in China is the information in regards to naturally giving birth to twins or triplets. If this situation arises, the family is allowed to keep the children because of the natural causes of this impregnation.

Family planning in China had its benefits, and its drawbacks. For example, it helped reduce the population by about 300 million people in its first 20 years. A drawback is that there are now millions of sibling-fewer people, and in China siblings are very important. Once the parent generation gets older, the children help take care of them, and the work is usually equally split among the siblings. Another benefit of the implementation of the one-child law is that it reduced the fertility rate from about 2.75 children born per woman, to about 1.8 children born per woman in the 1979.

Hong Kong

In Hong Kong, the Eugenics League was found in 1936, which became The Family Planning Association of Hong Kong in 1950. The organisation provides family planning advice, sex education, birth control services to the general public of Hong Kong. In the 1970s, due to the rapidly rising population, it launched the "Two Is Enough" campaign, which reduced the general birth rate through educational means.

The Family Planning Association of Hong Kong, Hong Kong's national family planning association, founded the International Planned Parenthood Federation with its counterparts in seven other countries.

India

Family planning in India is based on efforts largely sponsored by the Indian government. In the 1965-2009 period, contraceptive usage has more than tripled (from 13% of married women in 1970 to 48% in 2009) and the fertility rate has more than halved (from 5.7 in 1966 to 2.6 in 2009), but the national fertility rate is still high enough to cause long-term population growth. India adds up to 1,000,000 people to its population every 15 days.

Iran

While Iran's population grew at a rate of more than 3% per year between 1956 and 1986, the growth rate began to decline in the late 1980s and early 1990s after the government initiated a major population control program. By 2007 the growth rate had declined to 0.7 percent per year, with a birth rate of 17 per 1,000 persons and a death rate of 6 per 1,000. Reports by the UN show birth control policies in Iran to be effective with the country topping the list of greatest fertility decreases. UN's Population Division of the Department of Economic and Social Affairs says that between 1975 and 1980, the total fertility number was 6.5. The projected level for Iran's 2005 to 2010 birth rate is fewer than two.

In late July 2012, Supreme Leader Ali Khamenei described Iran's contraceptive services as "wrong," and Iranian authorities are slashing birth-control programs in what one Western newspaper (USA Today) describes as a "major reversal" of its long standing policy. Whether program cuts and high-level appeals for bigger families will be successful is still unclear.

Ireland

The sale of contraceptives was illegal in Ireland from 1935 until 1980, when it was legalized with strong restrictions, later loosened. It has been argued that the resulting demographic dividend played a role in the economic boom in Ireland that began in the 1990s and ended abruptly in 2008 (the Celtic tiger) was in part due to the legalisation of contraception in 1979 and subsequent decline in the fertility rate. In Ireland the ratio of workers to dependents increased due to lower fertility — the reality of which has been questioned — but was raised further by increased female labor market participation.

Pakistan

In agreement with the 1994 International Conference on Population and Development in Cairo,

Pakistan pledged that by 2010 it would provide universal access to family planning. Additionally, Pakistan's Poverty Reduction Strategy Paper has set specific national goals for increases in family planning and contraceptive use. In 2011 just one in five Pakistani women ages 15 to 49 uses modern birth control. Contraception is shunned under traditional social mores that are fiercely defended as fundamentalist Islam gains strength.

Russia

According to a 2004 study, current pregnancies were termed "desired and timely" by 58% of respondents, while 23% described them as "desired, but untimely", and 19% said they were "undesired". As of 2004, the share of women of reproductive age using hormonal or intrauterine birth control methods was about 46% (29% intrauterine, 17% hormonal). During the soviet era high quality contraceptives were difficult to obtain, and abortion became the most common way of preventing unwanted births. Since the dissolution of the Soviet Union abortion rates have fallen considerably, but they are still higher than rates in many developed countries.

Philippines

In the Philippines, the Responsible Parenthood and Reproductive Health Act of 2012 guarantees universal access to methods on contraception, fertility control, sexual education, and maternal care. While there is general agreement about its provisions on maternal and child health, there is great debate on its mandate that the Philippine government and the private sector will fund and undertake widespread distribution of family planning devices such as condoms, birth control pills, and IUDs, as the government continues to disseminate information on their use through all health care centers.

Singapore

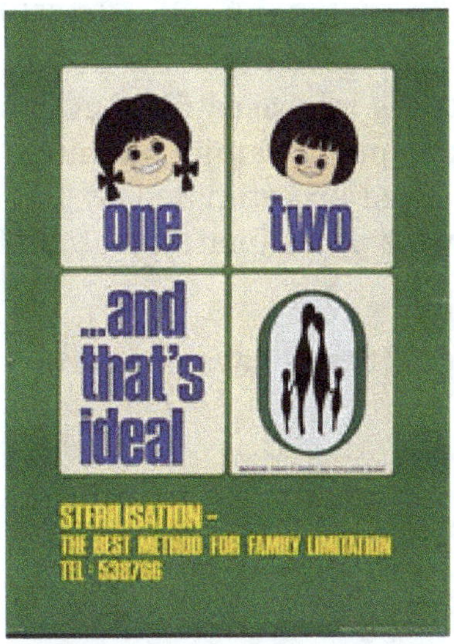

In the 1970s the Singaporean government encouraged much smaller families.

Population control in Singapore spans two distinct phases: first to slow and reverse the boom in births that started after World War II; and then, from the 1980s onwards, to encourage parents to have more children because birth numbers had fallen below replacement levels.

United Kingdom

Contraception has been available for free under the National Health Service since 1974, and 74% of reproductive-age women use some form of contraception. The levonorgestrel intrauterine system has been massively popular. Sterilization is popular in older age groups, among those 45–49, 29% of men and 21% of women have been sterilized. Female sterilization has been declining since 1996, when the intrauterine system was introduced. Emergency contraception has been available since the 1970s, a product was specifically licensed for emergency contraception in 1984, and emergency contraceptives became available over the counter in 2001. Since becoming available over the counter it has not reduced the use of other forms of contraception, as some moralists feared it might. In any year only 5% of women of childbearing age use emergency hormonal contraception.

Despite widespread availability of contraceptives, almost half of pregnancies were unintended in 2005. Abortion was legalized in 1967.

United States

Despite the availability of highly effective contraceptives, about half of U.S. pregnancies are unintended. Highly effective contraceptives, such as IUD, are underused in the United States. Increasing use of highly effective contraceptives could help meet the goal set forward in Healthy People 2020 to decrease unintended pregnancy by 10%. Cost to the user is one factor preventing many American women from using more effective contraceptives. Making contraceptives available without a copay increases use of highly effective methods, reduces unintended pregnancies, and may be instrumental in achieving the Healthy People 2020 goal.

In the United States, contraceptive use saves about $19 billion in direct medical costs each year. Title X of the Public Health Service Act, is a U.S. government program dedicated to providing family planning services for those in need. But funding for Title X as a percentage of total public funding to family planning client services has steadily declined from 44% of total expenditures in 1980 to 12% in 2006. Medicaid has increased from 20% to 71% in the same time. In 2006, Medicaid contributed $1.3 billion to public family planning. The 1.9 billion spent on publicly funded family planning in 2008 saved an estimated $7 billion in short-term Medicaid costs. Such services helped women prevent an estimated 1.94 million unintended pregnancies and 810,000 abortions.

About 3 out of 10 women in the United States have an abortion by the time they are 45 years old.

Uzbekistan

In Uzbekistan the government has pushed for uteruses to be removed from women in order to forcibly sterilize them.

Obstacles to Family Planning

There are many reasons as to why women do not use contraceptives. These reasons include logistical problems, limited access to transportation in order to access health clinics, lack of education and knowledge and opposition by partners, families or communities.

UNFPA says that "efforts to increase access must be sensitive to cultural and national contexts, and must consider economic, geographic and age disparities within countries."

UNFPA states that, "Poorer women and those in rural areas often have less access to family planning services. Certain groups — including adolescents, unmarried people, the urban poor, rural populations, sex workers and people living with HIV also face a variety of barriers to family planning. This can lead to higher rates of unintended pregnancy, increased risk of HIV and other STIs, limited choice of contraceptive methods, and higher levels of unmet need for family planning."

World Contraception Day

September 26 is designated as World Contraception Day, devoted to raising awareness of contraception and improving education about sexual and reproductive health, with a vision of "a world where every pregnancy is wanted". It is supported by a group of international NGOs, including:

Asian Pacific Council on Contraception, Centro Latinamericano Salud y Mujer, European Society of Contraception and Reproductive Health, German Foundation for World Population, International Federation of Pediatric and Adolescent Gynecology, International Planned Parenthood Federation, Marie Stopes International, Population Services International, The Population Council, The USAID, Women Deliver.

Infection Control

Infection control is the discipline concerned with preventing nosocomial or healthcare-associated infection, a practical (rather than academic) sub-discipline of epidemiology. It is an essential, though often underrecognized and undersupported, part of the infrastructure of health care. Infection control and hospital epidemiology are akin to public health practice, practiced within the confines of a particular health-care delivery system rather than directed at society as a whole. Anti-infective agents include antibiotics, antibacterials, antifungals, antivirals and antiprotozoals.

Infection control addresses factors related to the spread of infections within the healthcare setting (whether patient-to-patient, from patients to staff and from staff to patients, or among-staff), including prevention (via hand hygiene/hand washing, cleaning/disinfection/sterilization, vaccination, surveillance), monitoring/investigation of demonstrated or suspected spread of infection within a particular health-care setting (surveillance and outbreak investigation), and management (interruption of outbreaks). It is on this basis that the common title being adopted within health care is "infection prevention and control."

Infection Control in Healthcare Facilities

Aseptic technique is a key component of all invasive medical procedures. Similarly, infection control measures are most effective when Standard Precautions (health care) are applied because undiagnosed infection is common.

Hand Hygiene

Independent studies by Ignaz Semmelweis in 1846 in Vienna and Oliver Wendell Holmes, Sr. in 1843 in Boston established a link between the hands of health care workers and the spread of hospital-acquired disease. The U.S. Centers for Disease Control and Prevention (CDC) state that "It is well documented that the most important measure for preventing the spread of pathogens is effective handwashing." In the developed world, hand washing is mandatory in most health care settings and required by many different regulators.

In the United States, OSHA standards require that employers must provide readily accessible hand washing facilities, and must ensure that employees wash hands and any other skin with soap and water or flush mucous membranes with water as soon as feasible after contact with blood or other potentially infectious materials (OPIM).

In the UK healthcare professionals have adopted the 'Ayliffe Technique', based on the 6 step method developed by Graham Ayliffe, JR Babb and AH Quoraishi.

Mean percentage changes in bacterial numbers	
Method used	**Change in bacteria present**
Paper towels (2-ply 100% recycled).	- 48.4%
Paper towels (2-ply through-air dried, 50% recycled)	- 76.8%
Warm air dryer	+ 254.5%
Jet air dryer	+ 14.9%

Drying is an essential part of the hand hygiene process. In November 2008, a non-peer-reviewed study was presented to the European Tissue Symposium by the University of Westminster, London, comparing the bacteria levels present after the use of paper towels, warm air hand dryers, and modern jet-air hand dryers. Of those three methods, only paper towels reduced the total number of bacteria on hands, with "through-air dried" towels the most effective.

The presenters also carried out tests to establish whether there was the potential for cross-contamination of other washroom users and the washroom environment as a result of each type of drying method. They found that:

- the jet air dryer, which blows air out of the unit at claimed speeds of 400 mph, was capable of blowing micro-organisms from the hands and the unit and potentially contaminating other washroom users and the washroom environment up to 2 metres away
- use of a warm air hand dryer spread micro-organisms up to 0.25 metres from the dryer
- paper towels showed no significant spread of micro-organisms.

In 2005, in a study conducted by TUV Produkt und Umwelt, different hand drying methods were evaluated. The following changes in the bacterial count after drying the hands were observed:

Drying method	**Effect on bacterial count**
Paper towels and roll	Decrease of 24%
Hot-air drier	Increase of 117%

Sterilization

Sterilization is a process intended to kill all microorganisms and is the highest level of microbial kill that is possible. Sterilizers may be heat only, steam, or liquid chemical. Effectiveness of the sterilizer (e.g., a steam autoclave) is determined in three ways. First, mechanical indicators and gauges on the machine itself indicate proper operation of the machine. Second heat sensitive indicators or tape on the sterilizing bags change color which indicate proper levels of heat or steam. And, third (most importantly) is biological testing in which a microorganism that is highly heat and chemical resistant (often the bacterial endospore) is selected as the standard challenge. If the process kills this microorganism, the sterilizer is considered to be effective.

Sterilization, if performed properly, is an effective way of preventing bacteria from spreading. It should be used for the cleaning of the medical instruments or gloves, and basically any type of medical item that comes into contact with the blood stream and sterile tissues.

There are four main ways in which such items can be sterilized: autoclave (by using high-pressure steam), dry heat (in an oven), by using chemical sterilants such as glutaraldehydes or formaldehyde solutions or by radiation (with the help of physical agents). The first two are the most used methods of sterilizations mainly because of their accessibility and availability. Steam sterilization is one of the most effective types of sterilizations, if done correctly which is often hard to achieve. Instruments that are used in health care facilities are usually sterilized with this method. The general rule in this case is that in order to perform an effective sterilization, the steam must get into contact with all the surfaces that are meant to be disinfected. On the other hand, dry heat sterilization, which is performed with the help of an oven, is also an accessible type of sterilization, although it can only be used to disinfect instruments that are made of metal or glass. The very high temperatures needed to perform sterilization in this way are able to melt the instruments that are not made of glass or metal.

Steam sterilization is done at a temperature of 121 C (250 F) with a pressure of 209 kPa (15 lbs/in2). In these conditions, rubber items must be sterilized for 20 minutes, and wrapped items 134 C with pressure of 310 kPa for 7 minutes. The time is counted once the temperature that is needed has been reached. Steam sterilization requires four conditions in order to be efficient: adequate contact, sufficiently high temperature, correct time and sufficient moisture. Sterilization using steam can also be done at a temperature of 132 C (270 F), at a double pressure. Dry heat sterilization is performed at 170 C (340 F) for one hour or two hours at a temperature of 160 C (320 F). Dry heat sterilization can also be performed at 121 C, for at least 16 hours.

Chemical sterilization, also referred to as cold sterilization, can be used to sterilize instruments that cannot normally be disinfected through the other two processes described above. The items sterilized with cold sterilization are usually those that can be damaged by regular sterilization. Commonly, glutaraldehydes and formaldehyde are used in this process, but in different ways. When using the first type of disinfectant, the instruments are soaked in a 2-4% solution for at least 10 hours while a solution of 8% formaldehyde will sterilize the items in 24 hours or more. Chemical sterilization is generally more expensive than steam sterilization and therefore it is used for instruments that cannot be disinfected otherwise. After the instruments have been soaked in the chemical solutions, they are mandatory to be rinsed with sterile water which will remove the residues from the disinfectants. This is the reason why needles and syringes are not sterilized in this way, as the residues left by the chemical solution that has been used to disinfect them cannot be washed off with water and they may interfere with the administered treatment. Although formaldehyde is less expensive than glutaraldehydes, it is also more irritating to the eyes, skin and respiratory tract and is classified as a potential carcinogen.

Other sterilization methods exist, though their efficiency is still controversial. These methods include gas, UV, gas plasma, and chemical sterilization with agents such as peroxyacetic acid or paraformaldehyde.

Cleaning

Infections can be prevented from occurring in homes as well. In order to reduce their chances to contract an infection, individuals are recommended to maintain a good hygiene by washing their hands after every contact with questionable areas or bodily fluids and by disposing of garbage at regular intervals to prevent germs from growing.

Disinfection

Disinfection uses liquid chemicals on surfaces and at room temperature to kill disease causing microorganisms. Ultraviolet light has also been used to disinfect the rooms of patients infected with *Clostridium difficile* after discharge. Disinfection is less effective than sterilization because it does not kill bacterial endospores.

Personal Protective Equipment

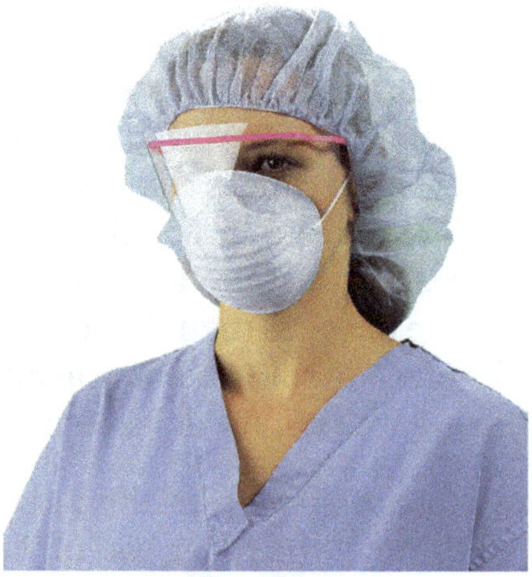

Disposable PPE

Personal protective equipment (PPE) is specialized clothing or equipment worn by a worker for protection against a hazard. The hazard in a health care setting is exposure to blood, saliva, or other bodily fluids or aerosols that may carry infectious materials such as Hepatitis C, HIV, or other blood borne or bodily fluid pathogen. PPE prevents contact with a potentially infectious material by creating a physical barrier between the potential infectious material and the healthcare worker.

The United States Occupational Safety and Health Administration (OSHA) requires the use of

Personal protective equipment (PPE) by workers to guard against blood borne pathogens if there is a reasonably anticipated exposure to blood or other potentially infectious materials.

Components of PPE include gloves, gowns, bonnets, shoe covers, face shields, CPR masks, goggles, surgical masks, and respirators. How many components are used and how the components are used is often determined by regulations or the infection control protocol of the facility in question. Many or most of these items are disposable to avoid carrying infectious materials from one patient to another patient and to avoid difficult or costly disinfection. In the US, OSHA requires the immediate removal and disinfection or disposal of a worker's PPE prior to leaving the work area where exposure to infectious material took place.

Antimicrobial Surfaces

Microorganisms are known to survive on non-antimicrobial in animate 'touch' surfaces (e.g., bedrails, over-the-bed trays, call buttons, bathroom hardware, etc.) for extended periods of time. This can be especially troublesome in hospital environments where patients with immunodeficiencies are at enhanced risk for contracting nosocomial infections.

Products made with antimicrobial copper alloy (brasses, bronzes, cupronickel, copper-nickel-zinc, and others) surfaces destroy a wide range of microorganisms in a short period of time. The United States Environmental Protection Agency has approved the registration of 355 different antimicrobial copper alloys and one synthetic copper-infused hard surface that kill *E. coli* O157:H7, methicillin-resistant *Staphylococcus aureus* (MRSA), *Staphylococcus*, *Enterobacter aerogenes,* and *Pseudomonas aeruginosa* in less than 2 hours of contact. Other investigations have demonstrated the efficacy of antimicrobial copper alloys to destroy *Clostridium difficile,* influenza A virus, adenovirus, and fungi. As a public hygienic measure in addition to regular cleaning, antimicrobial copper alloys are being installed in healthcare facilities in the U.K., Ireland, Japan, Korea, France, Denmark, and Brazil. The synthetic hard surface is being installed in the United States as well as in Israel.

Vaccination of Health Care Workers

Health care workers may be exposed to certain infections in the course of their work. Vaccines are available to provide some protection to workers in a healthcare setting. Depending on regulation, recommendation, the specific work function, or personal preference, healthcare workers or first responders may receive vaccinations for hepatitis B; influenza; measles, mumps and rubella; Tetanus, diphtheria, pertussis; N. meningitidis; and varicella.

Post-exposure Prophylaxis

In some cases where vaccines do not exist, post-exposure prophylaxis is another method of protecting the health care worker exposed to a life-threatening infectious disease. For example, the viral particles for HIV-AIDS can be precipitated out of the blood through the use of an antibody injection if given within four hours of a significant exposure.

Surveillance for Infections

Surveillance is the act of infection investigation using the CDC definitions. Determining the presence of a hospital acquired infection requires an infection control practitioner (ICP) to review a patient's chart and see if the patient had the signs and symptom of an infection. Surveillance definitions exist for infections of the bloodstream, urinary tract, pneumonia,surgical sites and gastroenteritis.

Surveillance traditionally involved significant manual data assessment and entry in order to assess preventative actions such as isolation of patients with an infectious disease. Increasingly, computerized software solutions are becoming available that assess incoming risk messages from microbiology and other online sources. By reducing the need for data entry, software can reduce the data workload of ICPs, freeing them to concentrate on clinical surveillance.

As of 1998, approximately one third of healthcare acquired infections were preventable. Surveillance and preventative activities are increasingly a priority for hospital staff. The *Study on the Efficacy of Nosocomial Infection Control* (SENIC) project by the U.S. CDC found in the 1970s that hospitals reduced their nosocomial infection rates by approximately 32 per cent by focusing on surveillance activities and prevention efforts.

Isolation and Quarantine

In the health care context, medical isolation refers to various physical measures taken to interrupt nosocomial spread of contagious diseases. Various forms of isolation exist, and are applied depending on the type of infection and agent involved, to address the likelihood of spread via airborne particles or droplets, by direct skin contact, or via contact with body fluids.

In cases where infection is merely suspected, individuals may be quarantined until the incubation period has passed and the disease manifests itself or the person remains healthy. Groups may undergo quarantine, or in the case of communities, a cordon sanitaire may be imposed to prevent infection from spreading beyond the community, or in the case of protective sequestration, into a community. Public health authorities may implement other forms of social distancing, such as school closings, to control an epidemic.

Outbreak Investigation

When an unusual cluster of illness is noted, infection control teams undertake an investigation to determine whether there is a true outbreak, a pseudo-outbreak (a result of contamination within the diagnostic testing process), or just random fluctuation in the frequency of illness. If a true outbreak is discovered, infection control practitioners try to determine what permitted the outbreak to occur, and to rearrange the conditions to prevent ongoing propagation of the infection. Often, breaches in good practice are responsible, although sometimes other factors (such as construction) may be the source of the problem.

Outbreaks investigations have more than a single purpose. These investigations are carried out in order to prevent additional cases in the current outbreak, prevent future outbreaks, learn about a new disease or learn something new about an old disease. Reassuring the public, minimizing the economic and social disruption as well as teaching epidemiology are some other obvious objectives of outbreak investigations.

According to the WHO, outbreak investigations are meant to detect what is causing the outbreak, how the pathogenic agent is transmitted, where it all started from, what is the carrier, what is the population at risk of getting infected and what are the risk factors.

The results of outbreak investigations are always made public in the means of a report in which the findings are communicated to the authorities, media, scientific community and so on. These reports are commonly used as pedagogical tools.

Training in Infection Control and Health Care Epidemiology

Practitioners can come from several different educational streams. Many begin as nurses, some as medical technologists (particularly in clinical microbiology), and some as physicians (typically infectious disease specialists). Specialized training in infection control and health care epidemiology are offered by the professional organizations described below. Physicians who desire to become infection control practitioners often are trained in the context of an infectious disease fellowship.

In the United States, Certification Board of Infection Control and Epidemiology is a private company that certifies infection control practitioners based on their educational background and professional experience, in conjunction with testing their knowledge base with standardized exams. The credential awarded is CIC, Certification in Infection Control and Epidemiology. It is recommended that one has 2 years of Infection Control experience before applying for the exam. Certification must be renewed every five years.

A course in hospital epidemiology (infection control in the hospital setting) is offered jointly each year by the Centers for Disease Control and Prevention (CDC) and the Society for Healthcare Epidemiology of America.

Standardization

Australia

In 2002, the Royal Australian College of General Practitioners published a revised standard for office-based infection control which covers the sections of managing immunisation, sterilisation and disease surveillance. However, the document on the personal hygiene of health workers is only limited to hand hygiene, waste and linen management, which may not be sufficient since some of the pathogens are air-born and could be spread through air flow.

United States

Currently, the federal regulation that describes infection control standards is found at 29 CFR Part 1910.1030 Bloodborne pathogens.

Injury Prevention

Injury prevention is an effort to prevent or reduce the severity of bodily injuries caused by external mechanisms, such as accidents, before they occur. Injury prevention is a component of safety and public health, and its goal is to improve the health of the population by preventing injuries and hence improving quality of life. Among laypersons, the term "accidental injury" is often used. However, "accidental" implies the causes of injuries are random in nature. Researchers use the term "unintentional injury" to refer to injuries that are nonvolitional but preventable. Within the field of public health, efforts are also made to prevent or reduce "intentional injury." Data from the U.S. Centers for Disease Control, for example, show unintentional injuries are the leading cause of death from early childhood until middle adulthood. During these years, unintentional injuries account for more deaths than the next nine leading causes of death combined.

Injury prevention strategies cover a variety of approaches, many of which are classified as falling under the "3 E's" of injury prevention: education, engineering modifications, and enforcement/ enactment. Some organizations, such as Safe Kids Worldwide, have expanded the list to six E's adding: evaluation, economic incentives and empowerment.

Measuring Effectiveness

Researching is challenging, because the usual outcome of interest is deaths or injuries prevented, and it is nearly impossible to measure how many people *did not* get hurt who otherwise would have. Education efforts can be measured by changes in knowledge, attitudes, beliefs and behaviors, before and after the intervention, however tying these changes back into reductions in morbidity and mortality is often problematic.

Examining trends in morbidity and mortality in the population is usually not difficult and may provide some indication of the effectiveness of injury prevention interventions. However, this approach suffers from the potential of ecological fallacy, where the data shows an association between an intervention and a change in the outcome, but there is actually no causal relationship.

Common Types

Traffic and Automobile Safety

Traffic safety and automobile safety are a major component of injury prevention because it is the leading cause of death for children and young adults into their mid 30s. Injury prevention efforts began in the early 1960s when activist Ralph Nader, exposed the automobiles as being more dangerous than necessary with his book Unsafe at Any Speed. This led to engineering changes in the way cars are designed to allow for more crush space between the vehicle and the occupant. The Centers for Disease Control and Prevention (CDC) also contributes much to automobile safety. The CDC Injury Prevention Champion, David Sleet, illustrated the importance of lowering the legal blood alcohol content limit to 0.08 percent for drivers; requiring disposable lighters to be child resistant; and using evidence to demonstrate the dangers of airbags to young children riding in the front seat of vehicles.

Engineering: vehicle crash worthiness, seat belts, airbags, locking seat belts for child seats.

Education: promote seat belt use, discourage impaired driving, promote child safety seats.

Enforcement and enactment: passage and enforcement of primary seat belt laws, speed limits, impaired driving enforcement.

Pedestrian Safety

Pedestrian safety is the focus of both epidemiological and psychological injury prevention research. Epidemiological studies typically focus on causes external to the individual such as traffic density, access to safe walking areas, socioeconomic status, injury rates, legislation for safety (e.g., traffic fines), or even the shape of vehicles which affects the severity of injuries resulting from a collision. Epidemiological data show children aged 1–4 are at greatest risk for injury in driveway and sidewalks. Children aged 5–14 are at greatest risk while attempting to cross streets.

The body of psychological research on pedestrian safety is currently much smaller than that in the epidemiological field, but is rapidly growing. Psychological pedestrian safety studies extend as far back as the mid-1980s when researchers began examining behavioral variables in children. Behavioral variables of interest include selection of crossing gaps in traffic, attention to traffic, the number of near hits or actual hits, or the routes children chose when crossing multiple streets such as while walking to school. Behavioral studies often collect such variables which imply risk of injury; e.g., children engaging in risky behaviors may be assumed to be at greater risk if actually crossing a street alone. The most common technique used in behavioral pedestrian research is the pretend road, in which a child stands some distance from the curb and watches traffic on the real road. The child then walks to the edge of the street when a crossing opportunity is chosen. Research is gradually shifting to more ecologically valid virtual reality techniques. Leading scientists in psychological pedestrian safety research are Dr. Benjamin Barton, Dr. David Schwebel and Dr. James Thomson.

Other

The following is an abbreviated topic list of some common focus areas of injury prevention efforts:

- Bicycle safety
- Boat and water safety
- Child passenger safety
- Consumer product safety
- Firearm safety
- Fire and burn safety
- Home safety
- Impaired driving
- Pedestrian safety
- Poison control
- Toy safety
- Traffic safety

- Sports injury safety
- Occupational safety and health

Oral Hygiene

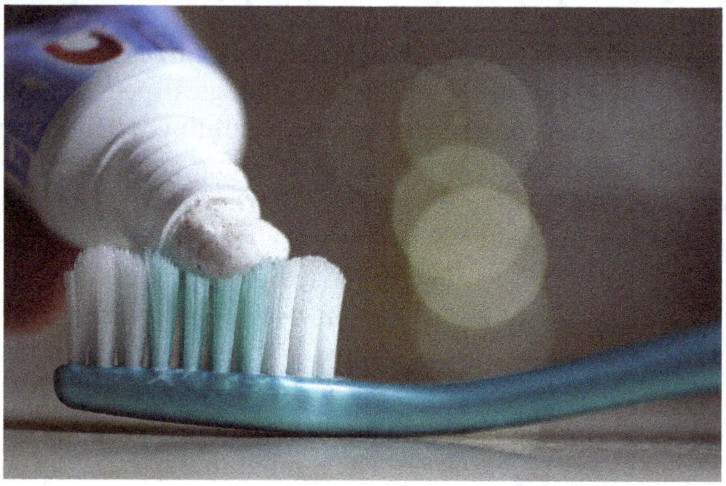

Proper oral hygiene requires regular brushing and flossing

Oral hygiene is an important part of a daily routine. It is the practice of keeping one's mouth clean and free of disease, by regular brushing and cleaning in between the teeth. It is important oral hygiene is completed on a regular basis, as it can prevent dental disease from occurring. The most common types of dental disease is dental decay (also known as dental caries), gingivitis and periodontitis. Regular brushing consists of brushing twice a day after breakfast and before going to bed. Cleaning in between your teeth is called interdental cleaning and it is equally important as tooth brushing. This is because a toothbrush cannot reach between your teeth, therefore only cleaning 50% of the surfaces. There are many tools to clean between the teeth, these include floss, flossettes, interdental brushes, wood sticks and gum picks. It is generally up to each individual to choose which tool they would prefer to use.

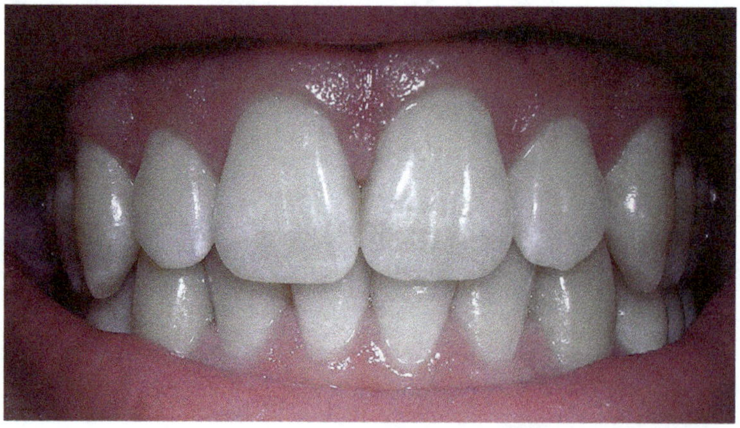

A healthy smile

Teeth

Teeth cleaning is the removal of dental plaque and tartar from teeth to prevent cavities, gingivitis, gum disease, and tooth decay. Severe gum disease causes at least one-third of adult tooth loss.

Tooth decay is the most common global disease. Over 80% of cavities occur inside fissures in teeth where brushing cannot reach food left trapped after every meal or snack and saliva or fluoride have no access to neutralise acid and remineralise demineralised teeth, unlike easy-to-clean parts of the tooth, where fewer cavities occur.

Dental sealants, which are applied by dentists, cover and protect fissures and grooves in the chewing surfaces of back teeth, preventing food from becoming trapped thus halting the decaying process. An elastomer strip has been shown to force sealant deeper inside opposing chewing surfaces and can also force fluoride toothpaste inside chewing surfaces to aid in remineralising demineralised teeth.

Since before recorded history, a variety of oral hygiene measures have been used for teeth cleaning. This has been verified by various excavations done throughout the world, in which chew sticks, tree twigs, bird feathers, animal bones and porcupine quills were recovered. Many people used different forms of teeth cleaning tools. Indian medicine (Ayurveda) has used the neem tree, or *daatun*, and its products to create teeth cleaning twigs and similar products; a person chews one end of the neem twig until it somewhat resembles the bristles of a toothbrush, and then uses it to brush the teeth. In the Muslim world, the miswak, or *siwak*, made from a twig or root, has antiseptic properties and has been widely used since the Islamic Golden Age. Rubbing baking soda or chalk against the teeth was also common, however this can have negative side effects over time.

Generally, dentists recommend that teeth be cleaned professionally at least twice per year. Professional cleaning includes tooth scaling, tooth polishing, and, if tartar has accumulated, debridement; this is usually followed by a fluoride treatment. However, the American Dental Hygienists' Association (ADHA) publicly stated in 1998 that there is an absence of evidence that scaling and polishing provides therapeutic value. The Cochrane Oral Health Group reviewed nine studies but found them to be of insufficient quality and not enough evidence to support the claims of the benefits of regular tooth scaling or tooth polishing.

Between cleanings by a dental hygienist, good oral hygiene is essential for preventing tartar build-up which causes the problems mentioned above. This is done through careful, frequent brushing with a toothbrush, combined with the use of dental floss to prevent accumulation of plaque on the teeth. Powered toothbrushes reduce dental plaque and gingivitis more than manual toothbrushing in both short and long term. Further evidence is needed to determine the clinical importance of these findings.

Dentist and dental hygienist are about preventing tooth loss and gum disease. The patient needs to be aware of the importance of brushing and flossing their teeth daily. New parents need to be educated to promote a healthy life and mouth for their children. At any age; a person should be notified about how to take care of their teeth and how they will be able to keep their teeth and not need dentures.

Plaque

Plaque is also widely known as dental biofilm, is a sticky, yellow film consisting of a wide range of bacteria which attaches to the tooth surfaces and can be visible around the gum line. It starts to reappear after the tooth surface has been cleaned, which is why regular brushing is encouraged . A high sugar diet influences the make-up of plaque. Sugar (fermentable carbohydrates), is converted into acid by the plaque. The acid is then responsible for the breakdown of the top layer of the teeth, eventually leading to tooth decay .

If plaque is left on the tooth surface undisturbed, not only is there an increased risk of tooth decay, but it will also go on to irritate the gums and make them appear red and swollen . Some bleeding may be noticed during tooth brushing or flossing. These are the signs of inflammation which indicate poor gum health .

Calculus

The longer that plaque stays on the tooth surface, the harder and more attached to the tooth it becomes. That is when it is referred to as 'calculus' and is required to be removed by a dental professional . If this is not treated, the inflammation will lead to the bone loss and eventually lead to the effected teeth to become lose . That is why it is important to clean away the plaque and prevent it from staying on the tooth surface for a long period of time.

Tooth Brushing

Routine tooth brushing is the principle method of preventing many oral diseases, and perhaps the most important activity an individual can practice to reduce plaque buildup. Controlling plaque reduces the risk of the individual suffering from plaque-associated diseases such as gingivitis, periodontitis, and caries – the three most common oral diseases in the world. The average brushing time for individuals is between just over 30 seconds to just over 60 seconds. Many oral health care professionals agree on the consensus that tooth brushing should take a minimum of 2 minutes, and be practiced at least twice a day. Brushing for at least 2 mins per session is optimal for preventing the most common oral diseases, and removes considerably more plaque than brushing only for 45 seconds

Dental dentifrices (toothpaste) with fluoride is an important tool to readily use when tooth brushing. The fluoride in the dentifrice is an important protective factor against caries, and an important supplement needed to remineralise already affected enamel. In preventing gum diseases, the use of dental dentifrices toothpaste does not assist the effectiveness of the activity with respect to amount of plaque removed.

Manual Tooth Brush

The modern manual tooth brush is a dental tool which consists of a head of nylon bristles attached to a long handle to help facilitate the manual action of tooth brushing. Furthermore, the handle aids in reaching as far back as teeth erupt in the oral cavity (mouth). The tooth brush is arguably a person's greatest tool at removing plaque from teeth, gums and the tongue, thus capable of preventing all plaque related diseases if used routinely, correctly and effectively. Oral health professionals recommend the use of a tooth brush with a small head and soft bristles as that is most effective against removing plaque without damaging the surrounding tissues .

Technique is crucial to the effectiveness of tooth brushing and its influence on disease prevention. Back and forth brushing is not effective in removing plaque surrounding the gum line. Brushing teeth should include systematic approach, whilst angling the bristles at a 45-degree angle towards the gums, and doing small circular motions at that angle . This action increases the effectiveness of the technique with respect to removing plaque at the gum line.

Electric Tooth Brush

Electric toothbrushes are toothbrushes with replaceable moving or vibrating bristle heads. The two main types of electric toothbrushes include the sonic range which has a vibrating head, and the oscillating-rotating range where the bristle head makes constant clockwise and anti-clockwise movements.

Sonic toothbrushes emit a high frequency of vibrations with a small amplitude, and a fluid turbulent activity that aids in plaque removal . The movements of the bristles and their vibrations help break up chains of bacteria up to 5mm below the gum line . The oscillating-rotating electric toothbrush on the other hand uses the same mechanical action produced by manual tooth brushing – removing plaque via mechanical disturbance of the biofilm – however at a higher frequency.

Using electric tooth brushes is less complex in regards to brushing technique, making it a viable option for children, and adults with conditions that may inhibit them from full dexterity. The bristle head should be guided from tooth to tooth slowly, following the contour of the gums and crowns of the tooth . The independent motions of the toothbrush head will take away from the need to manually wiggle the brush or to do circles.

Flossing

Tooth brushing alone will not remove plaque from all surfaces of the tooth as 40% of the surfaces are interdentally . One technique that can be used to access these areas is dental floss. When the proper technique is used, flossing can remove plaque and food particles from between the teeth and below the gums, The American Dental Association (ADA) even reports that up to 80% of plaque may be removed by this method . The ADA suggested cleaning between your teeth as part of a daily oral hygiene regime .

There are different types of floss available including:

- Unwaxed floss: Unbound nylon filaments that spread across the tooth and plaque/debris get trapped for easy removal.
- Waxed floss: less susceptible to tearing or shredding when used between tight contacts or areas with overhanging restorations.
- Polytetrafluoroethylene (PTFE): Slides easily through tight contacts and does not fray.

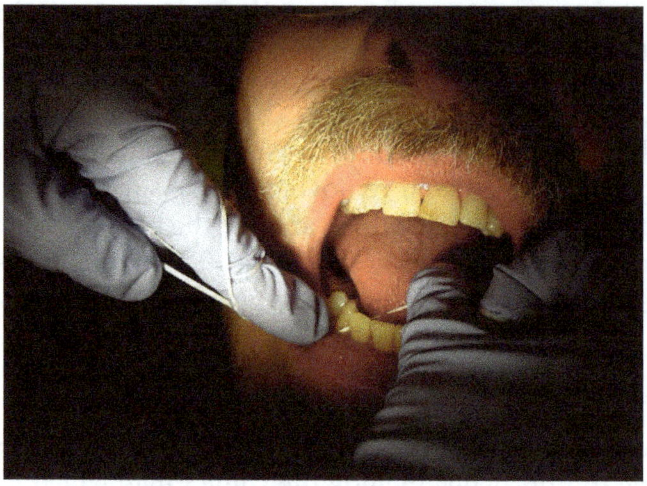

A dental hygienist demonstrates dental flossing.

The type of floss used is a personal preference, however without the proper technique, research has shown that it may not be effective. The correct technique to ensure maximum plaque is as follows:.

1. Floss length: 15 – 25cms wrapped around middle fingers.
2. For flossing on the maxilla, grasp the floss with thumb and forefinger, and with both forefingers when flossing the mandible. Ensure a length of roughly 2.5cms is left between the fingers.
3. Ease the floss gently between the teeth using a back and forth motion.
4. Position the floss in such a way that it becomes securely wrapped around the proximal surface of the tooth in a C shape.
5. Ensure that the floss is taken below the gingival margins using a back and forth motion apico-coronally.

There are a few different options on the market to choose from that can make flossing easier if dexterity or coordination is a barrier, or as a preference over normal floss. Floss threaders are ideal for cleaning between orthodontic appliances, and flossetts are ideal for those with poor dexterity.

Interdental Brushes

Interdental brushes come in a range of colours and sizes. It consists of a handle with a piece of wire covered in tapered bristles, designed to be placed into the interdental space, for interproximal plaque removal. Studies indicate that interdental brushes are equally or more effective then floss when removing plaque and reducing gingival inflammation.

The steps in using an interdental brush are as follows:

1. Identify the size required, the largest size that will fit without force is ideal Sometimes more than one size is required throughout the mouth.
2. Insert the bristles into the interdental space at a 90-degree angle.

3. Move the brush back and forth between the teeth.
4. Rinse under water to remove debris when necessary.
5. Rinse with warm soapy water once complete, and store in a clean dry area.
6. Replace once bristles are worn.

Tongue Scrapers

The tongue contains numerous bacteria which causes bad breath. Tongue cleaners are designed to remove the debris built up on the tongue. Using a toothbrush to clean the tongue is another possibility, however it might be hard to reach the back of the tongue and the bristles of the toothbrush may be too soft to remove the debris. Some may find it easier to use a tongue scraper instead because it does not tend to cause a gag reflex as readily as a toothbrush . Steps of using a tongue scraper:

- Rinse the tongue scraper in order to clean it and remove any present debris
- Start at the back of the tongue and gently scrape forwards
- Ensure to clean the sides of the tongue as well, not just the middle portion
- After the cleaning is completed, rinse the tongue scraper and any debris that is left behind
- Rinse the mouth

Oral Irrigation

Some dental professionals recommend oral irrigation as a way to clean teeth and gums.

Single-tufted Brushes

Single-tufted brushes are a tool in conjunction with tooth brushing. The tooth brush is designed to reach the 'hard to reach places' within the mouth. This tool is best used behind the lower front teeth, behind the back molars, crooked teeth and between spaces where teeth have been removed. The single- tufted brush design has an angled handle, a 4mm diameter and a rounded bristle tips.

Food and Drink

Foods that help muscles and bones also help teeth and gums. Breads and cereals are rich in vitamin B while fruits and vegetables contain vitamin C, both of which contribute to healthy gum tissue. Lean meat, fish, and poultry provide magnesium and zinc for teeth.

Eating a balanced diet and limiting snacks can prevent tooth decay and periodontal disease. The *Fédération dentaire internationale* (FDI World Dental Federation) has promoted foods such as raw vegetables, plain yogurt, cheese, or fruit as dentally beneficial—this has been echoed by the American Dental Association (ADA).

Beneficial Foods

Some foods may protect against cavities by naturally containing fluorine, from which fluoride is derived. Fluoride is naturally present in all water. Community water fluoridation is the addition of fluoride to adjust the natural fluoride concentration of a community's water supply to the level recommended for optimal dental health, approximately 1.0 ppm (parts per million). One ppm is the equivalent of 1 mg/L, or 1 inch in 16 miles. Fluoride is a primary protector against dental cavities. Fluoride makes the surface of teeth more resistant to acids during the process of remineralisation. Drinking fluoridated water is recommended by some dental professionals while others say that using toothpaste alone is enough. Milk and cheese are also rich in calcium and phosphate, and may also encourage remineralisation. All foods increase saliva production, and since saliva contains buffer chemicals this helps to stabilize the pH to near 7 (neutral) in the mouth. Foods high in fiber may also help to increase the flow of saliva and a bolus of fibre like celery string can force saliva into trapped food inside pits and fissures on chewing surfaces where over 80% of cavities occur, to dilute carbohydrate like sugar, neutralise acid and remineralise tooth like on easy to reach surfaces.

Harmful Foods

Sugars are commonly associated with dental cavities. Other carbohydrates, especially cooked starches, e.g. crisps/potato chips, may also damage teeth, although to a lesser degree (and indirectly) since starch has to be converted to sugars by salivary amylase (an enzyme in the saliva) first. Sugars that are higher in the stickiness index, such as toffee, are likely to cause more damage to teeth than those that are lower in the stickiness index, such as certain forms of chocolate or most fruits.

Sucrose (table sugar) is most commonly associated with cavities. The amount of sugar consumed at any one time is less important than how often food and drinks that contain sugar are consumed. The more frequently sugars are consumed, the greater the time during which the tooth is exposed to low pH levels, at which point demineralisation occurs (below 5.5 for most people). It is important therefore to try to encourage infrequent consumption of food and drinks containing sugar so that teeth have a chance to be repaired by remineralisation and fluoride. Limiting sugar-containing foods and drinks to meal times is one way to reduce the incidence of cavities. Sugars from fruit and fruit juices, e.g., glucose, fructose, and maltose seem equally likely to cause cavities.

Acids contained in fruit juice, vinegar and soft drinks lower the pH level of the oral cavity which causes the enamel to demineralize. Drinking drinks such as orange juice or cola throughout the day raises the risk of dental cavities tremendously.

Another factor which affects the risk of developing cavities is the stickiness of foods. Some foods or sweets may stick to the teeth and so reduce the pH in the mouth for an extended time, particularly if they are sugary. It is important that teeth be cleaned at least twice a day, preferably with a toothbrush and fluoride toothpaste, to remove any food sticking to the teeth. Regular brushing and the use of dental floss also removes the dental plaque coating the tooth surface.

Chewing Gum

Chewing gum assists oral irrigation between and around the teeth, cleaning and removing particles, but for teeth in poor condition it may damage or remove loose fillings as well. Dental chewing gums claim to improve dental health. Sugar-free chewing gum stimulates saliva production, and helps to clean the surface of the teeth.

Chewing Ice

When it comes to chewing ice, many might think it will do no harm since ice is made from water, and as many might know, water is great for the body. However, chewing on solid objects such as ice can have catastrophic consequences for your teeth. Chipping may occur and this can lead a pathway for greater teeth fractures in the future. Chewing on ice has been linked to symptoms of anemia. People with anemia tend to want to eat food with no nutritional value.

Alcohol

Drinking dark colored beverages such as wine or beer may stain the teeth leading to a not so white smile. Dryness is also another aftereffect of alcohol consumption leading to a dry mouth, preventing saliva to protect the teeth from plaque and bacteria.

Other

Smoking is one of the leading risk factors associated with periodontal diseases. It is thought that smoking impairs and alters normal immune responses, eliciting destructive processes while inhibiting reparative responses promoting the incidence and development of periodontal diseases.

Regular vomiting, as seen in bulimia nervosa and morning sickness also causes significant damage, due to acid erosion.

Mouthwash

There are three commonly used mouthwash; saline (salty water), Essential Oils (Listerine, Colgate Plax, Etc) and Chlorhexidine Gluconate.

Saline

Saline(warm salty water) is usually recommended after procedures like dental extractions. In a study completed in 2014, warm saline mouthrinse was compared to no mouthrinse in preventing alveolar osteitis (dry socket) post extraction. In the group that was instructed to rinse with saline, the prevalence of alveolar osteitis was less than in the group that did not.

Essential oils (EO) or Cetyl Pyridinium Chloride (CPC)

Essential oils, found in Listerine mouthwash, contains Eucalyptol, Menthol, Thymol, Methyl Calicylate. CPC containing mouthwash contains CetylPyridinium Chloride, found in brands such as Colgate Plax, Crest Pro Health, Oral B Pro Health Rinse. In a meta-analyses completed in 2016, EO and CPC mouthrinses were compared and it was found that plaque and gingivitis levels were lower with EO mouthrinse when used as an adjunct to mechanical plaque removal (toothbrushing and interdental cleaning)

Chlorhexidine

Chlorhexidine Gluconate is an antiseptic mouthrinse that can only be used in 2 week time periods due to brown staining on the teeth and tongue. Compared to Essential oils, it is more efficacious in controlling plaque levels, but has no better effect on gingivitis and is therefore generally used for post-surgical wound healing or the short-term control of plaque

Denture Care

Dentures, retainers, and other appliances must be kept extremely clean. It is recommended that dentures are cleaned mechanically twice a day with a soft bristled brush and denture cleansing paste. It is not recommended to use toothpaste, as it is too abrasive for acrylic, and will leave plaque retentive scratches in the surface.

Dentures should be taken out at night, as leaving them in whilst sleeping has been linked to poor oral health. Leaving a denture in during sleep reduces the protective cleansing and antibacterial properties of saliva against Candida Albicans (oral thrush) and denture stomatitis; the inflammation and redness of the oral mucosa underneath the denture . For the elderly, wearing a denture during sleep has been proven to greatly increase the risk of pneumonia .

It is now recommended that dentures should be stored in a dry container overnight, as keeping dentures dry for 8 hours significantly reduces the amount of candida albicans on an acrylic denture . Approximately once a week it is recommended to soak a denture overnight in an alkaline-peroxide denture cleansing tablet, as they have been proven to reduce bacterial mass and pathogenicity

Education

To become a dental hygienist, one must attend a college or university that is approved by The Commission of Dental Accreditation and take the National Board Dental Hygiene Examination. There are a few degrees one may receive. An associate's degree after attending community college is the most common and only takes at least two years to obtain one. After doing so, one may work in a dental office. There's also the option of receiving a bachelor's or master's degree if one plans to work in an educational institute either for teaching or research.

Oral Hygiene and Systemic Diseases

Several recent clinical studies suggest oral disease and inflammation (oral bacteria & oral infections) may be a potential risk factor for serious systemic diseases, such as:

- Cardiovascular Disease (Heart attack and Stroke)
- Bacterial Pneumonia: Oral hygiene care for critically ill patients has been reported to reduce the risk of ventilator associated pneumonia.
- Low birth weight/Extreme High Birth Weight
- Diabetes complications
- Osteoporosis

References

- "Women's Work: Gender Equality in Cuba and the Role of Women in Building Cuba's Future" (PDF). Center for Democracy in the Americas. Retrieved November 26, 2013
- Mokdad, A. H., Marks, J. S., Stroup, D. F., & Gerberding, J. L. (2004). Actual Causes of Death in the United States, 2000. Journal of the American Medical Association,291(10), 1238-1245
- World Cancer Report 2014. International Agency for Research on Cancer, World Health Organization. 2014. ISBN 978-92-832-0432-9
- "A prevention prescription for improving health and health care in America" (PDF). Bipartisan policy center. Retrieved March 24, 2016
- Cohen, J. T., Neumann, P. J., & Weinstein, M. C. (2008, February 14). Does Preventive Care Save Money? Health Economics and the Presidential Candidates. The New England Journal of Medicine, 358(7), 661-663
- David,, McDaid,; F.,, Sassi,; Sherry,, Merkur,; iLibrary., OECD. Promoting health, preventing disease : the economic case. ISBN 9780335262267. OCLC 973090310
- Frist, B (May 28, 2015). "US Healthcare reform should focus on prevention efforts to cut skyrocketing costs". US News and World Report. Retrieved 2016-03-24
- Effect of In Utero and Early-Life Conditions on Adult Health and Disease, Peter D. Gluckman et al., The New England Journal of Medicine, 359;1(2008)
- Bunton R, Macdonald G (2002). Health promotion: disciplines, diversity, and developments (2nd ed.). Routledge. ISBN 0-415-23569-3
- Cohen, Joshua. "The cost savings and cost-effectiveness of clinical preventative care. Robert Wood Johnson Foundation". THE SYNTHESIS PROJECT. Robert Wood Johnson Foundation. Retrieved March 24, 2016
- Kumanyika, S., Jeffery, R. W., Morabia, A., Ritenbaugh, C., & Antipatis, V. J. (2002). Obesity prevention: the case for action. International Journal of Obesity, 26, 425-436
- Tones K, Tilford S (2001). Health promotion: effectiveness, efficiency and equity (3rd ed.). Cheltenham UK: Nelson Thornes. ISBN 0-7487-4527-0
- Pincus, M. W., Rollings, P. K., Craft, A. B. and Green, B. (1991) Sunscreen use on Queenslands beaches. Australasian Journal of Dermatology, 32, 21–25
- Cohen, J.T., Neumann, P.J., & Weinstein, M.C. (2008). Does Preventive Care Save Money? Health Economics and the Presidential Candidates. New England Journal of Medicine, 358(7), 661 – 663
- Harrington, Scott E. (1 January 2010). "U. S. Health-care Reform: The Patient Protection and Affordable Care Act". The Journal of Risk and Insurance. 77 (3): 703–708
- "Estimating the Effects of Federal Policies Targeting Obesity: Challenges and Research Needs". Congressional Budget Office. Retrieved 2016-03-25
- Marshall, BJ (2 March 2012). "School based health promotion across Australia". Journal of School Health. 70: 251–252. doi:10.1111/j.1746-1561.2000.tb07430.x
- McQueen DV, Kickbusch I (2007). Health and modernity: the role of theory in health promotion. New York: Springer. p. 15. ISBN 978-0-387-37757-5
- Lindenberger, James H.; Bryant, Carol A. (2000). "Promoting Breastfeeding in the WIC Program: A Social Marketing Case Study". American Journal of Health Behavior. 24: 53–60. doi:10.5993/AJHB.24.1.8
- O'Grady, M. "Health-Care Cost Projections for Diabetes and other Chronic Diseases: The Current Context and Potential Enhancement." (PDF). Fight Chronic D\isease. Retrieved March 24, 2016

5

A Comprehensive Study of Health Care Systems

A health care system is a knowledge system that contains all information about the healthcare facilities and services of a nation, town or city. It is also an indicator of the access to medical facilities to a group of people. The exact kind of facilities varies from country to country. Some of themes discussed are first aid, health care ratings, geriatric care management and eHealth. This chapter discusses the methods of public health management in a critical manner providing key analysis to the subject matter.

Health System

A health system, also sometimes referred to as health care system or as healthcare system, is the organization of people, institutions, and resources that deliver health care services to meet the health needs of target populations.

There is a wide variety of health systems around the world, with as many histories and organizational structures as there are nations. Implicitly, nations must design and develop health systems in accordance with their needs and resources, although common elements in virtually all health systems are primary healthcare and public health measures. In some countries, health system planning is distributed among market participants. In others, there is a concerted effort among governments, trade unions, charities, religious organizations, or other co-ordinated bodies to deliver planned health care services targeted to the populations they serve. However, health care planning has been described as often evolutionary rather than revolutionary.

Goals

The World Health Organization (WHO), the directing and coordinating authority for health within the United Nations system, is promoting a goal of universal health care: to ensure that all people obtain the health services they need without suffering financial hardship when paying for them. According to WHO, healthcare systems' goals are good health for the citizens, responsiveness to the expectations of the population, and fair means of funding operations. Progress towards them depends on how systems carry out four vital functions: provision of health care services, resource generation, financing, and stewardship. Other dimensions for the evaluation of health systems include quality, efficiency, acceptability, and equity. They have also been described in the United States as "the five C's": Cost, Coverage, Consistency, Complexity, and Chronic Illness. Also, continuity of health care is a major goal.

Definitions

Often health system has been defined with a reductionist perspective, for example reducing it to healthcare system. In many publications, for example, both expressions are used interchangeably. Some authors have developed arguments to expand the concept of health systems, indicating additional dimensions that should be considered:

- Health systems should not be expressed in terms of their components only, but also of their interrelationships;
- Health systems should include not only the institutional or supply side of the health system, but also the population;
- Health systems must be seen in terms of their goals, which include not only health improvement, but also equity, responsiveness to legitimate expectations, respect of dignity, and fair financing, among others;
- Health systems must also be defined in terms of their functions, including the direct provision of services, whether they are medical or public health services, but also "other enabling functions, such as stewardship, financing, and resource generation, including what is probably the most complex of all challenges, the health workforce."

World Health Organization definition

The World Health Organization defines health systems as follows:

A health system consists of all organizations, people and actions whose primary intent is to promote, restore or maintain health. This includes efforts to influence determinants of health as well as more direct health-improving activities. A health system is therefore more than the pyramid of publicly owned facilities that deliver personal health services. It includes, for example, a mother caring for a sick child at home; private providers; behaviour change programmes; vector-control campaigns; health insurance organizations; occupational health and safety legislation. It includes inter-sectoral action by health staff, for example, encouraging the ministry of education to promote female education, a well known determinant of better health.

Providers

Healthcare providers are institutions or individuals providing healthcare services. Individuals including health professionals and allied health professions can be self-employed or working as an employee in a hospital, clinic, or other health care institution, whether government operated, private for-profit, or private not-for-profit (e.g. non-governmental organization). They may also work outside of direct patient care such as in a government health department or other agency, medical laboratory, or health training institution. Examples of health workers are doctors, nurses, midwives, dietitians, paramedics, dentists, medical laboratory technologists, therapists, psychologists, pharmacists, chiropractors, optometrists, community health workers, traditional medicine practitioners, and others.

Financial Resources

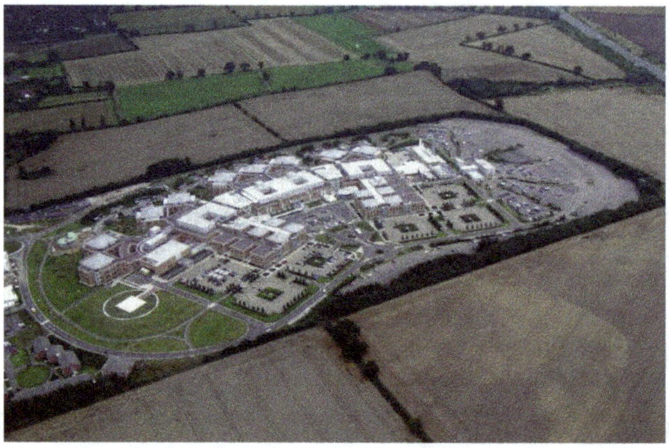

Norfolk and Norwich University Hospital, a National Health Service hospital in the United Kingdom.

There are generally five primary methods of funding health systems:

1. general taxation to the state, county or municipality
2. national health insurance
3. voluntary or private health insurance
4. out-of-pocket payments
5. donations to charities

Most countries' systems feature a mix of all five models. One study based on data from the OECD concluded that all types of health care finance "are compatible with" an efficient health system. The study also found no relationship between financing and cost control.

The term health insurance is generally used to describe a form of insurance that pays for medical expenses. It is sometimes used more broadly to include insurance covering disability or long-term nursing or custodial care needs. It may be provided through a social insurance program, or from private insurance companies. It may be obtained on a group basis (e.g., by a firm to cover its employees) or purchased by individual consumers. In each case premiums or taxes protect the insured from high or unexpected health care expenses.

By estimating the overall cost of health care expenses, a routine finance structure (such as a monthly premium or annual tax) can be developed, ensuring that money is available to pay for the health care benefits specified in the insurance agreement. The benefit is typically administered by a government agency, a non-profit health fund or a corporation operating seeking to make a profit.

Many forms of commercial health insurance control their costs by restricting the benefits that are paid by through deductibles, co-payments, coinsurance, policy exclusions, and total coverage limits and will severely restrict or refuse coverage of pre-existing conditions. Many government schemes also have co-payment schemes but exclusions are rare because of political pressure. The larger insurance schemes may also negotiate fees with providers.

Many forms of social insurance schemes control their costs by using the bargaining power of their community they represent to control costs in the health care delivery system. For example, by negotiating drug prices directly with pharmaceutical companies negotiating standard fees with the medical profession, or reducing unnecessary health care costs. Social schemes sometimes feature contributions related to earnings as part of a scheme to deliver universal health care, which may or may not also involve the use of commercial and non-commercial insurers. Essentially the more wealthy pay proportionately more into the scheme to cover the needs of the relatively poor who therefore contribute proportionately less. There are usually caps on the contributions of the wealthy and minimum payments that must be made by the insured (often in the form of a minimum contribution, similar to a deductible in commercial insurance models).

In addition to these traditional health care financing methods, some lower income countries and development partners are also implementing non-traditional or innovative financing mechanisms for scaling up delivery and sustainability of health care, such as micro-contributions, public-private partnerships, and market-based financial transaction taxes. For example, as of June 2011, UNITAID had collected more than one billion dollars from 29 member countries, including several from Africa, through an air ticket solidarity levy to expand access to care and treatment for HIV/AIDS, tuberculosis and malaria in 94 countries.

Payment Models

In most countries, wage costs for healthcare practitioners are estimated to represent between 65% and 80% of renewable health system expenditures. There are three ways to pay medical practitioners: fee for service, capitation, and salary. There has been growing interest in blending elements of these systems.

Fee-for-service

Fee-for-service arrangements pay general practitioners (GPs) based on the service. They are even more widely used for specialists working in ambulatory care.

There are two ways to set fee levels:

- By individual practitioners.
- Central negotiations (as in Japan, Germany, Canada and in France) or hybrid model (such as in Australia, France's sector 2, and New Zealand) where GPs can charge extra fees on top of standardized patient reimbursement rates.

Capitation

In *capitation payment systems*, GPs are paid for each patient on their "list", usually with adjustments for factors such as age and gender. According to OECD, "these systems are used in Italy (with some fees), in all four countries of the United Kingdom (with some fees and allowances for specific services), Austria (with fees for specific services), Denmark (one third of income with remainder fee for service), Ireland (since 1989), the Netherlands (fee-for-service for privately insured patients and public employees) and Sweden (from 1994). Capitation payments have become more frequent in "managed care" environments in the United States."

According to OECD, "Capitation systems allow funders to control the overall level of primary health expenditures, and the allocation of funding among GPs is determined by patient registrations. However, under this approach, GPs may register too many patients and under-serve them, select the better risks and refer on patients who could have been treated by the GP directly. Freedom of consumer choice over doctors, coupled with the principle of "money following the patient" may moderate some of these risks. Aside from selection, these problems are likely to be less marked than under salary-type arrangements."

Salary Arrangements

In several OECD countries, general practitioners (GPs) are employed on *salaries* for the government. According to OECD, "Salary arrangements allow funders to control primary care costs directly; however, they may lead to under-provision of services (to ease workloads), excessive referrals to secondary providers and lack of attention to the preferences of patients." There has been movement away from this system.

Information Resources

Sound information plays an increasingly critical role in the delivery of modern health care and efficiency of health systems. Health informatics – the intersection of information science, medicine and healthcare – deals with the resources, devices, and methods required to optimize the acquisition and use of information in health and biomedicine. Necessary tools for proper health information coding and management include clinical guidelines, formal medical terminologies, and computers and other information and communication technologies. The kinds of data processed may include patients' medical records, hospital administration and clinical functions, and human resources information.

The use of health information lies at the root of evidence-based policy and evidence-based management in health care. Increasingly, information and communication technologies are being utilised to improve health systems in developing countries through: the standardisation of health information; computer-aided diagnosis and treatment monitoring; informing population groups on health and treatment.

Management

The management of any health system is typically directed through a set of policies and plans adopted by government, private sector business and other groups in areas such as personal healthcare delivery and financing, pharmaceuticals, health human resources, and public health.

Public health is concerned with threats to the overall health of a community based on population health analysis. The population in question can be as small as a handful of people, or as large as all the inhabitants of several continents (for instance, in the case of a pandemic). Public health is typically divided into epidemiology, biostatistics and health services. Environmental, social, behavioral, and occupational health are also important subfields.

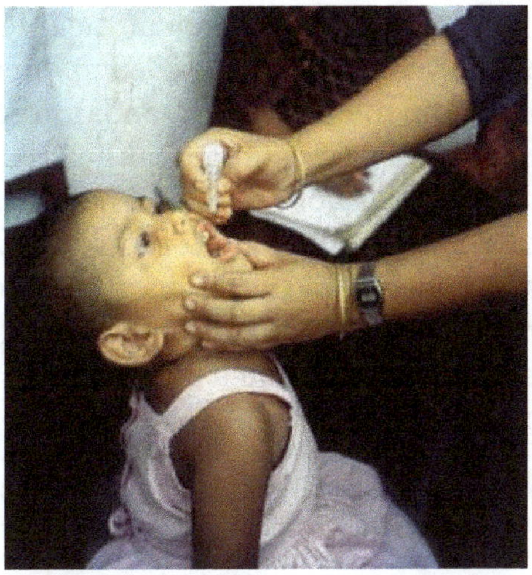

A child being immunized against polio.

Today, most governments recognize the importance of public health programs in reducing the incidence of disease, disability, the effects of ageing and health inequities, although public health generally receives significantly less government funding compared with medicine. For example, most countries have a vaccination policy, supporting public health programs in providing vaccinations to promote health. Vaccinations are voluntary in some countries and mandatory in some countries. Some governments pay all or part of the costs for vaccines in a national vaccination schedule.

The rapid emergence of many chronic diseases, which require costly long-term care and treatment, is making many health managers and policy makers re-examine their healthcare delivery practices. An important health issue facing the world currently is HIV/AIDS. Another major public health concern is diabetes. In 2006, according to the World Health Organization, at least 171 million people worldwide suffered from diabetes. Its incidence is increasing rapidly, and it is estimated that by the year 2030, this number will double. A controversial aspect of public health is the control of tobacco smoking, linked to cancer and other chronic illnesses.

Antibiotic resistance is another major concern, leading to the reemergence of diseases such as tuberculosis. The World Health Organization, for its World Health Day 2011 campaign, is calling for intensified global commitment to safeguard antibiotics and other antimicrobial medicines for future generations.

Health Systems Performance

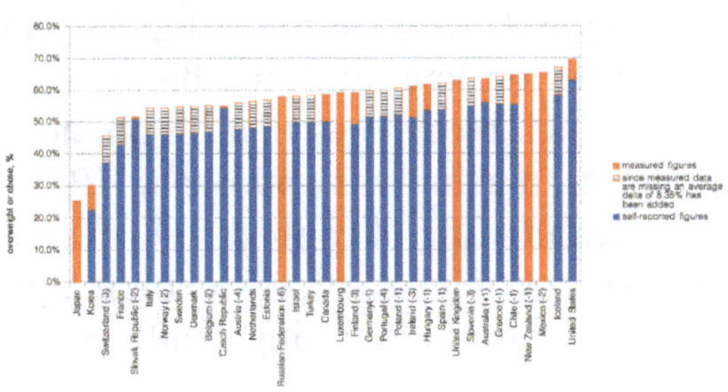

Percentage of overweight or obese population in 2010, Data source: OECD's iLibrary.

Since 2000, more and more initiatives have been taken at the international and national levels in order to strengthen national health systems as the core components of the global health system. Having this scope in mind, it is essential to have a clear, and unrestricted, vision of national health systems that might generate further progresses in global health. The elaboration and the selection of performance indicators are indeed both highly dependent on the conceptual framework adopted for the evaluation of the health systems performances. Like most social systems, health systems are complex adaptive systems where change does not necessarily follow rigid epidemiological models. In complex systems path dependency, emergent properties and other non-linear patterns are under-explored and unmeasured, which can lead to the development of inappropriate guidelines for developing responsive health systems.

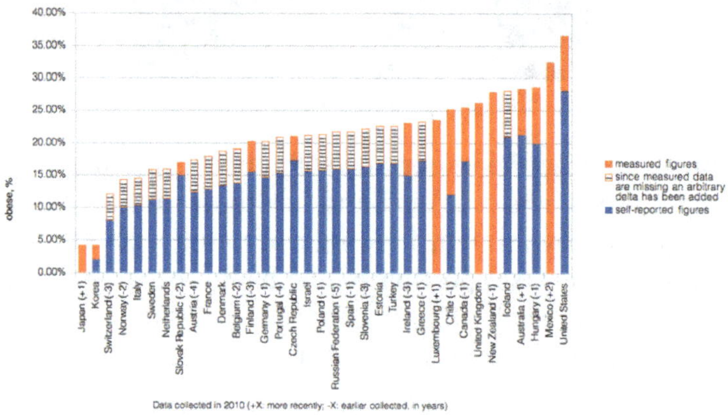

Percentage of obese population in 2010, Data source: OECD's iLibrary.

An increasing number of tools and guidelines are being published by international agencies and development partners to assist health system decision-makers to monitor and assess health systems strengthening including human resources development using standard definitions, indicators and measures. In response to a series of papers published in 2012 by members of the World Health Organization's Task Force on Developing Health Systems Guidance, researchers from the Future Health Systems consortium argue that there is insufficient focus on the 'policy implementation gap'. Recognizing the diversity of stakeholders and complexity of health systems is crucial to ensure that evidence-based guidelines are tested with requisite humility and without a rigid adherence to models dominated by a limited number of disciplines.

Health Policy and Systems Research (HPSR) is an emerging multidisciplinary field that challenges 'disciplinary capture' by dominant health research traditions, arguing that these traditions generate premature and inappropriately narrow definitions that impede rather than enhance health systems strengthening. HPSR focuses on low- and middle-income countries and draws on the relativist social science paradigm which recognises that all phenomena are constructed through human behaviour and interpretation. In using this approach, HPSR offers insight into health systems by generating a complex understanding of context in order to enhance health policy learning. HPSR calls for greater involvement of local actors, including policy makers, civil society and researchers, in decisions that are made around funding health policy research and health systems strengthening.

International Comparisons

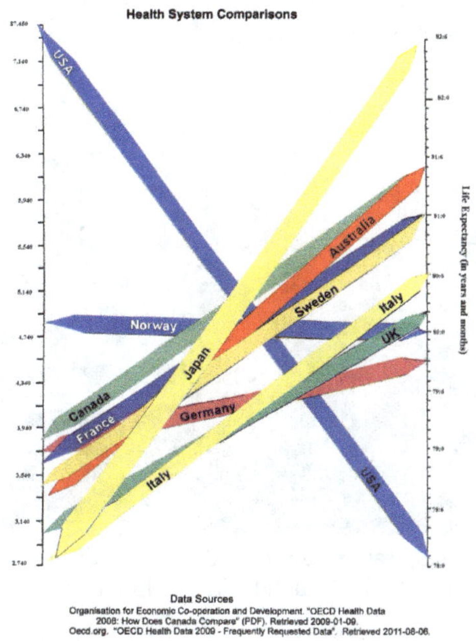

Chart comparing 2008 health care spending (left) vs. life expectancy (right) in OECD countries.

Health systems can vary substantially from country to country, and in the last few years, comparisons have been made on an international basis. The World Health Organization, in its *World Health Report 2000*, provided a ranking of health systems around the world according to criteria of the overall level and distribution of health in the populations, and the responsiveness and fair financing of health care services. The goals for health systems, according to the WHO's *World Health Report 2000 – Health systems: improving performance* (WHO, 2000), are good health, responsiveness to the expectations of the population, and fair financial contribution. There have been several debates around the results of this WHO exercise, and especially based on the country ranking linked to it, insofar as it appeared to depend mostly on the choice of the retained indicators.

Direct comparisons of health statistics across nations are complex. The Commonwealth Fund, in its annual survey, "Mirror, Mirror on the Wall", compares the performance of the health systems in Australia, New Zealand, the United Kingdom, Germany, Canada and the United States Its 2007 study found that, although the United States system is the most expensive, it consistently underperforms compared to the other countries. A major difference between the United States and the other countries in the study is that the United States is the only country without universal health care. The OECD also collects comparative statistics, and has published brief country profiles. Health Consumer Powerhouse makes comparisons between both national health care systems in the Euro health consumer index and specific areas of health care such as diabetes or hepatitis.

Health Care

Health care or healthcare is the maintenance or improvement of health via the diagnosis, treatment, and prevention of disease, illness, injury, and other physical and mental impairments in human beings. Healthcare is delivered by health professionals (providers or practitioners) in allied health professions, chiropractic, physicians, physician associates, dentistry, midwifery, nursing, medicine, optometry, pharmacy, psychology, and other health professions. It includes the work done in providing primary care, secondary care, and tertiary care, as well as in public health.

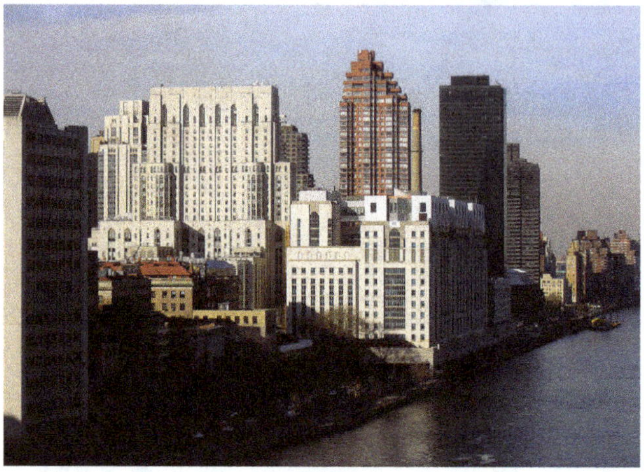

New York-Presbyterian Hospital in New York City is one of the world's busiest hospitals. Pictured is the Weill-Cornell facility (white complex at centre).

Access to healthcare varies across countries, groups, and individuals, largely influenced by social and economic conditions as well as the health policies in place. Countries and jurisdictions have different policies and plans in relation to the personal and population-based health care goals within their societies. Healthcare systems are organizations established to meet the health needs of target populations. Their exact configuration varies between national and subnational entities. In some countries and jurisdictions, healthcare planning is distributed among market participants, whereas in others, planning occurs more centrally among governments or other coordinating bodies. In all cases, according to the World Health Organization (WHO), a well-functioning healthcare system requires a robust financing mechanism; a well-trained and adequately-paid workforce; reliable information on which to base decisions and policies; and well maintained health facilities and logistics to deliver quality medicines and technologies.

Healthcare can contribute to a significant part of a country's economy. In 2011, the healthcare industry consumed an average of 9.3 percent of the GDP or US$ 3,322 (PPP-adjusted) per capita across the 34 members of OECD countries. The USA (17.7%, or US$ PPP 8,508), the Netherlands (11.9%, 5,099), France (11.6%, 4,118), Germany (11.3%, 4,495), Canada (11.2%, 5669), and Switzerland (11%, 5,634) were the top spenders, however life expectancy in total population at birth was highest in Switzerland (82.8 years), Japan and Italy (82.7), Spain and Iceland (82.4), France (82.2) and Australia (82.0), while OECD's average exceeds 80 years for the first time ever in 2011: 80.1 years, a gain of 10 years since 1970. The USA (78.7 years) ranges only on place 26 among the 34 OECD member countries, but has the highest costs by far. All OECD countries have achieved universal (or almost universal) health coverage, except Mexico and the USA.

Healthcare is conventionally regarded as an important determinant in promoting the general physical and mental health and well-being of people around the world. An example of this was the worldwide eradication of smallpox in 1980, declared by the WHO as the first disease in human history to be completely eliminated by deliberate health care interventions.

Delivery

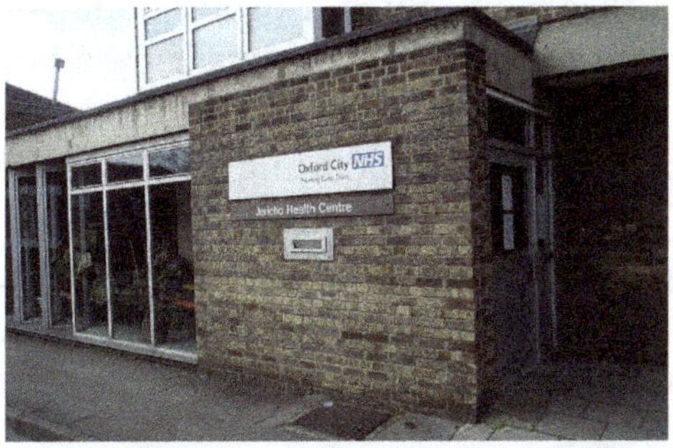

Primary care may be provided in community health centres.

The delivery of modern health care depends on groups of trained professionals and paraprofessionals coming together as interdisciplinary teams. This includes professionals in medicine, psychology, physiotherapy, nursing, dentistry, midwifery and allied health, plus many others such as public health practitioners, community health workers and assistive personnel, who systematically provide personal and population-based preventive, curative and rehabilitative care services.

While the definitions of the various types of health care vary depending on the different cultural, political, organizational and disciplinary perspectives, there appears to be some consensus that primary care constitutes the first element of a continuing health care process, that may also include the provision of secondary and tertiary levels of care. Healthcare can be defined as either public or private.

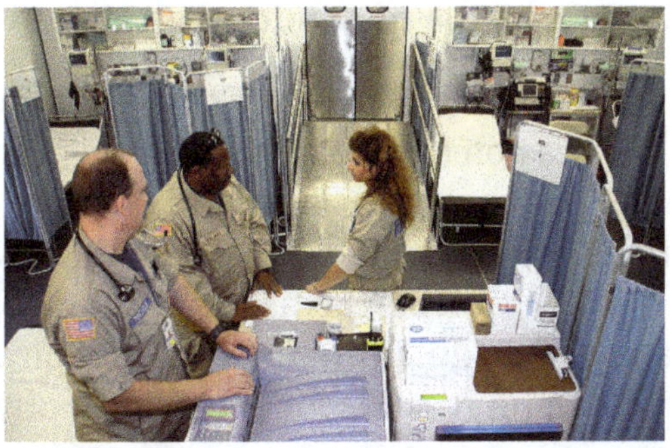

The emergency room is often a frontline venue for the delivery of primary medical care.

Primary Care

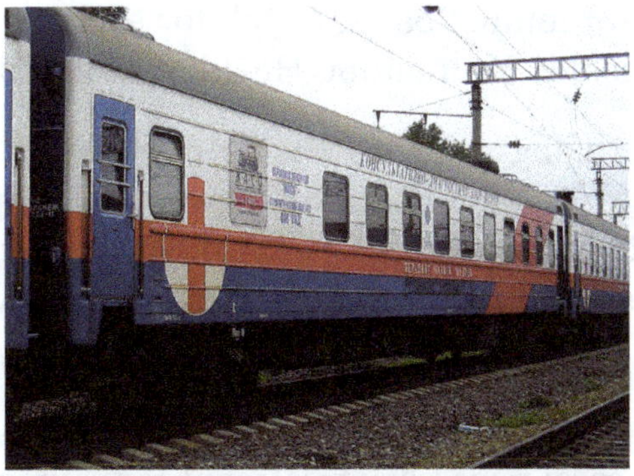

Medical train "Therapist Matvei Mudrov" in Khabarovsk, Russia

Primary care refers to the work of health professionals who act as a first point of consultation for all patients within the health care system. Such a professional would usually be a primary care physician, such as a general practitioner or family physician, a licensed independent practitioner such as a physiotherapist, or a non-physician primary care provider (mid-level provider) such as a physician assistant or nurse practitioner. Depending on the locality, health system organization, and sometimes at the patient's discretion, they may see another health care professional first, such as a pharmacist, a nurse (such as in the United Kingdom), a clinical officer (such as in parts of Africa), or an Ayurvedic or other traditional medicine professional (such as in parts of Asia). Depending on the nature of the health condition, patients may then be referred for secondary or tertiary care.

Primary care is often used as the term for the health care services which play a role in the local community. It can be provided in different settings, such as Urgent care centres which provide services to patients same day with appointment or walk-in bases.

Primary care involves the widest scope of health care, including all ages of patients, patients of all socioeconomic and geographic origins, patients seeking to maintain optimal health, and patients with all manner of acute and chronic physical, mental and social health issues, including multiple chronic diseases. Consequently, a primary care practitioner must possess a wide breadth of knowledge in many areas. Continuity is a key characteristic of primary care, as patients usually prefer to consult the same practitioner for routine check-ups and preventive care, health education, and every time they require an initial consultation about a new health problem. The International Classification of Primary Care (ICPC) is a standardized tool for understanding and analyzing information on interventions in primary care by the reason for the patient visit.

Common chronic illnesses usually treated in primary care may include, for example: hypertension, diabetes, asthma, COPD, depression and anxiety, back pain, arthritis or thyroid dysfunction. Primary care also includes many basic maternal and child health care services, such as family planning services and vaccinations. In the United States, the 2013 National Health Interview Survey found that skin disorders (42.7%), osteoarthritis and joint disorders (33.6%), back problems (23.9%), disorders of lipid metabolism (22.4%), and upper respiratory tract disease (22.1%, excluding asthma) were the most common reasons for accessing a physician.

In the United States, primary care physicians have begun to deliver primary care outside of the managed care (insurance-billing) system through direct primary care which is a subset of the more familiar concierge medicine. Physicians in this model bill patients directly for services, either on a pre-paid monthly, quarterly, or annual basis, or bill for each service in the office. Examples of direct primary care practices include Foundation Health in Colorado and Qliance in Washington.

In context of global population aging, with increasing numbers of older adults at greater risk of chronic non-communicable diseases, rapidly increasing demand for primary care services is expected in both developed and developing countries. The World Health Organization attributes the provision of essential primary care as an integral component of an inclusive primary health care strategy.

Secondary Care

Secondary care includes acute care: necessary treatment for a short period of time for a brief but serious illness, injury or other health condition, such as in a hospital emergency department. It also includes skilled attendance during childbirth, intensive care, and medical imaging services.

The term "secondary care" is sometimes used synonymously with "hospital care". However, many secondary care providers do not necessarily work in hospitals, such as psychiatrists, clinical psychologists, occupational therapists, most dental specialties or physiotherapists (physiotherapists are also primary care providers, and a referral is not required to see a physiotherapist), and some primary care services are delivered within hospitals. Depending on the organization and policies of the national health system, patients may be required to see a primary care provider for a referral before they can access secondary care.

For example, in the United States, which operates under a mixed market health care system, some physicians might voluntarily limit their practice to secondary care by requiring patients to see a primary care provider first, or this restriction may be imposed under the terms of the payment agreements in private or group health insurance plans. In other cases medical specialists may see patients without a referral, and patients may decide whether self-referral is preferred.

In the United Kingdom and Canada, patient self-referral to a medical specialist for secondary care is rare as prior referral from another physician (either a primary care physician or another specialist) is considered necessary, regardless of whether the funding is from private insurance schemes or national health insurance.

Allied health professionals, such as physical therapists, respiratory therapists, occupational therapists, speech therapists, and dietitians, also generally work in secondary care, accessed through either patient self-referral or through physician referral.

Tertiary Care

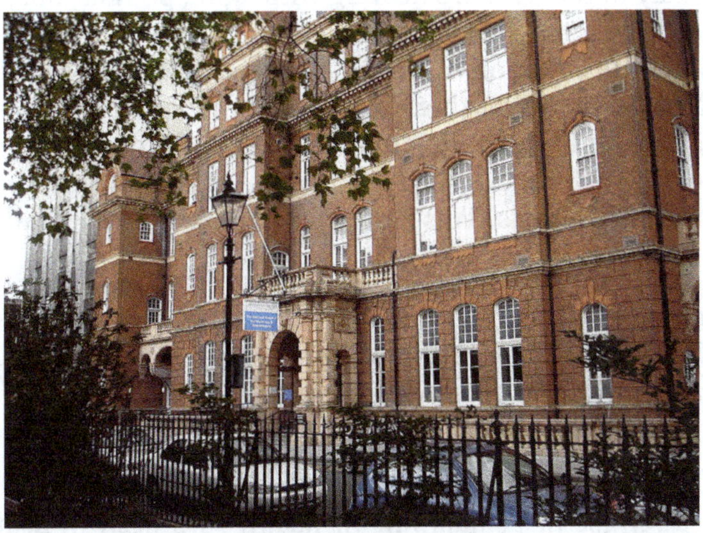

The National Hospital for Neurology and Neurosurgery in London, United Kingdom is a specialist neurological hospital.

Tertiary care is specialized consultative health care, usually for inpatients and on referral from a primary or secondary health professional, in a facility that has personnel and facilities for advanced medical investigation and treatment, such as a tertiary referral hospital.

Examples of tertiary care services are cancer management, neurosurgery, cardiac surgery, plastic surgery, treatment for severe burns, advanced neonatology services, palliative, and other complex medical and surgical interventions.

Quaternary Care

The term quaternary care is sometimes used as an extension of tertiary care in reference to advanced levels of medicine which are highly specialized and not widely accessed. Experimental medicine and some types of uncommon diagnostic or surgical procedures are considered quaternary care. These services are usually only offered in a limited number of regional or national health care centres. This term is more prevalent in the United Kingdom, but just as applicable in the United States. A quaternary care hospital may have virtually any procedure available, whereas a tertiary care facility may not offer a sub-specialist with that training.

Home and Community Care

Many types of health care interventions are delivered outside of health facilities. They include many interventions of public health interest, such as food safety surveillance, distribution of condoms and needle-exchange programmes for the prevention of transmissible diseases.

They also include the services of professionals in residential and community settings in support of self care, home care, long-term care, assisted living, treatment for substance use disorders and other types of health and social care services.

Community rehabilitation services can assist with mobility and independence after loss of limbs or loss of function. This can include prosthesis, orthotics or wheelchairs.

Many countries, especially in the west are dealing with aging populations, and one of the priorities of the health care system is to help seniors live full, independent lives in the comfort of their own homes. There is an entire section of health care geared to providing seniors with help in day-to-day activities at home, transporting them to doctor's appointments, and many other activities that are so essential for their health and well-being. Although they provide home care for older adults in cooperation, family members and care workers may harbor diverging attitudes and values towards their joint efforts. This state of affairs presents a challenge for the design of ICT for home care.

With obesity in children rapidly becoming a major concern, health services often set up programs in schools aimed at educating children in good eating habits; making physical education compulsory in school; and teaching young adolescents to have positive self-image.

Ratings

Health care ratings are ratings or evaluations of health care used to evaluate process of care, healthcare structures and/or outcomes of a healthcare services. This information is translated into report cards that are generated by quality organizations, nonprofit, consumer groups and media. This evaluation of quality can be based on:

- Measures of Hospital quality

- Measures of Health Plan Quality
- Measures of Physician Quality
- Measures of Quality for Other Health Professionals
- Measures of Patient Experience

Related Sectors

Health care extends beyond the delivery of services to patients, encompassing many related sectors, and set within a bigger picture of financing and governance structures.

Health System

A health system, also sometimes referred to as health care system or healthcare system is the organization of people, institutions, and resources to deliver health care services to meet the health needs of target populations.

Health Care Industry

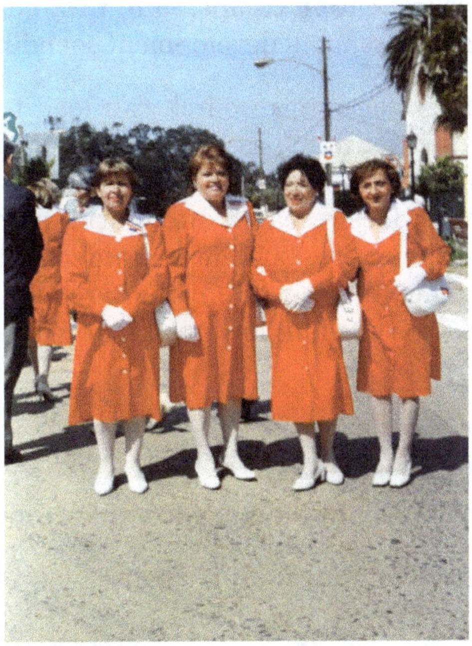

A group of Chilean 'Damas de Rojo' volunteering at their local hospital

The health care industry incorporates several sectors that are dedicated to providing health care services and products. As a basic framework for defining the sector, the United Nations' International Standard Industrial Classification categorizes health care as generally consisting of hospital activities, medical and dental practice activities, and "other human health activities". The last class involves activities of, or under the supervision of, nurses, midwives, physiotherapists, scientific or diagnostic laboratories, pathology clinics, residential health facilities, patient advocates, or other allied health professions, e.g. in the field of optometry, hydrotherapy, medical massage, yoga therapy, music therapy, occupational therapy, speech therapy, chiropody, homeopathy, chiropractics, acupuncture, etc.

In addition, according to industry and market classifications, such as the Global Industry Classification Standard and the Industry Classification Benchmark, health care includes many categories of medical equipment, instruments and services as well as biotechnology, diagnostic laboratories and substances, and drug manufacturing and delivery.

For example, pharmaceuticals and other medical devices are the leading high technology exports of Europe and the United States. The United States dominates the biopharmaceutical field, accounting for three-quarters of the world's biotechnology revenues.

Health Care Research

The quantity and quality of many health care interventions are improved through the results of science, such as advanced through the medical model of health which focuses on the eradication of illness through diagnosis and effective treatment. Many important advances have been made through health research, including biomedical research and pharmaceutical research, which form the basis for evidence-based medicine and evidence-based practice in health care delivery.

For example, in terms of pharmaceutical research and development spending, Europe spends a little less than the United States (€22.50bn compared to €27.05bn in 2006). The United States accounts for 80% of the world's research and development spending in biotechnology.

In addition, the results of health services research can lead to greater efficiency and equitable delivery of health care interventions, as advanced through the social model of health and disability, which emphasizes the societal changes that can be made to make population healthier. Results from health services research often form the basis of evidence-based policy in health care systems. Health services research is also aided by initiatives in the field of AI for the development of systems of health assessment that are clinically useful, timely, sensitive to change, culturally sensitive, low burden, low cost, involving for the patient and built into standard procedures.

Health Care Financing

There are generally five primary methods of funding health care systems:

1. general taxation to the state, county or municipality
2. social health insurance
3. voluntary or private health insurance
4. out-of-pocket payments
5. donations to health charities

In most countries, the financing of health care services features a mix of all five models, but the exact distribution varies across countries and over time within countries. In all countries and jurisdictions, there are many topics in the politics and evidence that can influence the decision of a government, private sector business or other group to adopt a specific health policy regarding the financing structure.

For example, social health insurance is where a nation's entire population is eligible for health care coverage, and this coverage and the services provided are regulated. In almost every jurisdiction with a government-funded health care system, a parallel private, and usually for-profit, system is allowed to operate. This is sometimes referred to as two-tier health care or universal health care.

For example, in Poland, the costs of health services borne by the National Health Fund (financed by all citizens that pay health insurance contributions) in 2012 amounted to 60.8 billion PLN (approximately 20 billion USD). The right to health services in Poland is granted to 99.9% of the population (also registered unemployed persons and their spouses).

Health Care Administration and Regulation

The management and administration of health care is another sector vital to the delivery of health care services. In particular, the practice of health professionals and operation of health care institutions is typically regulated by national or state/provincial authorities through appropriate regulatory bodies for purposes of quality assurance. Most countries have credentialing staff in regulatory boards or health departments who document the certification or licensing of health workers and their work history.

Health Information Technology

Health information technology (HIT) is "the application of information processing involving both computer hardware and software that deals with the storage, retrieval, sharing, and use of health care information, data, and knowledge for communication and decision making." Technology is a broad concept that deals with a species' usage and knowledge of tools and crafts, and how it affects a species' ability to control and adapt to its environment. However, a strict definition is elusive; "technology" can refer to material objects of use to humanity, such as machines, hardware or utensils, but can also encompass broader themes, including systems, methods of organization, and techniques. For HIT, technology represents computers and communications attributes that can be networked to build systems for moving health information. Informatics is yet another integral aspect of HIT.

Health information technology can be divided into further components like Electronic Health Record (EHR), Electronic Medical Record (EMR), Personal Health Record (PHR), Practice Management System (PMS), Health Information Exchange (HIE) and many more. There are multiple purposes for the use of HIT within the health care industry. Further, the use of HIT is expected to improve the quality of health care, reduce medical errors, improve the health care service efficiency and reduce health care costs.

Self-care

In health care, self-care is any necessary human regulatory function which is under individual control, deliberate and self-initiated.

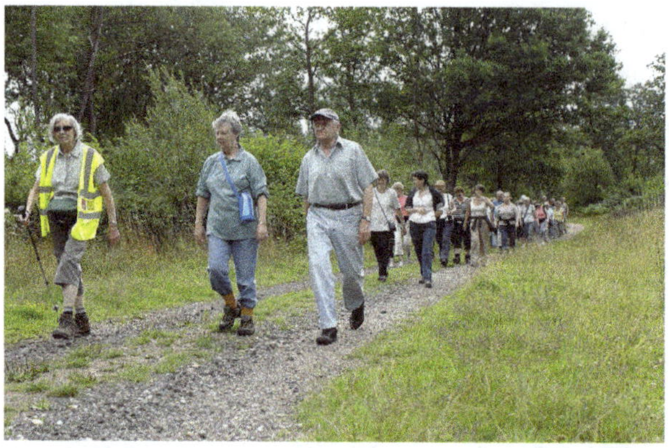

Walking for Health.

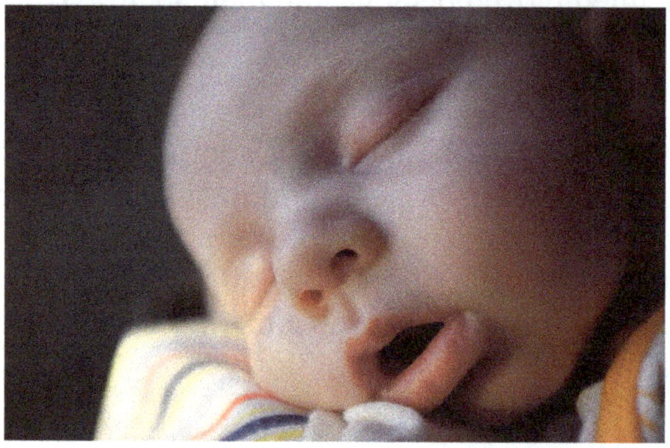

Sleep is a fundamental human need

Some place self-care on a continuum with health care providers at the opposite end to self-care. In modern medicine, preventive medicine aligns most closely with self-care. A lack of adherence to medical advice and the onset of a mental disorder can make self-care difficult. Self-care is seen as a partial solution to the global rise in health care costs placed on governments. The notion that self-care is a fundamental pillar of health and social care means it is an essential component of a modern health care system governed by regulations and statutes.

Self-care is considered a primary form of care for patients with chronic conditions who make many day-to-day decisions, or self-manage, their illness. Self-management is critical and self-management education complements traditional patient education in primary care to support patients to live the best possible quality of life with their chronic condition. Self-care is learned, purposeful and continuous. In philosophy, self-care refers to the care and cultivation of self in a comprehensive sense, focusing in particular on the soul and the knowledge of self.

Universal Requisites

There are a number of self-care requisites applicable to all humans across all ages and necessary to fundamental human needs. For example, as humans we need to intake sufficient air, water and food; care also needs to be taken with the process of elimination and excrement. There must be a balance between rest and activity as well as between solitude and social activities. The prevention and avoidance of human hazards and participation in social groups are also requisites. Maturity requires the autonomous performance of self-care duties.

Self-care Maintenance

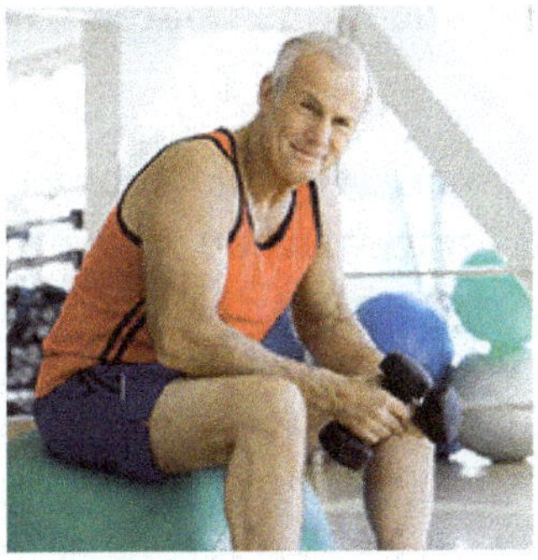

Maintaining fitness at an elderly age

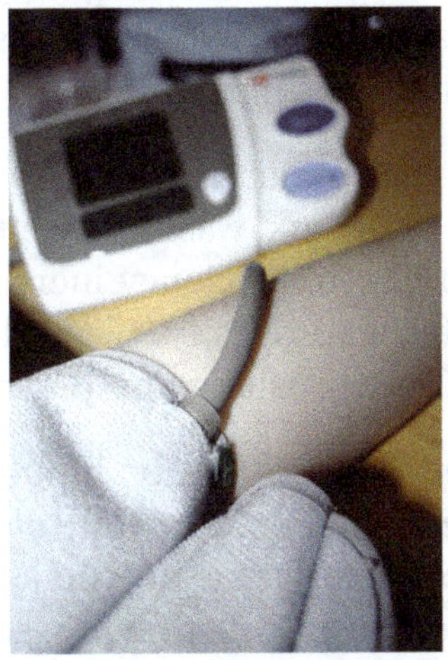

Checking blood pressure at home with an electronic sphygmomanometer.

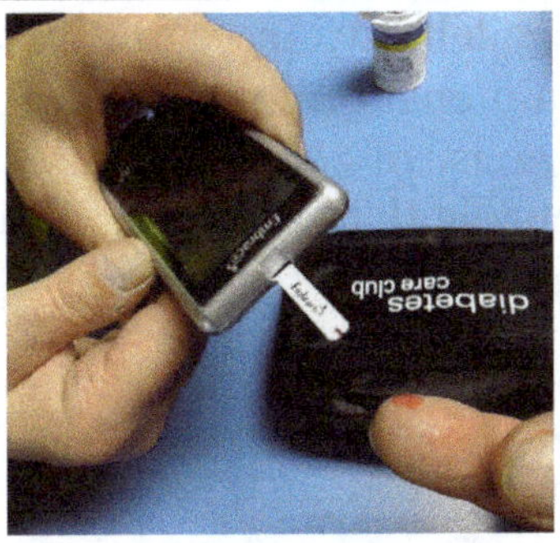

Blood sugar testing for diabetes

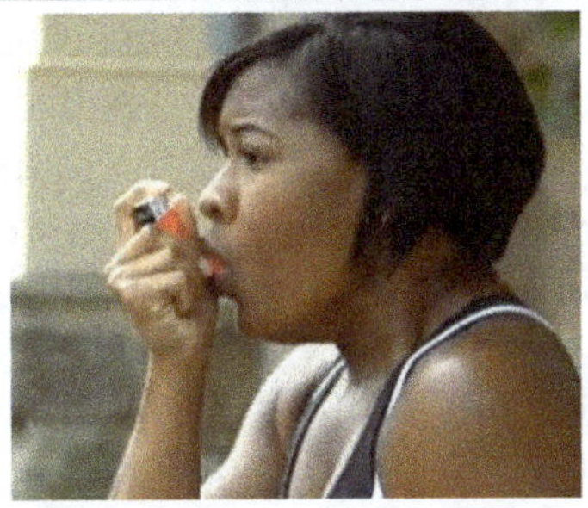

Asthma inhalers contain a medication that treats the symptoms of asthma

Self-care includes all health decisions people (as individuals or consumers) make for themselves and their families to ensure they are physically and mentally fit.

Self-care Maintenance Behaviors

Self-care maintenance behaviors include illness prevention, illness behaviors, and proper hygiene. Illness prevention measures include tobacco avoidance, exercise, and diet. Tobacco use is the largest preventable cause of death and disease in the US. By avoiding or quitting tobacco use, overall health and quality of life are improved and risk of disease and premature death are reduced. The benefits of regular physical activity include weight control, reduced risk of chronic disease, strengthened bones and muscles, improved mental health, improved ability to participate in daily activities, and increased chance of living longer. The Center for Disease Control and Prevention (CDC) recommends 2 hours and thirty minutes of moderate activity each week. Examples of this include brisk walking, swimming, dancing, riding a bike, and even jumping rope. Another important aspect to self care includes eating fresh fruits and vegetables, lean meats and other proteins. Processed foods should be limited. Limiting saturated fats, trans fats, sugars, and sodium will also contribute to a healthy diet.

Illness behaviors include taking medicines as prescribed and getting vaccinations. When medicines are not taken as prescribed, complications can occur. These complications include disease progression, reduced functional abilities, lower quality of life, and increased hospital visits. Vaccinations helps protect individuals from serious illnesses and complications related to vaccine-preventable diseases like pneumonia.

Hygiene is another important part of self-care maintenance. Hygiene behaviors include adequate sleep, regular oral care, and hand washing. Getting 7–8 hours of sleep each night can protect physical and mental health. Sleep deficiency increases the risk of heart disease, kidney disease, high blood pressure, diabetes, and obesity. Sleep deficiency can also lead to depression, suicide, and risk-taking behavior. Teeth brushing and personal hygiene can prevent infection.

Self-care maintenance behaviors can be influenced by external factors, such as access to healthcare and living environments. Social determinants of health play a huge role in how people take care of themselves. Access to care is one major determinant of one's ability to carry out self-care maintenance behaviors.This includes having access to transportation to visit a health care service, availability of open hours of offices/clinics, and whether or not the care is affordable. These external factors can determine a person's ability to perform self-care maintenance because a person may not be able to perform a behavior based on its availability. Access within a one's living environment is another factor that influences self-care maintenance. An individual's environment determines whether they are able to go to the gym to exercise or go to a grocery store to buy healthy food. Living in a food desert or having limited resources that allow for physical activity would decrease the likelihood of participating in self-care maintenance behaviors.

Internal factors, such as motivation, emotions, and cognitive abilities also influence self-care maintenance behaviors. Motivation is often the driving force behind performing self-care maintenance behaviors. A person who is motivated to stay healthy and managing and/or prevent a chronic illness is more likely to be interested in performing maintenance behaviors, such as those mentioned above. Emotions are also indicative of whether a person is going to perform such behaviors. A person with depression is more likely to have a poor dietary intake low in fruits and vegetables, reduced physical activity, and poor medication adherence. An individual with impaired cognitive or functional abilities also has a diminished ability to performing self-care maintenance behaviors. Some of these behaviors, such as medication adherence, require the ability to maintain a schedule, but someone with memory impairment may have difficulty completing tasks based on memory.

Skills are also a significant aspect that influences an individual's ability to perform self-care behaviors. Individuals need to be able to plan, set goals, and make appropriate decisions regarding their health needs. In addition, self-care is influenced by an individual's attitude and belief in his or her self-efficacy. Having the confidence to perform an action and to overcome barriers is indicative of success in performing self-care behaviors. Cultural beliefs and values may also influence self-care. Self-care may be viewed as highly important in some countries or within certain cultures that value independence, but in other cultures, self-care may contradict their beliefs and values.

Social supports also influence how an individual performs self-care maintenance. Social supports include family, friends, and support groups. Support groups can be through religious groups, groups that manage chronic illnesses, or a community group. These supports can help by having people to talk to or help make decisions about your care. Individuals who live with chronic illness acknowledge that shared care can help make living with a chronic illness less stressful. If you are suffering from a chronic illness and would like to join a support group, there are resources that could be found online or offered by your primary care provider.

Living with one or more chronic illnesses can be very difficult. There are numerous medications, different specialists, and self-care maintenance behaviors that are necessary. With all of these working parts, it can be difficult to keep track of everything. The presence of co-morbid conditions makes performing self-care maintenance behaviors harder to complete. Pill burden is a huge factor in self-care maintenance of multiple chronic illnesses because many people may complain of not wanting to take all the medication or get confused regarding the schedule of their medications. As an example, a patient with diabetes would need to exercise, but if they also have COPD they easily develop shortness of breath which would cause them to stop exercising. It is important to address all the symptoms of each chronic illness an individual suffers from so that individuals with chronic illnesses can successfully perform self-care maintenance behaviors.

The benefits of living a healthy lifestyle were analyzed in the Caerphilly Heart Disease Study. Evidence showed a risk reduction in chronic diseases (including dementia and cognitive impairment) to be significantly associated with healthy lifestyles.

Self-care is also taking care of minor ailments, long term conditions, or one's own health after discharge from secondary and tertiary health care. For instances of neck pain, for example, self-care is the recommended treatment.

Patients who are better informed and more educated possess greater motivation for self-care. Individuals conduct self-care and experts and professionals support self-care to enable individuals to undertake enhanced self-care. The recognition and evaluation of symptoms is a key aspect of self-care. The main issues involved with self-care and the onset of illness are medically related such managing drug side effects, emotions and psychological issues, changes to lifestyle and knowledge acquisition to assist in decision-making.

Self-care support has crucial enabling value and considerable scope in developing countries with an already overburdened health care system. But it also has an essential role to play in affluent countries where people are becoming more conscious about their health and want to have a greater role in taking care of themselves.

To enable people to do enhanced self-care, they can be supported in various ways and by different service providers.

Methods Used to Improve Self-Care

Multifaceted interventions that tailor education to the individual are more effective than patient education alone. Approaches used to improve self-care are summarized here.

- "Teach-back" is used to gauge how much information is retained after patient teaching. Teach-back occurs when patients are asked to repeat information that was given to them. The educator checks for gaps in the patient's understanding, reinforces messages, and creates a collaborative conversation with the patient. It is important for individuals with a chronic illness to comprehend and recall information received about their condition. Teach-back education can both educate patients and assess learning. One example of how a provider can initiate teach-back is by asking, "I want to make sure that I explained everything clearly. If you were talking to your neighbor, what would you tell her/him we talked about today". This phrase protects the patient's self-esteem while placing responsibility for understanding on both the provider and patient. One study performed showed that patients with heart failure who received teach-back education had a 12% lower readmission rate compared to patients who did not receive teach-back. Although the teach-back method is effective in the short-term, there is little evidence to support its long-term effect. Long-term knowledge retention is crucial for self-care, so further research is needed on this approach.

- Habits are automatic responses to commonly encountered situations. One example of a habit is hand washing after restroom use. The main characteristic of a habit is automaticity. A habit is formed when environmental cues result in a behavior with very little conscious deliberation.
- Behavioral economics is a subset of the study of economics that examines how cognitive, social, and emotional factors play in role in an individual's economic decisions. Behavioral economics is now influencing the design of healthcare interventions aimed at improving self-care maintenance. Because humans do not always make rational decisions when it comes to self-care, behavioral economics takes into account the complexity and irrationality of human behavior.
- Motivational Interviewing is a way to engage people in critically thinking about their self-care needs. MI uses an interviewing style that focuses on the individual's goals and can be used in any context. MI is based on three psychological theories: cognitive dissonance, self-perception, and the transtheoretical model of change. MI is intended to enhance intrinsic motivation for change.
- Health coaching is another method of promoting motivation to initiate and maintain behavior change. The health coach facilitates behavior change by emphasizing personal goals, life experiences, and values.

Self-Care Monitoring

Self-care monitoring is the process of surveillance that involves measurement and perception of bodily changes. Effective self-care monitoring also requires being able to label and interpret changes in the body as normal or abnormal. Listening to your body and recognizing signs and symptoms, increasing factual knowledge towards disease or illness are all important factors. Being able to interpret and label your symptoms, understanding the process of your disease, and knowing how to act and treat accordingly allows competency in knowing when to seek further medical help.

Self-care monitoring consists of both the perception and measurement of symptoms. Symptom perception is the process of monitoring one's body for signs of changing health. This includes body awareness or body listening, recognizing symptoms relevant to health, and interpreting and labeling these symptoms. For example, a patient with diabetes may use body listening to perceive feelings of shakiness and sweating. These feelings are labeled as symptoms of low blood sugar, and the patient will decide how to act based on this information. Prompt and accurate recognition of symptoms is a necessary part of a patient's management of their health. In heart attack patients, delays in seeking treatment for worsening symptoms have been found to contribute to poor health outcomes.

Changes in health status or body function can be monitored with various tools and technologies. The range and complexity of medical devices used in both hospital and homecare settings are increasing. Certain devices are specific to a common need of a disease process. For example, various types of glucose monitors are used by patients with diabetes to track their blood sugar levels. Other devices can provide a more general set of information, such as a weight scale, blood pressure cuff, pulse oximeter, etc. Less technological tools can include organizers, charts, and diagrams to trend or keep track of things such as amount of calories, mood, vital sign measurements, and more.

Barriers to self-care Monitoring

A patient's ability to engage in self-care monitoring greatly impacts the progression of his/her disease. Barriers to monitoring can go unrecognized and end up interfering with effective self-care. Barriers can include knowledge deficits, undesirable self-care regimens, different instructions from multiple providers, and limitations to access related to income or disability. Psychosocial factors such as motivation, anxiety, depression, confidence can also serve as barriers.

- Cost of equipment - This is a common barrier to self-care monitoring. Certain equipment is needed to monitor symptoms, such as test strips and needles in blood glucose monitoring. The cost of equipment can be expensive for some individuals, so they are less motivated and less likely to keep track of symptoms.
- Lack of knowledge - With monitoring, it is important to understand what you're looking for and why you're doing it. For example, some individuals may not understand the implications of high blood sugars or high blood pressure. Thus, they don't feel the need to monitor it. Also, if you don't understand the importance of the monitoring, you will not do it.
- Fear of outcomes/fear of using equipment - In the example of blood glucose monitoring, some people may be afraid of needles, which will deter them from doing fingersticks to read their blood sugar. Other people may have a fear or anxiety of how results may turn out and may avoid them. For example, a person who did not follow a diet to maintain their blood pressure or blood sugar may have a fear that it is already high and thus, does not want to monitor it.
- Familial/social support (or lack thereof) - Monitoring something implies doing it on a regular/frequent basis. Doing anything consistently sometimes requires reminders or a little encouragement from others.

Improving Self-care Monitoring

Because self-care monitoring is conducted primarily by patients and their caregivers, it is necessary to work with patients closely on this topic. Providers should assess the current self-care monitoring regimen and build off this to create an individualized plan of care. Knowledge and education specifically designed for the patient's level of understating is central to self-care monitoring. When patients understand the symptoms that correspond with their disease, they can learn to recognize these symptoms early on. Then they can self-manage their disease and prevent complications.

Additional research to improve self-care monitoring is underway in the following fields:

- Mindfulness: Mindfulness and meditation, when incorporated into a one-day education program for diabetic patients, have been shown to improve diabetic control in a 3-month follow-up in comparison to those who received the education without a focus on mindfulness.
- Decision-making: How a patient's decision making capacity can be encouraged/improved with the support of their provider, leading to better self-care monitoring and outcomes.
- Self-efficacy: Self-efficacy has been shown to be more closely linked to a patient's ability to perform self-care than health literacy or knowledge.
- Wearable technology: How self-care monitoring is evolving with technology like wearable activity monitors.

Self-care Management

Self-care management is defined as the response to signs and symptoms when they occur. Self-care management involves the evaluation of physical and emotional changes and deciding if these changes need to be addressed. Changes may occur because of illness, treatment, or the environment. Once treatment is done, it needs to be evaluated to judge whether it would be useful to do again in the future. Treatments are based on the signs and symptoms experienced. Treatments are usually specific to the illness.

Self-care Management Behaviors

Self-care management includes recognizing symptoms, treating the symptoms, and evaluating the treatment. Self-care management behaviors are symptom- and disease-specific. For example, a patient with asthma may recognize the symptom of shortness of breath. This patient can manage the symptom by using an inhaler and seeing if their breathing improves. A patient with heart failure manages their condition by recognizing symptoms such as swelling and shortness of breath. Self-care management behaviors for heart failure may include taking a water pill, limiting fluid and salt intake, and seeking help from a healthcare provider.

Regular self-care monitoring is needed to identify symptoms early and judge the effectiveness of treatments. Some examples include:

- Inject insulin in response to high blood sugar and then re-check to evaluate if blood glucose lowered
- Use social support and healthy leisure activities to fight feelings of social isolation. This has been shown to be effective for patients with chronic lung disease

Unique Factors Influencing Self-care Management

Access to care: Access to care is a major barrier affecting self-care management. Treatment of symptoms might require consultation with a healthcare provider. Access to the health care system is largely influenced by providers. Many people suffering from a chronic illness do not have access to providers within the health care system for several reasons. Three major barriers to care include: insurance coverage, poor access to services, and being unable to afford costs. Without access to trained health care providers, outcomes are typically worse.

Financial constraints: Financial barriers impact self-care management. The majority of insurance coverage is provided by employers. Loss of employment is frequently accompanied by loss of health insurance and inability to afford health care. In patients with diabetes and chronic heart disease, financial barriers are associated with poor access to care, poor quality of care, and vascular disease. As a result, these patients have reduced rates of medical assessments, measurements of Hemoglobin A1C (a marker that assesses blood glucose levels over the last 3 months), cholesterol measurements, eye and foot examinations, diabetes education, and aspirin use. Research has found that people in higher social classes are better at self-care management of chronic conditions. In addition, people with lower levels of education often lack resources to effectively engage in self-management behaviors.

Age: Elderly patients are more likely to rate their symptoms differently and delay seeking care longer when they have symptoms. For example, an elderly person with heart failure may experience the symptom of shortness of breath differently than someone with heart failure who is younger. There are many reasons contributing to this difference in symptom experience. Providers should be aware of the potential delay in provider-seeking behavior in elderly patients which could worsen their overall condition.

Prior experience: Prior experience contributes to the development of skills in self-care management. Experience helps the patient develop cues and patterns that they can remember and follow, leading to reasonable goals and actions in repeat situations(. A patient who has skills in self-management knows what to do during repeated symptomatic events. This could lead to them recognizing their symptoms earlier, and seeking a provider sooner.

Health care literacy: Health care literacy is another factor affecting self-care management. Health care literacy is the amount of basic health information people are able to understand. Health care literacy is the major variable contributing to differences in patient ratings of self-management support. Successful self-care involves understanding the meaning of changes in one's body. Individuals who can identify changes in their body are then able to come up with options and decide on a course of action(. Health education at the patient's literacy level can increase the patient's ability to problem solve, set goals, and acquire skills in applying practical information. A patient's literacy can also affect their rating of healthcare quality. A poor healthcare experience may cause a patient to avoid returning to that same provider. This creates a delay in acute symptom management. Providers must consider health literacy when designing treatment plans that require self-management skills.

Co-morbid conditions: A patient with multiple chronic illnesses may experience compounding effects of their illnesses. This can include worsening of one condition by the symptoms or treatment of another. People tend to prioritize one of their conditions. This limits the self-care management of their other illnesses. One condition may have more noticeable symptoms than others. Or the patient may be more emotionally connected to one illness, for example, the one they have had for a long time. If providers are unaware of the effect of having multiple illnesses, the patient's overall health may fail to improve or worsen as a result of therapeutic efforts.

Ways to Improve Self-care Management

There are many ways for patients and healthcare providers to work together to improve the patient's self-care management. Stoplight and skill teaching allow patients and providers to work together to develop decision-making strategies.

1. Stoplight is an action plan for the daily treatment of a patient's chronic illness created by the healthcare team and the patient. It makes decision making easier by categorizing signs and symptoms and determining the appropriate actions for each set. It separates signs and symptoms into three zones:

- *Green* is the safe zone, meaning the patient's signs and symptoms are what is typically expected. The patient should continue with their daily self-care tasks, such as taking daily medications and eating a healthy diet.
- *Yellow* is the caution zone, meaning the patient's signs and symptoms should be monitored as they are abnormal, but they are not yet dangerous. Some actions may need to be taken in this zone in order to go back to the green zone, for instance taking an additional medication. The patient may need to contact their healthcare team for advice.
- *Red* is the danger zone, meaning the patient's signs and symptoms show that something is dangerously wrong. If in this category the patient needs to take actions to return to the green category, such as taking an emergency medication, as well as contact their healthcare team immediately. They may also need to contact emergency medical assistance.

The stoplight plan helps patients to make decisions about what actions to take for different signs and symptoms and when to contact their healthcare team with a problem. The patient and their provider will customize certain signs and symptoms that fit in each stoplight category.

2. Skills teaching is a learning opportunity between a healthcare provider and a patient where a patient learns a skill in self-care unique to his or her chronic illness. Some of these skills may be applied to the daily management of the symptoms of a chronic illness. Other skills may be applied when there is an exacerbation of a symptom. An exacerbation of a symptom means that the symptom is in a worsened state or is different from what the patient normally experiences. The patient should not only learn the purpose of self-care skills. It is also important to learn when to apply skills in daily management of a chronic illness and how the skill might be modified or changed when the patient experiences an exacerbation of a symptom.

For example, a patient newly diagnosed with persistent asthma might learn about taking an oral medicine for daily management, control of chronic symptoms and prevention of an asthma attack. However, there may come a time when the patient might be exposed to an environmental trigger or stress that causes an asthma attack. The patient starts to experience shortness of breath, chest tightness or wheezing. When this unexpected symptom occurs, the skill of taking daily medicines and the medicine that is taken may change. Rather than taking an oral medicine daily, a different medication is needed for quick rescue and relief of symptoms. The rescue medication works quickly with an inhaler. Knowing to choose the right medication and knowing how to take the medicine with an inhaler is a skill that is learned for the self-care management of asthma.

In skills teaching, it is important for the patient and provider to discuss skills and address any lingering questions. It is important for the patient to know when and how a skill is to be implemented, and how the skill may need to be changed when the symptom is different from normal. Learning self-care management skills for the first time in the care of a chronic illness is not easy, but with patience, practice, persistence and experience, personal mastery of self-care skills can be achieved.

Support

Self-care support can include the following:

- Self-care information on health and human body systems, lifestyle and healthy eating.
- Support to capture, manage, interpret, and report observations of daily living (ODLs), the tracking of trends, and the use of the resulting information as clues for self-care action and decision making.
- Information prescriptions providing personalised information and instructions to enable an individual to self-care and take control of their health
- Self-care and self-monitoring devices and assistive technology
- Self-care skills and life skills training programmes and courses for people
- Aid from spiritual care givers
- Advice from licensed counselors, clinical social workers, psychotherapists, pharmacists, physiotherapists and complementary therapists
- Self-care support networks which can be face to face or virtual, and made up of peers or people who want to provide support to others or receive support and information from others (including a self-care primer for provider/consumer convergence.)
- Being attuned to one's spirituality

Approaches

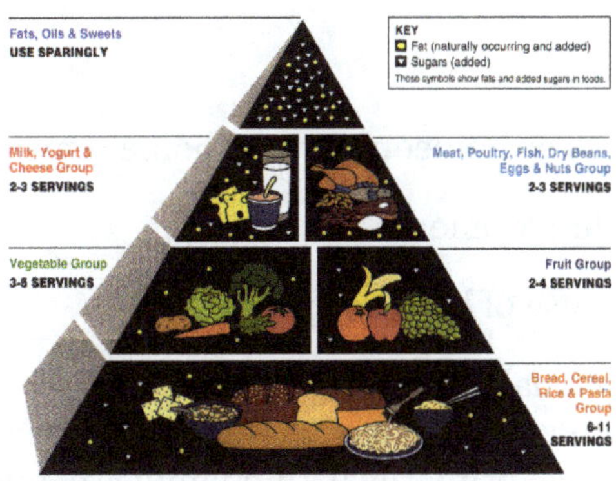

Food pyramid

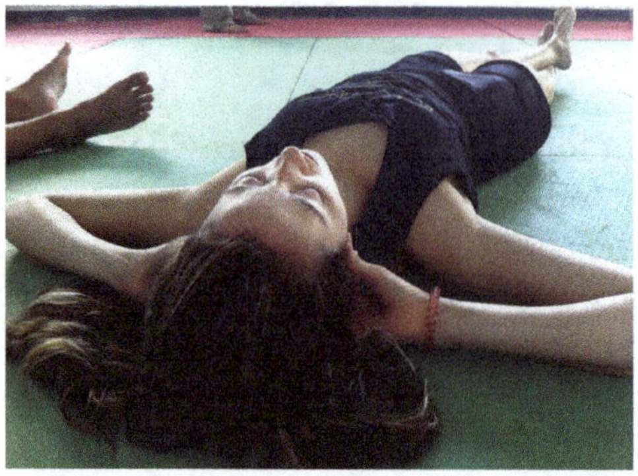

Self-massage

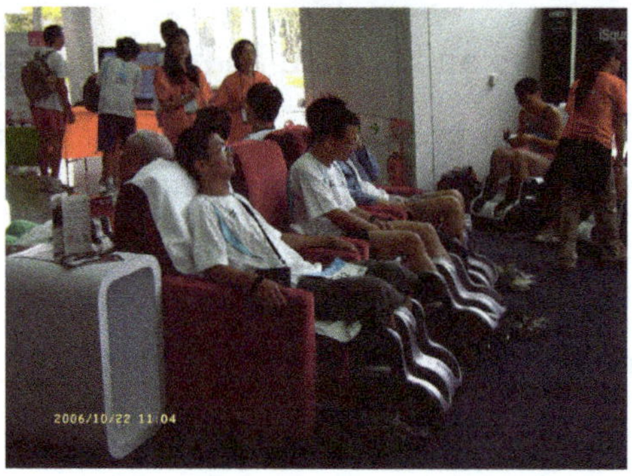

Massage with robotic massage chairs.

Self-care practices are shaped by what are seen as the proper lifestyle choices of local communities. Health-related self-care topics include:

- General fitness training and physical exercise
- Healthy diet, meals, diet foods and fasting
- Smoking cessation and avoiding alcohol abuse
- Personal hygiene
- Life extension
- Pain management
- Stress management
- Alternative medicine such as homeopathy and home remedies
- Self-help and personal development
- Self-care portals and the use of health apps

A lack of self-care in terms of personal health, hygiene and living conditions is referred to as self-neglect. The use of caregivers and Personal Care Assistants may be needed. An aging population is seeking greater self-care knowledge primarily within families connections and with responsibility usually belonging to the mother.

Philosophy

Michel Foucault understood the art of living (French *art de vivre*, Latin *ars vivendi*) and the care of self (French *le souci de soi*) to be central to philosophy. The third volume of his three-volume study *The History of Sexuality* is dedicated to this notion. For Foucault, the notion of *care of self* (*epimeleia heautou*) of Ancient Greek and Roman philosophy comprises an attitude towards the self, others and the world, as well as a certain form of attention. For Foucault, the pursuit of the care for one's own well-being also comprises self-knowledge (gnōthi seauton).

The self-care deficit nursing theory was developed by Dorothea Orem between 1959 and 2001. The positively viewed theory explores the use professional care and an orientation towards resources. Under Orem's model self-care has limits when its possibilities have been exhausted therefore making professional care legitimate. These deficits in self-care are seen as shaping the best role a nurse may provide. There are two phases in Orem's self-care; the investigative and decision-making phase and the production phase.

Health Professional

A health professional, health practitioner or healthcare provider (sometimes simply "provider") is an individual who provides preventive, curative, promotional or rehabilitative health care services in a systematic way to people, families or communities.

A health professional may operate within all branches of health care, including medicine, surgery, dentistry, midwifery, pharmacy, psychology, nursing or allied health professions. A health professional may also be a public/community health expert working for the common good of the society.

Practitioners and Professionals

Healthcare practitioners include physicians, dentists, pharmacists, pharmacy technicians, physician assistants, nurses, advanced practice registered nurses, surgeons, surgeon's assistant, athletic trainers, surgical technologist, midwives, dietitians, therapists, psychologists, chiropractors, clinical officers, social workers, phlebotomists, occupational therapists, optometrists, physical therapists, radiographers, radiotherapists, respiratory therapists, audiologists, speech pathologists, operating department practitioners, emergency medical technicians, paramedics, medical laboratory scientists, medical prosthetic technicians and a wide variety of other human resources trained to provide some type of health care service. They often work in hospitals, healthcare centres, and other service delivery points, but also in academic training, research, and administration. Some provide care and treatment services for patients in private homes. Many countries have a large number of community health workers who work outside formal healthcare institutions. Managers of healthcare services, health information technicians, and other assistive personnel and support workers are also considered a vital part of health care teams.

Healthcare practitioners are commonly grouped into health professions. Within each field of expertise, practitioners are often classified according to skill level and skill specialization. "Health professionals" are highly skilled workers, in professions that usually require extensive knowledge including university-level study leading to the award of a first degree or higher qualification. This category includes physicians, physician assistants, dentists, midwives, radiographers, registered nurses, pharmacists, physiotherapists, optometrists, operating department practitioners and others. Allied health professionals, also referred to as "health associate professionals" in the International Standard Classification of Occupations, support implementation of health care, treatment and referral plans usually established by medical, nursing, and other health professionals, and usually require formal qualifications to practice their profession. In addition, unlicensed assistive personnel assist with providing health care services as permitted.

Another way to categorize healthcare practitioners is according to the sub-field in which they practice, such as mental health care, pregnancy and childbirth care, surgical care, rehabilitation care, or public health.

Mental Health Practitioners

A mental health practitioner is a health worker who offers services for the purpose of improving the mental health of individuals or treating mental illness. These include psychiatrists, clinical psychologists, clinical social workers, psychiatric-mental health nurse practitioners, marriage and family therapists, mental health counselors, as well as other health professionals and allied health professions. These health care providers often deal with the same illnesses, disorders, conditions, and issues; however their scope of practice often differs. The most significant difference across categories of mental health practitioners is education and training.

Maternal and Newborn Health Practitioners

A maternal and newborn health practitioner is a health worker who deals with the care of women and their children before, during and after pregnancy and childbirth. Such health practitioners include obstetricians, midwives, obstetrical nurses and many others. One of the main differences between these professions is in the training and authority to provide surgical services and other life-saving interventions. In some developing countries, traditional birth attendants, or traditional midwives, are the primary source of pregnancy and childbirth care for many women and families, although they are not certified or licensed.

Geriatric Care Practitioners

A geriatric care practitioner plans and coordinates the care of the elderly and/or disabled to promote their health, improve their quality of life, and maintain their independence for as long as possible. They include geriatricians, adult-gerontology nurse practitioners, clinical nurse specialists, geriatric clinical pharmacists, geriatric nurses, geriatric care managers, geriatric aides,Nursing aides, Caregivers and others who focus on the health and psychological care needs of older adults.

Surgical Practitioners

A surgical practitioner is a healthcare professional who specializes in the planning and delivery of a patient's perioperative care, including during the anaesthetic, surgical and recovery stages. They may include general and specialist surgeons, surgeon's assistant, assistant surgeon, surgical assistant, anesthesiologists, anesthesiologist assistant, nurse anesthetists, surgical nurses, clinical officers, operating department practitioners, anaesthetic technicians, perioperative nursing, surgical technologists, and others.

Rehabilitation Care Practitioners

A rehabilitation care practitioner is a health worker who provides care and treatment which aims to enhance and restore functional ability and quality of life to those with physical impairments or disabilities. These include physiatrists, rehabilitation nurses, clinical nurse specialists, nurse practitioners, physiotherapists, orthotists, prosthetists, occupational therapists, recreational therapists, audiologists, speech and language pathologists, respiratory therapists, rehabilitation counsellors, physical rehabilitation therapists, athletic trainers, physiotherapy technicians, orthotic technicians, prosthetic technicians, personal care assistants, and others.

Eye Care Practitioners

Care and treatment for the eye and the adnexa may be delivered by ophthalmologists specializing in surgical/medical care, or optometrists specializing in refractive management and medical/therapeutic care.

Medical Diagnosis Providers

Medical diagnosis providers are health workers responsible for the process of determining which disease or condition explains a person's symptoms and signs. It is most often referred to as diagnosis with the medical context being implicit. This usually involves a team of healthcare providers in various diagnostic units. These include radiographers, radiologists, medical laboratory scientists, pathologists, and related professionals.

Oral Care Practitioners

A dental care practitioner is a health worker who provides care and treatment to promote and restore oral health. These include dentists and dental surgeons, dental assistants, dental auxiliaries, dental hygienists, dental nurses, dental technicians, dental therapists, and related professionals.

Foot Care Practitioners

Care and treatment for the foot, ankle, and lower leg may be delivered by podiatrists, pedorthists, foot health practitioners, podiatric medical assistants, podiatric nurse and others.

Public Health Practitioners

A public health practitioner focuses on improving health among individuals, families and communities through the prevention and treatment of diseases and injuries, surveillance of cases, and promotion of healthy behaviors. This category includes community and preventive medicine specialists, public health nurses, clinical nurse specialists, dietitians, environmental health officers, paramedics, epidemiologists, health inspectors, and others.

Alternative Medicine Practitioners

In many societies, practitioners of alternative medicine have contact with a significant number of people, either as integrated within or remaining outside the formal health care system. These include practitioners in acupuncture, Ayurveda, herbalism, homeopathy, naturopathy, Siddha medicine, traditional Chinese medicine, traditional Korean medicine, and Unani. In some countries such as Canada, chiropractors and osteopaths (are different than doctors of osteopathic medicine in the United States) are considered alternative medicine practitioners.

Practice Conditions and Regulations

Shortages of Health Professionals

Many jurisdictions report shortfalls in the number of trained health human resources to meet population health needs and/or service delivery targets, especially in medically underserved areas. For example, in the United States, the 2010 federal budget invested $330 million to increase the number of doctors, nurses, and dentists practicing in areas of the country experiencing shortages of trained health professionals. The Budget expands loan repayment programs for physicians, nurses, and dentists who agree to practice in medically underserved areas. This funding will enhance the capacity of nursing schools to increase the number of nurses. It will also allow states to increase access to oral health care through dental workforce development grants. The Budget's new resources will sustain the expansion of the health care workforce funded in the Recovery Act. There were 15.7 million health care professionals in the US as of 2011.

In Canada, the 2011 federal budget announced a Canada Student Loan forgiveness program to encourage and support new family physicians, nurse practitioners and nurses to practice in underserved rural or remote communities of the country, including communities that provide health services to First Nations and Inuit populations.

In Uganda, the Ministry of Health reports that as many as 50% of staffing positions for health workers in rural and underserved areas remain vacant. As of early 2011, the Ministry was conducting research and costing analyses to determine the most appropriate attraction and retention packages for medical officers, nursing officers, pharmacists, and laboratory technicians in the country's rural areas.

At the international level, the World Health Organization estimates a shortage of almost 4.3 million doctors, midwives, nurses, and support workers worldwide to meet target coverage levels of essential primary health care interventions. The shortage is reported most severe in 57 of the poorest countries, especially in sub-Saharan Africa.

Occupational Hazards

Occupational stress and occupational burnout are highly prevalent among health professionals. Some studies suggest that workplace stress is pervasive in the health care industry because of inadequate staffing levels, long work hours, exposure to infectious diseases and hazardous substances leading to illness or death, and in some countries threat of malpractice litigation. Other stressors include the emotional labor of caring for ill people and high patient loads. The consequences of this stress can include substance abuse, suicide, major depressive disorder, and anxiety, all of which occur at higher rates in health professionals than the general working population. Elevated levels of stress are also linked to high rates of burnout, absenteeism and diagnostic errors, and to reduced rates of patient satisfaction. In Canada, a national report (*Canada's Health Care Providers*) also indicated higher rates of absenteeism due to illness or disability among health care workers compared to the rest of the working population, although those working in health care reported similar levels of good health and fewer reports of being injured at work. There is some evidence that cognitive-behavioral therapy, relaxation training and therapy (including meditation and massage), and modifying schedules can reduce stress and burnout among multiple sectors of health care providers. Research is ongoing in this area, especially with regards to physicians, whose occupational stress and burnout is less researched compared to other health professions.

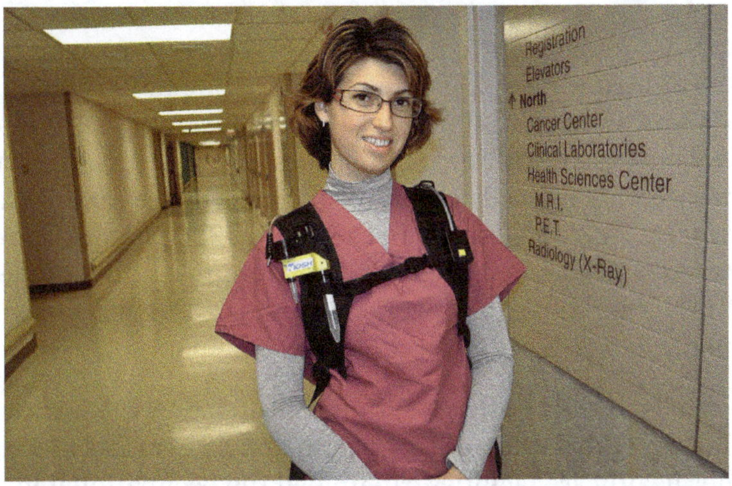

A healthcare professional wears an air sampling device to investigate exposure to airborne influenza

Exposure to respiratory infectious diseases like tuberculosis (caused by *Mycobacterium tuberculosis*) and influenza can be reduced with the use of respirators; this exposure is a significant occupational hazard for health care professionals. Exposure to dangerous chemicals, including chemotherapy drugs, is another potential occupational risk. These drugs can cause cancer and other health conditions. Healthcare workers are also at risk for diseases that are contracted through extended contact with a patient, including scabies. Health professionals are also at risk for contracting blood-borne diseases like hepatitis B, hepatitis C, and HIV/AIDS through needlestick injuries or through contact with bodily fluids. This risk can be mitigated with vaccination when there is a vaccine available, like with hepatitis B. In epidemic situations, such as the 2014-2016 West African Ebola virus epidemic or the 2003 SARS outbreak, healthcare workers are at even greater risk, and were disproportionately affected in both the Ebola and SARS outbreaks. In general, appropriate personal protective equipment (PPE) is the first-line mode of protection for healthcare workers from infectious diseases. For it to be effective against highly contagious diseases, personal protective equipment must be watertight and prevent the skin and mucous membranes from contacting infectious material. Different levels of personal protective equipment created to unique standards are used in situations where the risk of infection is different. Practices such as triple gloving and multiple respirators do not provide a higher level of protection and present a burden to the worker, who is additionally at increased risk of exposure when removing the PPE. Compliance with appropriate personal protective equipment rules may be difficult in certain situations, such as tropical environment or low-resource settings. A 2016 Cochrane systematic review found low quality evidence that using more breathable fabric in PPE, double gloving, and active training reduce the risk of contamination.

Female health care workers may face specific types of workplace-related health conditions and stress. According to the World Health Organization, women predominate in the formal health workforce in many countries, and are prone to musculoskeletal injury (caused by physically demanding job tasks such as lifting and moving patients) and burnout. Female health workers are exposed to hazardous drugs and chemicals in the workplace which may cause adverse reproductive outcomes such as spontaneous abortion and congenital malformations. In some contexts, female health workers are also subject to gender-based violence including from coworkers and patients.

Healthcare workers are at higher risk of on-the-job injury due to violence. Drunk, confused, and hostile patients and visitors are a continual threat to providers attempting to treat patients. Frequently, assault and violence in a healthcare setting goes unreported and is wrongly assumed to be part of the job. Violent incidents typically occur during one-on-one care; being alone with patients increases healthcare workers' risk of assault. In the United States, healthcare workers suffer ⅔ of nonfatal workplace violence incidents. Psychiatric units represent the highest proportion of violent incidents, at 40%; they are followed by geriatric units (20%) and the emergency department (10%). Workplace violence can also cause psychological trauma.

The Occupational Health Safety Network is a system developed by the National Institute for Occupational Safety and Health (NIOSH) to address health and safety risks among health care providers. Hospitals and other healthcare facilities can upload the occupational injury data they already collect to the secure database for analysis and benchmarking with other de-identified facilities from throughout the U.S. NIOSH works with OHSN participants in identifying and implementing timely and targeted interventions. OHSN modules currently focus on three high risk and preventable events that can lead to injuries or musculoskeletal disorders among healthcare providers: musculoskeletal injuries from patient handling activities; slips, trips, and falls; and workplace violence. Slips, trips, and falls are the second-most common cause of worker's compensation claims in the US, and cause 21% of work absences due to injury. These injuries most commonly result in strains and sprains; women, those older than 45, and those who have been working less than a year in a healthcare setting are at the highest risk.

Health care professionals are also likely to experience sleep deprivation due to their jobs. Many health care professionals are on a shift work schedule, and therefore experience misalignment of their work schedule and their circadian rhythm. In 2007, 32% of healthcare workers were found to get fewer than 6 hours of sleep a night. Sleep deprivation also predisposes healthcare professionals to make mistakes that may potentially endanger a patient.

Regulation and Registration of Professionals

Practicing without a license that is valid and current is typically illegal. In most jurisdictions, the provision of health care services is regulated by the government. Individuals found to be providing medical, nursing or other professional services without the appropriate certification or license may face sanctions and criminal charges leading to a prison term. The number of professions subject to regulation, requisites for individuals to receive professional licensure, and nature of sanctions that can be imposed for failure to comply vary across jurisdictions.

In the United States, under Michigan state laws, an individual is guilty of felony if identified as practicing in the health profession without a valid personal license or registration. Health professionals can also be imprisoned if found guilty of practicing beyond the limits allowed by their licences and registration. The state laws define the scope of practice for medicine, nursing, and a number of allied health professions. In Florida, practicing medicine without the appropriate license is a crime classified as a third degree felony, which may give imprisonment up to five years. Practicing a health care profession without a license which results in serious bodily injury classifies as a second degree felony, providing up to 15 years' imprisonment.

In the United Kingdom, healthcare professionals are regulated by the state; the UK Health and Care Professions Council (HCPC) protects the 'title' of each profession it regulates. For example, it is illegal for someone to call himself an Occupational Therapist or Radiographer if they are not on the register held by the HCPC.

Primary Care

Primary care is the day-to-day healthcare given by a health care provider. Typically this provider acts as the first contact and principal point of continuing care for patients within a healthcare system, and coordinates other specialist care that the patient may need. Patients commonly receive primary care from professionals such as a primary care physician (general practitioner or family physician), a nurse practitioner (adult-gerontology nurse practitioner, family nurse practitioner, or pediatric nurse practitioner), or a physician assistant. In some localities such a professional may be a registered nurse, a pharmacist, a clinical officer (as in parts of Africa), or a Ayurvedic or other traditional medicine professional (as in parts of Asia). Depending on the nature of the health condition, patients may then be referred for secondary or tertiary care.

Background

The World Health Organization attributes the provision of essential primary care as an integral component of an inclusive primary healthcare strategy. Primary care involves the widest scope of healthcare, including all ages of patients, patients of all socioeconomic and geographic origins, patients seeking to maintain optimal health, and patients with all manner of acute and chronic physical, mental and social health issues, including multiple chronic diseases. Consequently, a primary care practitioner must possess a wide breadth of knowledge in many areas. Continuity is a key characteristic of primary care, as patients usually prefer to consult the same practitioner for routine check-ups and preventive care, health education, and every time they require an initial consultation about a new health problem. Collaboration among providers is a desirable characteristic of primary care.

The International Classification of Primary Care (ICPC) is a standardized tool for understanding and analyzing information on interventions in primary care by the reason for the patient visit. Common chronic illnesses usually treated in primary care may include, for example: hypertension, angina, diabetes, asthma, COPD, depression and anxiety, back pain, arthritis or thyroid dysfunction. Primary care also includes many basic maternal and child health care services, such as family planning services and vaccinations.

In context of global population ageing, with increasing numbers of older adults at greater risk of chonic non-communicable diseases, rapidly increasing demand for primary care services is expected around the world, in both developed and developing countries.

Primary Care by Country

United Kingdom

In the United Kingdom, patients can access primary care services through their local general practice, community pharmacy, optometrist, dental surgery and community hearing care providers. Services are generally provided free-of-charge through the National Health Service. In the UK, unlike many other countries, patients do not normally have direct access to hospital consultants and the GP controls access to secondary care. This practice is referred to as "gatekeeping"; the future of this role has been questioned by researchers who conclude "*Gatekeeping policies should be revisited to accommodate the government's aim to modernise the NHS in terms of giving patients more choice and facilitate more collaborative work between GPs and specialists. At the same time, any relaxation of gatekeeping should be carefully evaluated to ensure the clinical and non-clinical benefits outweigh the costs*".

599 GP practices closed between 2010–11 and 2014–15, while 91 opened and average practice list size increased from 6,610 to 7,171.

According to the Local Government Association 57 million GP consultations in England in 2015 were for minor conditions and illnesses, 5.2 million of them for blocked noses.

Canada

In Canada, access to primary and other healthcare services are guaranteed for all citizens through the Canada Health Act.

Nigeria

In Nigeria, healthcare is a concurrent responsibility of three tiers of government. Local governments focus on the delivery of primary care (e.g. through a system of dispensaries), state governments manage the various general hospitals (secondary care), while the federal government's role is mostly limited to coordinating the affairs of the Federal Medical Centres and university teaching hospitals (tertiary care).

United States

A 2009 report by the New England Healthcare Institute determined that an increased demand on primary care by older, sicker patients and decreased supply of primary care practitioners has led to a crisis in primary care delivery. The research identified a set of innovations that could enhance the quality, efficiency and effectiveness of primary care in the United States.

On March 23, 2010 President Obama signed the Patient Protection and Affordable Care Act (ACA) into law. The law is estimated to have expanded health insurance coverage by 20 million people by early 2016 and is expected to expand health care to 34 million people by 2021. The success of the expansion of health insurance under the ACA in large measure depends on the availability of primary care physicians. Unfortunately, The ACA has drastically exacerbated the projected deficit of primary care physicians needed to ensure care for insured Americans. According to the Association of American Medical Colleges (AAMC) without the ACA, the United States would have been short roughly 64,000 physicians by 2020; with the implementation of the ACA, it will be 91,000 physicians short. According to the AAMC's November 2009 physician work force report, nationally, the rate of physicians providing primary care is 79.4 physicians per 100,000 residents.

Primary healthcare results in better health outcomes, reduced health disparities and lower spending, including on avoidable emergency room visits and hospital care. With that being said, primary care physicians are an important component in ensuring that the healthcare system as a whole is sustainable. However, despite their importance to the healthcare system, the primary care position has suffered in terms of its prestige in part due to the differences in salary when compared to doctors that decide to specialize. In a 2010 national study of physician wages conducted by the UC Davis Health System found that specialists are paid as much as 52 percent more than primary care physicians, even though primary care physicians see far more patients.

Primary care physicians earn $60.48 per hour; specialists on average earn $88.34. A follow up study conducted by the UC Davis Health System found that earnings over the course of the careers of primary care physicians averaged as much as $2.8 million less than the earnings of their specialist colleagues. This discrepancy in pay has potentially made primary care a less attractive choice for medical school graduates. In 2015, almost 19,000 doctors graduated from American medical schools and only 7 percent of graduates chose a career in primary care. The average age of a primary care physician in the United States is 47 years old, and one quarter of all primary care physicians are nearing retirement. Fifty years ago roughly half of the physicians in America practiced primary care; today, fewer than one third of them do.

US Strategies to Address the Primary Care Shortage

The Patient Protection Affordable Care Act contains a number of provisions to increase primary care capacity. These provisions are directed towards medical school graduates and include payment reform, student loan forgiveness programs and increased primary care residency positions The PPACA also provides funding and mandates to increase the role of physician extenders like nurse practitioners and physician assistants to enhance the primary care workforce. The PPCA is projected to increase patient demand for primary care services. Through the adoption of new patient care delivery models that include physicians working in tandem with nurse practitioners and physician assistants, demand for future primary care services could be met. Consumer surveys have found the American public to be open to a greater role for physician extenders in the primary care setting. Policies and laws, primarily at the state level, would need to redefine and reallocate the roles and responsibilities for non-physician licensed providers to optimize these new models of care.

Primary Healthcare

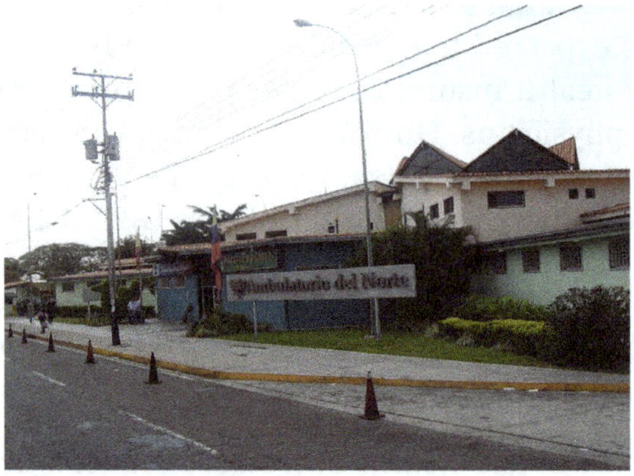

Public ambulatory care facility in Maracay, Venezuela, providing primary care for ambulatory care sensitive conditions.

Primary healthcare (PHC) refers to "essential health care" that is based on scientifically sound and socially acceptable methods and technology, which make universal health care accessible to all individuals and families in a community. It is through their full participation and at a cost that the community and the country can afford to maintain at every stage of their development in the spirit of self-reliance and self-determination". In other words, PHC is an approach to health beyond the traditional health care system that focuses on health equity-producing social policy. PHC includes all areas that play a role in health, such as access to health services, environment and lifestyle. Thus, primary healthcare and public health measures, taken together, may be considered as the cornerstones of universal health systems.

This ideal model of healthcare was adopted in the declaration of the International Conference on Primary Health Care held in Alma Ata, Kazakhstan in 1978 (known as the "Alma Ata Declaration"), and became a core concept of the World Health Organization's goal of *Health for all*. The Alma-Ata Conference mobilized a "Primary Health Care movement" of professionals and institutions, governments and civil society organizations, researchers and grassroots organizations that undertook to tackle the "politically, socially and economically unacceptable" health inequalities in all countries. There were many factors that inspired PHC; a prominent example is the Barefoot doctors of China.

Goals and Principles

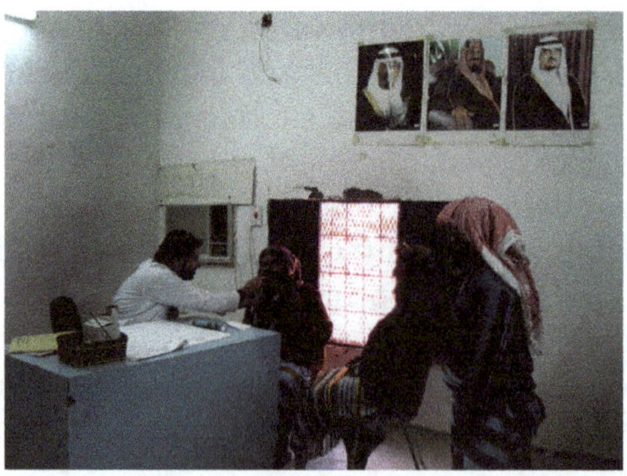

A primary health care worker in Saudi Arabia, 2008

The ultimate goal of primary healthcare is the attainment of better health services for all. It is for this reason that World Health Organization (WHO), has identified five key elements to achieving this goal:

- reducing exclusion and social disparities in health (universal coverage reforms);
- organizing health services around people's needs and expectations (service delivery reforms);
- integrating health into all sectors (public policy reforms);
- pursuing collaborative models of policy dialogue (leadership reforms); and
- increasing stakeholder participation.

Behind these elements lies a series of basic principles identified in the Alma Ata Declaration that should be formulated in national policies in order to launch and sustain PHC as part of a comprehensive health system and in coordination with other sectors:

- Equitable distribution of health care – according to this principle, primary care and other services to meet the main health problems in a community must be provided equally to all individuals irrespective of their gender, age, caste, color, urban/rural location and social class.
- Community participation – in order to make the fullest use of local, national and other available resources. Community participation was considered sustainable due to its grass roots nature and emphasis on self-sufficiency, as opposed to targeted (or vertical) approaches dependent on international development assistance.
- Health workforce development – comprehensive healthcare relies on adequate number and distribution of trained physicians, nurses, allied health professions, community health workers and others working as a health team and supported at the local and referral levels.
- Use of appropriate technology – medical technology should be provided that is accessible, affordable, feasible and culturally acceptable to the community. Examples of appropriate technology include refrigerators for vaccine cold storage. Less appropriate could include, in many settings, body scanners or heart-lung machines, which benefit only a small minority concentrated in urban areas. They are generally not accessible to the poor, but draw a large share of resources.
- Multi-sectional approach – recognition that health cannot be improved by intervention within just the formal health sector; other sectors are equally important in promoting the health and self-reliance of communities. These sectors include, at least: agriculture (e.g. food security); education; communication (e.g. concerning prevailing health problems and the methods of preventing and controlling them); housing; public works (e.g. ensuring an adequate supply of safe water and basic sanitation); rural development; industry; community organizations (including Panchayats or local governments, voluntary organizations, etc.).

In sum, PHC recognizes that healthcare is not a short-lived intervention, but an ongoing process of improving people's lives and alleviating the underlying socioeconomic conditions that contribute to poor health. The principles link health and development, advocating political interventions, rather than passive acceptance of economic conditions.

Approaches

The hospital ship USNS *Mercy* (T-AH-19) in Manado, Indonesia, during Pacific Partnership 2012.

The primary health care approach has seen significant gains in health were applied even when adverse economic and political conditions prevail.

Although the declaration made at the Alma-Ata conference deemed to be convincing and plausible in specifying goals to PHC and achieving more effective strategies, it generated numerous criticisms and reactions worldwide. Many argued the declaration did not have clear targets, was too broad, and was not attainable because of the costs and aid needed. As a result, PHC approaches have evolved in different contexts to account for disparities in resources and local priority health problems; this is alternatively called the Selective Primary Health Care (SPHC) approach.

Selective PHC

After the year 1978 Alta Alma Conference, the Rockefeller Foundation held a conference in 1979 at its Bellagio conference center in Italy to address several concerns. Here, the idea of Selective Primary Health Care was introduced as a strategy to complement comprehensive PHC. It was based on a paper by Julia Walsh and Kenneth S. Warren entitled "Selective Primary Health Care, an Interim Strategy for Disease Control in Developing Countries". This new framework advocated a more economically feasible approach to PHC by only targeting specific areas of health, and choosing the most effective treatment plan in terms of cost and effectiveness. One of the foremost examples of SPHC is "GOBI" (growth monitoring, oral rehydration, breastfeeding, and immunization), focusing on combating the main diseases in developing nations.

GOBI-FFF

Selective PHC approach consists of techniques known collectively under the acronym "GOBI-FFF". It focuses on severe population health problems in certain developing countries, where a few diseases are responsible for high rates of infant and child mortality. Health care planning is employed to see which diseases require most attention and, subsequently, which intervention can be most effectively applied as part of primary care in a least-cost method. The targets and effects of Selective PHC are specific and measurable. The approach aims to prevent most health and nutrition problems before they begin:

- Growth monitoring: the monitoring of how much infants grow within a period, with the goal to understand needs for better early nutrition.
- Oral rehydration therapy: to combat dehydration associated with diarrhea
- Breastfeeding

- Immunization
- Family planning (birth spacing)
- Female education
- Food supplementation: for example, iron and folic acid fortification/supplementation to prevent deficiencies in pregnant women.

PHC and Population Aging

Given global demographic trends, with the numbers of people age 60 and over expected to double by 2025, PHC approaches have taken into account the need for countries to address the consequences of population ageing. In particular, in the future the majority of older people will be living in developing countries that are often the least prepared to confront the challenges of rapidly ageing societies, including high risk of having at least one chronic non-communicable disease, such as diabetes and osteoporosis. According to WHO, dealing with this increasing burden requires health promotion and disease prevention intervention at community level as well as disease management strategies within health care systems.

PHC and Mental Health

Some jurisdictions apply PHC principles in planning and managing their healthcare services for the detection, diagnosis and treatment of common mental health conditions at local clinics, and organizing the referral of more complicated mental health problems to more appropriate levels of mental health care.

Background and Controversies

Barefoot Doctors

The "Barefoot doctors" of China were an important inspiration for PHC because they illustrated the effectiveness of having a healthcare professional at the community level with community ties. Barefoot doctors were a diverse array of village health workers who lived in rural areas and received basic healthcare training. They stressed rural rather than urban healthcare, and preventive rather than curative services. They also provided a combination of western and traditional medicines. They had close community ties, were relatively low-cost, and perhaps most importantly they encouraged self-reliance through advocating prevention and hygiene practices. The program experienced a massive expansion of rural medical services in China, with the number of barefoot doctors increasing dramatically between the early 1960s and the Cultural Revolution (1964-1976).

Criticisms

Although many countries were keen on the idea of primary healthcare after the Alma Ata conference, the Declaration itself was criticized for being too "idealistic" and "having an unrealistic time table". More specific approaches to prevent and control diseases - based on evidence of prevalence, morbidity, mortality and feasibility of control (cost-effectiveness) - were subsequently proposed. The best known model was the Selective PHC approach (described above). Selective PHC favoured short-term goals and targeted health investment, but it did not address the social causes of disease. As such, the SPHC approach has been criticized as not following Alma Ata's core principle of everyone's entitlement to healthcare and health system development.

In Africa, the PHC system has been extended into isolated rural areas through construction of health posts and centers that offer basic maternal-child health, immunization, nutrition, first aid, and referral services. Implementation of PHC is said to be affected after the introduction of structural adjustment programs by the World Bank.

eHealth

eHealth (also written e-health) is a relatively recent term for healthcare practice supported by electronic processes and communication, dating back to at least 1999. Usage of the term varies. A study in 2005 found 51 unique definitions. Some argue that it is interchangeable with health informatics with a broad definition covering electronic/digital processes in health while others use it in the narrower sense of healthcare practice using the Internet. It can also include health applications and links on mobile phones, referred to as mHealth or m-Health. Since about 2011, the increasing recognition of the need for better cyber-security and regulation may result in the need for these specialized resources to develop safer eHealth solutions that can withstand these growing threats.

Types

The term can encompass a range of services or systems that are at the edge of medicine/healthcare and information technology, including:

- Electronic health record: enabling the communication of patient data between different healthcare professionals (GPs, specialists *etc.*);
- Computerized physician order entry: a means of requesting diagnostic tests and treatments electronically and receiving the results
- ePrescribing: access to prescribing options, printing prescriptions to patients and sometimes electronic transmission of prescriptions from doctors to pharmacists
- Clinical decision support system: providing information electronically about protocols and standards for healthcare professionals to use in diagnosing and treating patients
- Telemedicine: physical and psychological diagnosis and treatments at a distance, including telemonitoring of patients functions;
- Consumer health informatics: use of electronic resources on medical topics by healthy individuals or patients;
- Health knowledge management: *e.g.* in an overview of latest medical journals, best practice guidelines or epidemiological tracking (examples include physician resources such as Medscape and MDLinx);

- Virtual healthcare teams: consisting of healthcare professionals who collaborate and share information on patients through digital equipment (for transmural care);
- mHealth or m-Health: includes the use of mobile devices in collecting aggregate and patient level health data, providing healthcare information to practitioners, researchers, and patients, real-time monitoring of patient vitals, and direct provision of care (via mobile telemedicine);
- Medical research using grids: powerful computing and data management capabilities to handle large amounts of heterogeneous data.
- Health informatics / healthcare information systems: also often refer to software solutions for appointment scheduling, patient data management, work schedule management and other administrative tasks surrounding health.

Contested Definition

Several authors have noted the variable usage in the term, from being specific to the use of the Internet in healthcare to being generally around any use of computers in healthcare. Various authors have considered the evolution of the term and its usage and how this maps to changes in health informatics and healthcare generally. Oh *et al.*, in a 2005 systematic review of the term's usage, offered the definition of eHealth as a set of technological themes in health today, more specifically based on commerce, activities, stakeholders, outcomes, locations, or perspectives. One thing that all sources seem to agree on is that e-Health initiatives do not originate with the patient, though the patient may be a member of a patient organization that seeks to do this.

Data Exchange

One of the factors blocking the use of e-Health tools from widespread acceptance is the concern about privacy issues regarding patient records, most specifically the EPR (Electronic patient record). This main concern has to do with the confidentiality of the data. There is also concern about non-confidential data however. Each medical practise has its own jargon and diagnostic tools. To standardize the exchange of information, various coding schemes may be used in combination with international medical standards. Systems that deal with these transfers are often referred to as Health Information Exchange (HIE). Of the forms of e-Health already mentioned, there are roughly two types; front-end data exchange and back-end exchange.

Front-end exchange typically involves the patient, while back-end exchange does not. A common example of a rather simple front-end exchange is a patient sending a photo taken by mobile phone of a healing wound and sending it by email to the family doctor for control. Such an actions may avoid the cost of an expensive visit to the hospital.

A common example of a back-end exchange is when a patient on vacation visits a doctor who then may request access to the patient's health records, such as medicine prescriptions, x-ray photographs, or blood test results. Such an action may reveal allergies or other prior conditions that are relevant to the visit.

Thesaurus

Successful e-Health initiatives such as e-Diabetes have shown that for data exchange to be facilitated either at the front-end or the back-end, a common thesaurus is needed for terms of reference. Various medical practises in chronic patient care (such as for diabetic patients) already have a well defined set of terms and actions, which makes standard communication exchange easier, whether the exchange is initiated by the patient or the caregiver.

In general, explanatory diagnostic information (such as the standard ICD-10) may be exchanged insecurely, and private information (such as personal information from the patient) must be secured. E-health manages both flows of information, while ensuring the quality of the data exchange.

Early Adopters

Patients living with long term conditions (also called Chronic conditions) over time often acquire a high level of knowledge about the processes involved in their own care, and often develop a routine in coping with their condition. For these types of routine patients, front-end e-Health solutions tend to be relatively easy to implement.

E-mental Health

E-mental health is frequently used to refer to internet based interventions and support for mental health conditions. However, it can also refer to the use of information and communication technologies that also includes the use of social media, landline and mobile phones. E-mental health services can include information; peer support services, computer and internet based programs, virtual applications and games as well as real time interaction with trained clinicians. Programs can also be delivered using telephones and interactive voice response (IVR)

Mental disorders includes a range of conditions such as alcohol and drug use disorders, mood disorders such as depression, dementia and Alzheimer's disease, delusional disorders such as schizophrenia and anxiety disorders. The majority of e-mental health interventions have focused on the treatment of depression and anxiety. There are, however, programs also for problems as diverse as smoking cessation gambling and post-disaster mental health.

Advantages and Disadvantages

E-mental health has a number of advantages such as being low cost, easily accessible and providing anonymity to users. However, there are also a number of disadvantages such as concerns regarding treatment credibility, user privacy and confidentiality. Online security involves the implementation of appropriate safeguards to protect user privacy and confidentiality. This includes appropriate collection and handling of user data, the protection of data from unauthorized access and modification and the safe storage of data.

E-mental health has been gaining momentum in the academic research as well as practical arenas in a wide variety of disciplines such as psychology, clinical social work, family and marriage therapy, and mental health counseling. Testifying to this momentum, the E-Mental Health movement has its own international organization, The International Society for Mental Health Online.

Programs

There are at least four programs currently available to treat anxiety and depression. Two programs have been identified by the UK National Institute for Health and Care Excellence as cost effective for use in primary care. The first is *Fearfighter* which is a text based cognitive behavioral therapy program to treat people with phobias and the second is *Beating the Blues*, an interactive text, cartoon and video CBT program for anxiety and depression. Two programs have been supported for use in primary care by the Australian Government. The first is *Anxiety Online*, a text based program for the anxiety, depressive and eating disorders, and the second is *THIS WAY UP*, a set of interactive text, cartoon and video programs for the anxiety and depressive disorders.

There are a number of online programs relating to smoking cessation. *QuitCoach* is a personalised quit plan based on the users response to questions regarding giving up smoking and tailored individually each time the user logs into the site. *Freedom From Smoking* takes users through lessons that are grouped into modules that provide information and assignments to complete. The modules guide participants through steps such as preparing to quit smoking, stopping smoking and preventing relapse.

Other internet programs have been developed specifically as part of research into treatment for specific disorders. For example, an online self-directed therapy for problem gambling was developed to specifically test this as a method of treatment. All participants were given access to a website. The treatment group was provided with behavioural and cognitive strategies to reduce or quit gambling. This was presented in the form of a workbook which encouraged participants to self-monitor their gambling by maintaining an online log of gambling and gambling urges. Participants could also use a smartphone application to collect self-monitoring information. Finally participants could also choose to receive motivational email or text reminders of their progress and goals.

An internet based intervention was also developed for use after Hurricane Ike in 2009. During this study, 1,249 disaster-affected adults were randomly recruited to take part in the intervention. Participants were given a structured interview then invited to access the web intervention using a unique password. Access to the website was provided for a four-month period. As participants accessed the site they were randomly assigned to either the intervention. those assigned to the intervention were provided with modules consisting of information regarding effective coping strategies to manage mental health and health risk behaviour.

Cybermedicine

Cybermedicine is the use of the Internet to deliver medical services, such as medical consultations and drug prescriptions. It is the successor to telemedicine, wherein doctors would consult and treat patients remotely via telephone or fax.

Cybermedicine is already being used in small projects where images are transmitted from a primary care setting to a medical specialist, who comments on the case and suggests which intervention might benefit the patient. A field that lends itself to this approach is dermatology, where images of an eruption are communicated to a hospital specialist who determines if referral is necessary.

The field has also expanded to include online “ask the doctor” services that allow patients direct, paid access to consultations (with varying degrees of depth) with medical professionals (examples include Bundoo.com, Doctor Spring, Teladoc, and Ask The Doctor).

A Cyber Doctor, known in the UK as a Cyber Physician, is a medical professional who does consultation via the internet, treating virtual patients, who may never meet face to face. This is a new area of medicine which has been utilized by the armed forces and teaching hospitals offering online consultation to patients before making their decision to travel for unique medical treatment only offered at a particular medical facility.

Self-monitoring Healthcare Devices

Self-monitoring is the use of sensors or tools which are readily available to the general public to track and record personal data. The sensors are usually wearable devices and the tools are digitally available through mobile device applications. Self-monitoring devices were created for the purpose of allowing personal data to be instantly available to the individual to be analyzed. As of now, fitness and health monitoring are the most popular applications for self-monitoring devices. The biggest benefit to self-monitoring devices is the elimination of the necessity for third party hospitals to run tests, which are both expensive and lengthy. These devices are an important advancement in the field of personal health management.

Currently, self-monitoring healthcare devices exist in many forms. An example is the Nike+ Fuelband, which is a modified version of the original pedometer. This device is wearable on the wrist and allows one to set a personal goal for a daily energy burn. It records the calories burned and the number of steps taken for each day while simultaneously functioning as a watch. To add to the ease of the user interface, it includes both numeric and visual indicators of whether or not the individual has achieved his or her daily goal. Finally, it is also synced to an iPhone app which allows for tracking and sharing of personal record and achievements.

Other monitoring devices have more medical relevance. A well-known device of this type is the blood glucose monitor. The use of this device is restricted to diabetic patients and allows users to measure the blood glucose levels in their body. It is extremely quantitative and the results are available instantaneously. However, this device is not as independent of a self-monitoring device as the Nike+ Fuelband because it requires some patient education before use. One needs to be able to make connections between the levels of glucose and the effect of diet and exercise. In addition, the users must also understand how the treatment should be adjusted based on the results. In other words, the results are not just static measurements.

The demand for self-monitoring health devices is skyrocketing, as wireless health technologies have become especially popular in the last few years. In fact, it is expected that by 2016, self-monitoring health devices will account for 80% of wireless medical devices. The key selling point for these devices is the mobility of information for consumers. The accessibility of mobile devices such as smartphones and tablets has increased significantly within the past decade. This has made it easier for users to access real-time information in a number of peripheral devices.

There are still many future improvements for self-monitoring healthcare devices. Although most of these wearable devices have been excellent at providing direct data to the individual user, the biggest task which remains at hand is how to effectively use this data. Although the blood glucose monitor allows the user to take action based on the results, measurements such as the pulse rate, EKG signals, and calories do not necessarily serve to actively guide an individual's personal health-care management. Consumers are interested in qualitative feedback in addition to the quantitative measurements recorded by the devices.

Evaluation

Knowledge of the socio-economic performance of eHealth is limited, and findings from evaluations are often challenging to transfer to other settings. Socio-economic evaluations of some narrow types of mHealth can rely on health economic methodologies, but larger scale eHealth may have too many variables, and tortuous, intangible cause and effect links may need a wider approach. Why Do Evaluations of eHealth Programs Fail? An Alternative Set of Guiding Principles describes one way to do this.

In Developing Countries

eHealth in general, and telemedicine in particular, is a vital resource to remote regions of emerging and developing countries but is often difficult to establish because of the lack of communications infrastructure. For example, in Benin, hospitals often can become inaccessible due to flooding during the rainy season and across Africa, the low population density, along with severe weather conditions and the difficult financial situation in many African states, has meant that the majority of the African people are badly disadvantaged in medical care. In many regions there is not only a significant lack of facilities and trained health professionals, but also no access to eHealth because there is also no internet access in remote villages, or even a reliable electricity supply.

Internet connectivity, and the benefits of eHealth, can be brought to these regions using satellite broadband technology, and satellite is often the only solution where terrestrial access may be limited, or poor quality, and one that can provide a fast connection over a vast coverage area.

First Aid

First aid is the assistance given to any person suffering a sudden illness or injury, with care provided to preserve life, prevent the condition from worsening, and/or promote recovery. It includes initial intervention in a serious condition prior to professional medical help being available, such as performing CPR while awaiting an ambulance, as well as the complete treatment of minor conditions, such as applying a plaster to a cut. First aid is generally performed by the layperson, with many people trained in providing basic levels of first aid, and others willing to do so from acquired knowledge. Mental health first aid is an extension of the concept of first aid to cover mental health.

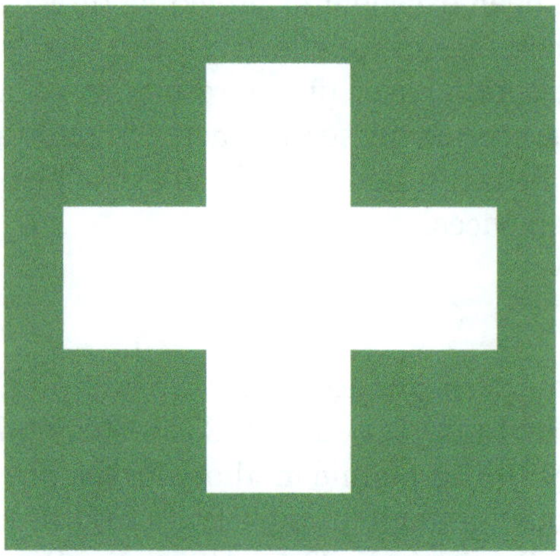

The universal first aid symbol

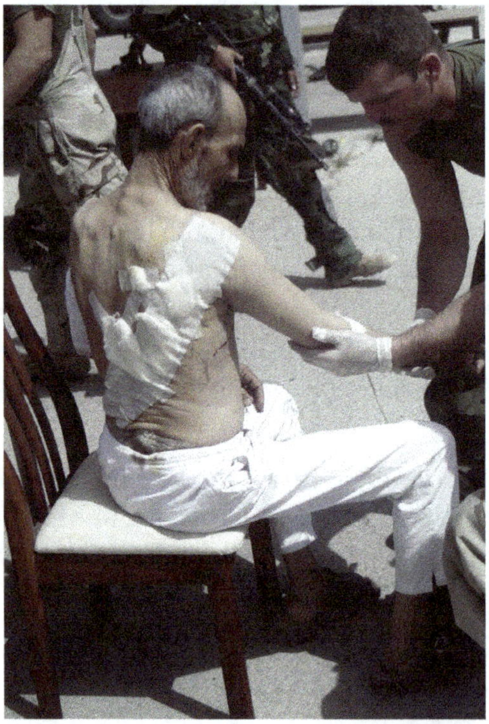

A US Navy corpsman gives first aid to an injured Iraqi citizen.

There are many situations which may require first aid, and many countries have legislation, regulation, or guidance which specifies a minimum level of first aid provision in certain circumstances. This can include specific training or equipment to be available in the workplace (such as an Automated External Defibrillator), the provision of specialist first aid cover at public gatherings, or mandatory first aid training within schools. First aid, however, does not necessarily require any particular equipment or prior knowledge, and can involve improvisation with materials available at the time, often by untrained persons.

First aid can be performed on all mammals, although this article relates to the care of human patients.

History

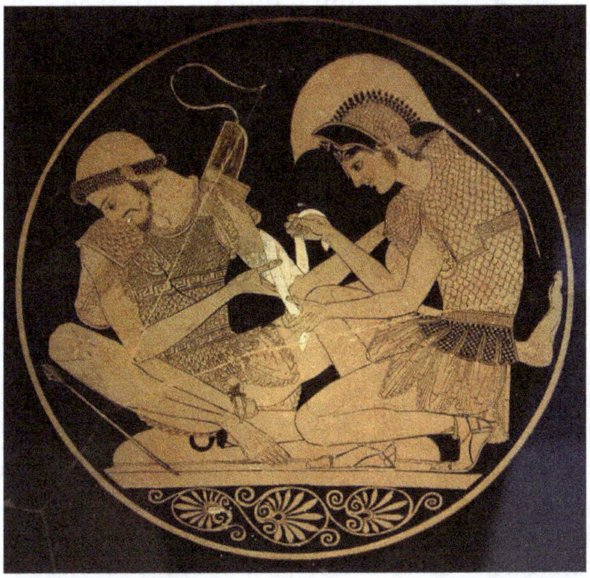

The binding of a battlefield wound depicted on ancient Greek pottery

Early History and Warfare

Skills of what is now known as first aid have been recorded throughout history, especially in relation to warfare, where the care of both traumatic and medical cases is required in particularly large numbers. The Ancient Egyptians (aka people of KMT) were the first to use bandages including the high genius doctor Imhotep. They not only used them to create mummies but also as part of the treatments for surgical patients. Most ancient Greek doctors, philosophers, etc studied in ancient Egypt and then returned to Greece. The bandaging of battle wounds is shown on Classical Greek pottery from circa 500 BCE, whilst the parable of the Good Samaritan includes references to binding or dressing wounds. There are numerous references to first aid performed within the Roman army, with a system of first aid supported by surgeons, field ambulances, and hospitals. Roman legions had the specific role of capsarii, who were responsible for first aid such as bandaging, and are the forerunners of the modern combat medic.

Further examples occur through history, still mostly related to battle, with examples such as the Knights Hospitaller in the 11th century CE, providing care to pilgrims and knights in the Holy Land.

Formalization of Life Saving Treatments

During the late 18th century, drowning as a cause of death was a major concern amongst the population. In 1767, a society for the preservation of life from accidents in water was started in Amsterdam, and in 1773, physician William Hawes began publicizing the power of artificial respiration as means of resuscitation of those who appeared drowned. This led to the formation, in 1774, of the Society for the Recovery of Persons Apparently Drowned, later the Royal Humane Society, who did much to promote resuscitation.

Napoleon's surgeon, Baron Dominique-Jean Larrey, is credited with creating an ambulance corps (the ambulance volantes), which included medical assistants, tasked to administer first aid in battle.

In 1859 Jean-Henri Dunant witnessed the aftermath of the Battle of Solferino, and his work led to the formation of the Red Cross, with a key stated aim of "aid to sick and wounded soldiers in the field". The Red Cross and Red Crescent are still the largest provider of first aid worldwide.

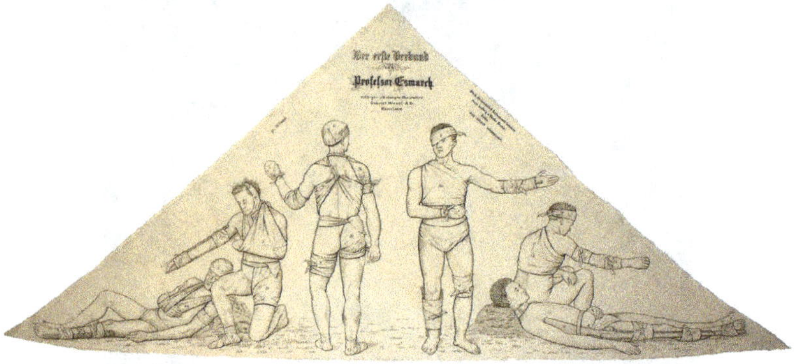

Esmarch bandage showing soldiers how to perform first aid

In 1870, Prussian military surgeon Friedrich von Esmarch introduced formalized first aid to the military, and first coined the term "erste hilfe" (translating to 'first aid'), including training for soldiers in the Franco-Prussian War on care for wounded comrades using pre-learnt bandaging and splinting skills, and making use of the Esmarch bandage which he designed. The bandage was issued as standard to the Prussian combatants, and also included aide-memoire pictures showing common uses.

In 1872, the Order of Saint John of Jerusalem in England changed its focus from hospice care, and set out to start a system of practical medical help, starting with making a grant towards the establishment of the UK's first ambulance service. This was followed by creating its own wheeled transport litter in 1875 (the St John Ambulance), and in 1877 established the St John Ambulance Association (the forerunner of modern-day St John Ambulance) "to train men and women for the benefit of the sick and wounded".

Also in the UK, Surgeon-Major Peter Shepherd had seen the advantages of von Esmarch's new teaching of first aid, and introduced an equivalent programme for the British Army, and so being the first user of "first aid for the injured" in English, disseminating information through a series of lectures. Following this, in 1878, Shepherd and Colonel Francis Duncan took advantage of the newly charitable focus of St John, and established the concept of teaching first aid skills to civilians. The first classes were conducted in the hall of the Presbyterian school in Woolwich (near Woolwich barracks where Shepherd was based) using a comprehensive first aid curriculum.

First aid training began to spread through the British Empire through organisations such as St John, often starting, as in the UK, with high risk activities such as ports and railways.

Aims

The key aims of first aid can be summarised in three key points, sometimes known as 'the three P's':-

- Preserve life: The overriding aim of all medical care which includes first aid, is to save lives and minimize the threat of death.

- Prevent further harm: Prevent further harm also sometimes called prevent the condition from worsening, or danger of further injury, this covers both external factors, such as moving a patient away from any cause of harm, and applying first aid techniques to prevent worsening of the condition, such as applying pressure to stop a bleed becoming dangerous.
- Promote recovery: First aid also involves trying to start the recovery process from the illness or injury, and in some cases might involve completing a treatment, such as in the case of applying a plaster to a small wound.

Key Skills

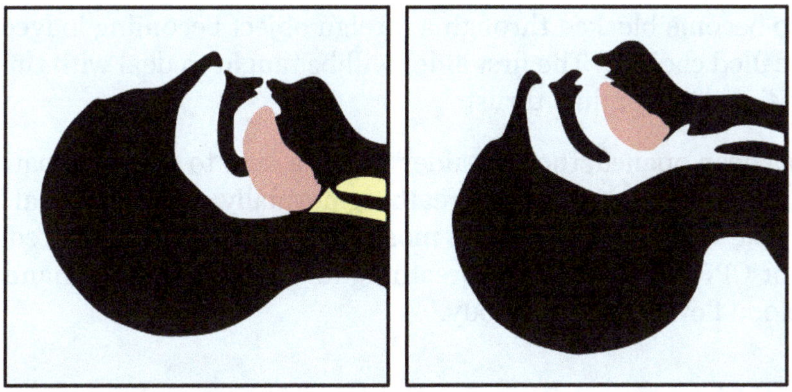

In case of tongue fallen backwards, blocking the airway, it is necessary to hyperextend the head and pull up the chin, so that the tongue lifts and clears the airway.

Certain skills are considered essential to the provision of first aid and are taught ubiquitously. Particularly the "ABC"s of first aid, which focus on critical life-saving intervention, must be rendered before treatment of less serious injuries. ABC stands for *Airway*, *Breathing*, and *Circulation*. The same mnemonic is used by all emergency health professionals. Attention must first be brought to the airway to ensure it is clear. Obstruction (choking) is a life-threatening emergency. Following evaluation of the airway, a first aid attendant would determine adequacy of breathing and provide rescue breathing if necessary. Assessment of circulation is now not usually carried out for patients who are not breathing, with first aiders now trained to go straight to chest compressions (and thus providing artificial circulation) but pulse checks may be done on less serious patients.

Some organizations add a fourth step of "D" for *Deadly bleeding* or *Defibrillation*, while others consider this as part of the *Circulation* step. Variations on techniques to evaluate and maintain the ABCs depend on the skill level of the first aider. Once the ABCs are secured, first aiders can begin additional treatments, as required. Some organizations teach the same order of priority using the "3Bs": *Breathing*, *Bleeding*, and *Bones* (or "4Bs": *Breathing*, *Bleeding*, *Burns*, and *Bones*). While the ABCs and 3Bs are taught to be performed sequentially, certain conditions may require the consideration of two steps simultaneously. This includes the provision of both artificial respiration and chest compressions to someone who is not breathing and has no pulse, and the consideration of cervical spine injuries when ensuring an open airway.

Preserving Life

In order to stay alive, all persons need to have an open airway—a clear passage where air can move in through the mouth or nose through the pharynx and down into the lungs, without obstruction. Conscious people will maintain their own airway automatically, but those who are unconscious (with a GCS of less than 8) may be unable to maintain a patent airway, as the part of the brain which automatically controls breathing in normal situations may not be functioning.

If the patient was breathing, a first aider would normally then place them in the recovery position, with the patient leant over on their side, which also has the effect of clearing the tongue from the pharynx. It also avoids a common cause of death in unconscious patients, which is choking on regurgitated stomach contents.

The airway can also become blocked through a foreign object becoming lodged in the pharynx or larynx, commonly called choking. The first aider will be taught to deal with this through a combination of 'back slaps' and 'abdominal thrusts'.

Once the airway has been opened, the first aider would assess to see if the patient is breathing. If there is no breathing, or the patient is not breathing normally, such as agonal breathing, the first aider would undertake what is probably the most recognized first aid procedure—cardiopulmonary resuscitation or CPR, which involves breathing for the patient, and manually massaging the heart to promote blood flow around the body.

Promoting Recovery

The first aider is also likely to be trained in dealing with injuries such as cuts, grazes or bone fracture. They may be able to deal with the situation in its entirety (a small adhesive bandage on a paper cut), or may be required to maintain the condition of something like a broken bone, until the next stage of definitive care (usually an ambulance) arrives.

Training

Basic principles, such as knowing to use an adhesive bandage or applying direct pressure on a bleed, are often acquired passively through life experiences. However, to provide effective, life-saving first aid interventions requires instruction and practical training. This is especially true where it relates to potentially fatal illnesses and injuries, such as those that require cardiopulmonary resuscitation (CPR); these procedures may be invasive, and carry a risk of further injury to the patient and the provider. As with any training, it is more useful if it occurs *before* an actual emergency, and in many countries, emergency ambulance dispatchers may give basic first aid instructions over the phone while the ambulance is on the way.

Training is generally provided by attending a course, typically leading to certification. Due to regular changes in procedures and protocols, based on updated clinical knowledge, and to maintain skill, attendance at regular refresher courses or re-certification is often necessary. First aid training is often available through community organizations such as the Red Cross and St. John Ambulance, or through commercial providers, who will train people for a fee. This commercial training is most common for training of employees to perform first aid in their workplace. Many community organizations also provide a commercial service, which complements their community programmes.

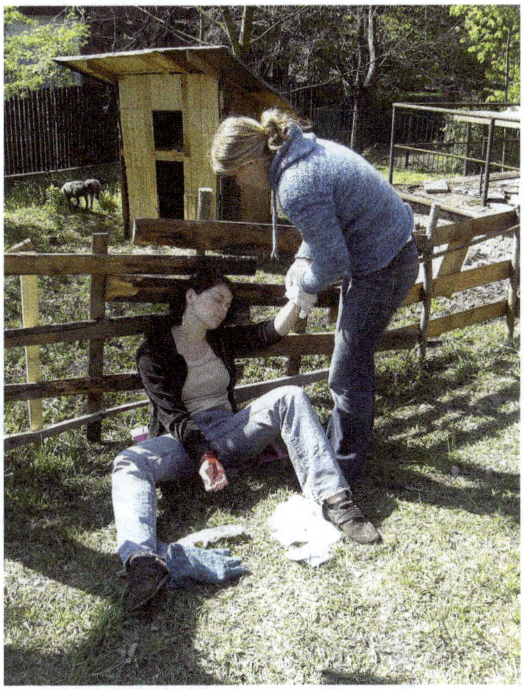

First aid scenario training in progress

Specific Disciplines

There are several types of first aid (and first aider) which require specific additional training. These are usually undertaken to fulfill the demands of the work or activity undertaken.

- Aquatic/Marine first aid is usually practiced by professionals such as lifeguards, professional mariners or in diver rescue, and covers the specific problems which may be faced after water-based rescue and/or delayed MedEvac.
- Battlefield first aid takes into account the specific needs of treating wounded combatants and non-combatants during armed conflict.
- Hyperbaric first aid may be practiced by SCUBA diving professionals, who need to treat conditions such as the bends.
- Oxygen first aid is the providing of oxygen to casualties who suffer from conditions resulting in hypoxia.
- Wilderness first aid is the provision of first aid under conditions where the arrival of emergency responders or the evacuation of an injured person may be delayed due to constraints of terrain, weather, and available persons or equipment. It may be necessary to care for an injured person for several hours or days.
- Mental health first aid is taught independently of physical first aid. How to support someone experiencing a mental health problem or in a crisis situation. Also how to identify the first signs of someone developing mental ill health and guide people towards appropriate help.

First Aid Services

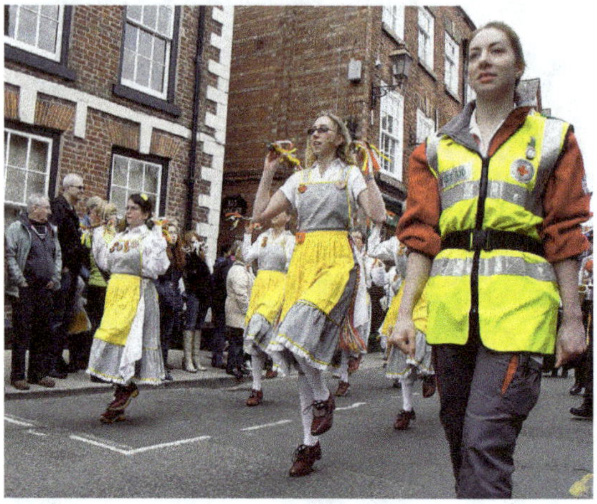

First aider of the British Red Cross accompanies parade of morris dancers at the Knutsford Royal May Day 2012

Some people undertake specific training in order to provide first aid at public or private events, during filming, or other places where people gather. They may be designated as a first aider, or use some other title. This role may be undertaken on a voluntary basis, with organisations such as the Red Cross and St John Ambulance, or as paid employment with a medical contractor.

People performing a first aid role, whether in a professional or voluntary capacity, are often expected to have a high level of first aid training and are often uniformed.

Symbols

Although commonly associated with first aid, the symbol of a red cross is an official protective symbol of the Red Cross. According to the Geneva Conventions and other international laws, the use of this and similar symbols is reserved for official agencies of the International Red Cross and Red Crescent, and as a protective emblem for medical personnel and facilities in combat situations. Use by any other person or organization is illegal, and may lead to prosecution.

The internationally accepted symbol for first aid is the white cross on a green background shown below.

Some organizations may make use of the Star of Life, although this is usually reserved for use by ambulance services, or may use symbols such as the Maltese Cross, like the Order of Malta Ambulance Corps and St John Ambulance. Other symbols may also be used.

St. Andrew's First Aid Badge	Emblem of the Red Cross	Star of life

Conditions that Often Require First Aid

- Altitude sickness, which can begin in susceptible people at altitudes as low as 5,000 feet, can cause potentially fatal swelling of the brain or lungs.
- Anaphylaxis, a life-threatening condition in which the airway can become constricted and the patient may go into shock. The reaction can be caused by a systemic allergic reaction to allergens such as insect bites or peanuts. Anaphylaxis is initially treated with injection of epinephrine.
- Battlefield first aid—This protocol refers to treating shrapnel, gunshot wounds, burns, bone fractures, etc. as seen either in the 'traditional' battlefield setting or in an area subject to damage by large-scale weaponry, such as a bomb blast.
- Bone fracture, a break in a bone initially treated by stabilizing the fracture with a splint.
- Burns, which can result in damage to tissues and loss of body fluids through the burn site.
- Cardiac Arrest, which will lead to death unless CPR preferably combined with an AED is started within minutes. There is often no time to wait for the emergency services to arrive as 92 percent of people suffering a sudden cardiac arrest die before reaching hospital according to the American Heart Association.
- Choking, blockage of the airway which can quickly result in death due to lack of oxygen if the patient's trachea is not cleared, for example by the Heimlich Maneuver.
- Childbirth.
- Cramps in muscles due to lactic acid build up caused either by inadequate oxygenation of muscle or lack of water or salt.
- Diving disorders, drowning or asphyxiation.
- Gender-specific conditions, such as dysmenorrhea and testicular torsion.
- Heart attack, or inadequate blood flow to the blood vessels supplying the heart muscle.
- Heat stroke, also known as sunstroke or hyperthermia, which tends to occur during heavy exercise in high humidity, or with inadequate water, though it may occur spontaneously in some chronically ill persons. Sunstroke, especially when the victim has been unconscious, often causes major damage to body systems such as brain, kidney, liver, gastric tract. Unconsciousness for more than two hours usually leads to permanent disability. Emergency treatment involves rapid cooling of the patient.
- Hair tourniquet a condition where a hair or other thread becomes tied around a toe or finger tightly enough to cut off blood flow.
- Heat syncope, another stage in the same process as heat stroke, occurs under similar conditions as heat stroke and is not distinguished from the latter by some authorities.
- Heavy bleeding, treated by applying pressure (manually and later with a pressure bandage) to the wound site and elevating the limb if possible.

- Hyperglycemia (diabetic coma) and Hypoglycemia (insulin shock).
- Hypothermia, or Exposure, occurs when a person's core body temperature falls below 33.7 °C (92.6 °F). First aid for a mildly hypothermic patient includes rewarming, which can be achieved by wrapping the affected person in a blanket, and providing warm drinks, such as soup, and high energy food, such as chocolate. However, rewarming a severely hypothermic person could result in a fatal arrhythmia, an irregular heart rhythm.
- Insect and animal bites and stings.
- Joint dislocation.
- Poisoning, which can occur by injection, inhalation, absorption, or ingestion.
- Seizures, or a malfunction in the electrical activity in the brain. Three types of seizures include a grand mal (which usually features convulsions as well as temporary respiratory abnormalities, change in skin complexion, etc.) and petit mal (which usually features twitching, rapid blinking, and/or fidgeting as well as altered consciousness and temporary respiratory abnormalities).
- Muscle strains and Sprains, a temporary dislocation of a joint that immediately reduces automatically but may result in ligament damage.
- Stroke, a temporary loss of blood supply to the brain.
- Toothache, which can result in severe pain and loss of the tooth but is rarely life-threatening, unless over time the infection spreads into the bone of the jaw and starts osteomyelitis.
- Wounds and bleeding, including lacerations, incisions and abrasions, Gastrointestinal bleeding, avulsions and Sucking chest wounds, treated with an occlusive dressing to let air out but not in.

First Aid Kit

Many accidents can happen at home, office, schools, laboratories etc. which require immediate attention before the patient is attended by the doctor.

Making of the First Aid Kit

Though professional first aid kits are readily available one can make a simple kit easily at home. Still ready made First Aid kits/boxes/pouches/cases are recommended as they have well organized compartments. To make a First Aid kit, a strong, durable bag or transparent plastic box should be taken and a white cross in a green square placed on the sides and on the top. This will make for easy identification of the box to any user. The kit should be kept such that it is within reach in case of an emergency.

A First Aid Kit should have the following contents:

- first-aid manual different sizes
- adhesive tape
- adhesive bandages in severe sizes

- elastic bandage
- a splint
- antiseptic wipes
- soap
- antibiotic ointment
- antiseptic solution (like hydrogen peroxide or saline)
- hydrocortisone cream (1%)
- acetaminophen and ibuprofen
- extra prescription medications (if the family is going on vacation)
- tweezers
- sharp scissors
- safety pins
- disposable instant cold packs
- calamine lotion
- alcohol wipes or ethyl alcohol
- thermometer
- tooth preservation kit
- plastic non-latex gloves(at least 2 pairs)
- flashlight and extra batteries
- thermal shock blanket
- mouthpiece for administering CPR (can be obtained from your local Red Cross)
- blanket (stored nearby)
- First Aid Card containing emergency personal information, phone numbers, medications, manual,

Health Care Ratings

Health care ratings are ratings or evaluations of health care.

Technological advances played a key role in facilitating the data collection and number crunching needed to generate health care ratings.

Health care ratings are coming of age in a time of rising levels of consumer health literacy.

Surveys consistently show that consumers rely heavily on friends and family when making healthcare decisions. With social networking and global connectivity, some of these family and friend referrals will include a wider network and will increasingly rely on quality data retrieved from multiple sources. Government, non-profit and private organizations are building public-private collaborations focused on the development of a nationwide system in the United States.

Types of Measures

Quality measures are standards that are used to assess the various aspects of the healthcare system. Using the Donabidien framework, these measures evaluate process of care, healthcare structures and/or outcomes of a healthcare services. This information is translated into report cards that are generated by quality organizations, nonprofit,consumer groups and media. This evaluation of quality is based on:

Measures of Hospital quality

Measures of Health Plan Quality

Measures of Physician Quality

Measures of Quality for Other Health Professionals

Measures of Patient Experience

Reporting Organizations

Measures are collected and disseminated by a number of quality reporting organizations.

Consumer Assessment of Health Professionals and Systems(CAHPS)

The Joint Commission

The National Quality Forum (NQF)

National Quality Measures Clearinghouse

The Robert Wood Johnson Foundation (RWJF), the largest philanthropy in the United States dedicated to improving health and health care, provides support for multiple efforts dedicated to increasing public awareness of the performance of health professionals:

- Aligning Forces for Quality is a national initiative that is focused on improving the overall quality of care in local communities. As part of this initiative, collaborative teams in 16 targeted communities work to make information about hospital and physician performance available to the public.
- Consumer-Purchaser Disclosure Project is a collaboration of leading consumer, employer and labor organizations working to ensure that all Americans have access to publicly reported health care performance information.

- National Quality Forum is a nonprofit membership organization created to develop and implement a national strategy for health care quality measurement and reporting.

Possible Benefits

Organizations are sensitive to public reporting As the healthcare system moves from supply driven to demand driven, transparency of such quality reporting is important for informed decision making and efficiency improvements

A 2001 retrospective cohort study found that health plans voluntarily generating public reports had higher quality ratings than those that chose not to publicly report. Another retrospective study of HMO's yielded similar results, revealing that HMOs with lower quality scores were more likely to stop public reporting while higher performing HMOs continued to publicly report. Analysis of hospital performance reporting and consumer selection found mixed results about public perception and market share. A 1997 study "reported that releasing hospital-specific mortality rates was associated with small but statistically significant effects on utilization, whereas press reports of single, unexpected deaths were associated with a relatively large effect."

More recent studies have identified the potential of public disclosure of performance in encouraging providers to focus on gaps in quality and stimulate performance improvement In addition, from a consumer perspective, health quality reports can encourage patients to preferentially choose high quality healthcare such as best health plans or assess the performance of providers

Possible Challenges

Low Use of Ratings

A 2007 survey of factors impacting individual consumer health professional selections found that only 11 percent of American adults looked for a new primary care physician. Of those 11% went online for information, 38% used doctor or healthplan information. Nearly 40% used multiple sources. 28 percent needed a new specialist physician and 16 percent underwent a medical procedure at a new facility. Few of those relied on price or quality information and relied almost exclusively on physician referrals. Only 3% of patients undergoing procedures and 7% choosing a specialist went online for information.

A 2008 survey of public awareness and use of healthcare quality reports reported that: 20% of Americans surveyed said they had seen quality information about hospitals and only 7% said they used the information to make a decision. 12% of Americans surveyed said they had seen quality information about doctors and only 6% said they used the information to make a decision.

Although public reporting has taken center stage in qualitative and health policy research, there has been a slow uptake. Barriers identified are related to consumer behaviors and challenges with the conceptual framework. Health literacy is a key component to comprehend and use performance data. However, complexity of the performance data, technicality and presentation of the quality data makes the quality reports difficult to understand. Another impediment to the development of health quality reports is the challenge associated with measuring performance at the individual physician level (due to inadequate sample sizes, difficulty adjusting for the severity of patients medical condition) . This has led to group-level reporting which makes these reports less useful for consumers.

Thus, given the changing healthcare landscape, further research to understand consumer behaviors will be important to inform the development and increased uptake of health grade reports.

Accessibility

There appears to be a breakdown in creative use of technology to get the information in the hands of those interested in using it. As pointed out by Kristen Madison, Senior Fellow at the Leonard Davis Institute of Health Economics, searching the Internet for "the term 'hospital quality' or' hospital report card' does not always turn up relevant report cards, even if they do exist". To make these reports more accessible, large philanthropies, including the Robert Wood Johnson Foundation, have funded major initiatives that are focused on performance measurement like the Aligning Forces for Quality program.

History of Health Quality Reporting

The earliest efforts to report on health professionals or facilities date to the mid-1980s when the Health Care Financing Administration (HCFA) – now the Centers for Medicare and Medicaid Services (CMS) – published nationwide hospital-specific mortality data. The information was controversial at the time and HCFA ended publication of the mortality information in the early 1990s.

The media, state governments and the employer community have also contributed to the development of public reporting. Newsday published mortality rates for heart bypass surgery for 140 New York surgeons in December, 1991. The information resulted from a Freedom of Information lawsuit seeking data from the New York State Department of Health. State agencies in California, New York and Pennsylvania also published cardiac surgery hospital and physician information in the early-mid-1990s. Some states also report on other types of hospital and physician information in their licensing and regulatory roles. Information on complaints, sanctions and other disciplinary actions has slowly become available through state licensing boards and Departments of Health. The Cleveland Health Quality Choice Coalition was an early collaborative effort between hospitals, physicians and purchasers that provided public information on hospital quality, though it is no longer in operation.

Largely at the urging of employers implementing managed care plans in the late 1980s and early 1990s, the development of health plan measures and reports began to emerge. Prompted by concerns about possible quality of care problems in managed care plans, the National Committee for Quality Assurance's (NCQA) Healthcare Effectiveness Data and Information Set (HEDIS) was developed to capture information about health plan quality of care. This measure set has been widely used by large employers, states and the Federal government as the basis for accrediting plans and for public reporting. At the same time, the Agency for Healthcare Research and Quality (AHRQ) funded the development of a survey instrument to assess patient experience with receiving care from their managed care plan. The tool, the Consumer Assessment of Healthcare Providers and Systems (CAHPS) has been widely embraced and was embedded in NCQA's health plan accreditation program. The CAHPS program has expanded over time to include a suite of survey tools to assess patient experience, including the CAHPS Hospital Survey (H-CAHPS) and the Clinician and Group CAHPS Survey.

The federal government re-entered the public reporting field in the late 1990s and the early years of the 21st century with the launch of the Compare websites , including Health Plan Compare and Nursing Home Compare, and subsequently Home Health Compare and Dialysis Compare. During the same period, AHRQ was building on its quality indicator work through the Hospital Care and Utilization Project (HCUP) (now Healthcare Cost and Utilization Project) with the development of the AHRQ Quality Indicators in 2001 and the AHRQ Patient Safety measures in 2002. Starting in 2007, AHRQ launched a learning network of community collaboratives (i.e., the Charter Value Exchanges), which were committed to measuring and publicly reporting on provider performance in their communities. Those efforts were supplemented by the regional collaborative work of the Robert Wood Johnson Foundation's Aligning Forces for Quality in 17 communities nationwide.

Other key organizations were also forming or expanding their portfolio to include measure development – particularly related to hospitals. The National Quality Forum (NQF) became operational in 2000 with the mission of standardizing health care performance measurement and strategies. Following on the release of the Institute of Medicine report To Err is Human, employers formed the Leapfrog Group, whose mission was to push hospitals to adopt safe practices. Leapfrog asked hospitals to voluntarily complete an annual survey to report on their safety practices, and these results were made public and, in some cases, became embedded in pay-for-performance programs. The Joint Commission was incorporating performance measurement into their accreditation process and multi-stakeholder groups such as the Hospital Quality Alliance (HQA) were working with Centers for Medicare and Medicaid Services on the development of Medicare's Hospital Compare.

Measure development and reporting on the physician side lagged measurement efforts at the plan and hospital level. In part due to methodological challenges involved in reporting given smaller sample sizes at the physician level, and also due to provider resistance. Recognizing increased pressure to measure performance and reduce variation, physician organizations began their own efforts to develop a set of performance measures. In 2000, the American Medical Association convened the Physician Consortium for Performance Improvement.page (PCPI) to develop, test and maintain physician performance measures. In September 2004, the American Academy of Family Physicians, the American College of Physicians, America's Health Insurance Plans and AHRQ created the Ambulatory Care Quality Alliance (AQA) to implement performance measurement at the physician level. Legislation in 2006 created the Physician Quality Reporting Initiative (PQRI), now termed as the Physician Quality Reporting System (PQRS), sponsored by Centers for Medicare and Medicaid Services. This "pay-for-reporting" program provides incentive payments to physicians who report quality data; however, to date individual physician performance results are not publicly available for use by consumers. Similar to the hospital compare website, the new Physician Compare website, provides information on physicians and other healthcare professionals who are currently enrolled in Medicare. Data on their affiliation, certification status and participation in CMS quality improvement programs is also made available to the Medicare beneficiaries

In the last decade the eHealth world for consumers has exploded with the growth of online advocacy and support groups.

The Patient Protection and Affordable Care Act passed in 2010 also calls for more public reporting of information about health professionals. As efforts by employers and health plans to assess the performance of both the quality and efficiency of individual physicians have grown, physicians have challenged these efforts for lack of transparency on the methods used to score them. In response to a settlement by the New York Attorney General, a coalition of purchasers and consumer groups developed the Patient Charter for Physician Performance Measurement, Reporting and Tiering (The Patient Charter"), which was released in 2008. The Patient Charter provided a process for reviewing the methods used to score providers and a framework for making the methods transparent.

Today, there are hundreds of public reporting activities across many types of health facilities and professionals including hospitals, physician groups, nursing homes, home health agencies, dialysis facilities, hospices and nurses. Some of these reporting activities result from government action, some from internal health professional or facility efforts to become more transparent, some from investigative journalism, some from community collaboratives, and others from employer or consumer groups. The ability to publish and update information through the Internet has facilitated the dissemination of information about health care performance. However, the information available to any given patient or family member still varies substantially in terms of its breadth, relevance and accessibility.

Geriatric Care Management

Geriatric care management (also known as "elder care management", "senior health care management" and "professional care management") is the process of planning and coordinating care of the elderly and others with physical and/or mental impairments to meet their long term care needs, improve their quality of life, and maintain their independence for as long as possible. It entails working with persons of old age and their families in managing, rendering and referring various types of health and social care services. Geriatric care managers accomplish this by combining a working knowledge of health and psychology, human development, family dynamics, public and private resources and funding sources, while advocating for their clients throughout the continuum of care. For example, they may assist families of older adults and others with chronic needs such as those suffering from Alzheimer's disease or other dementia.

Overview

Geriatric care management integrates health care and psychological care with other needed services such as: housing, home care services, nutritional services, assistance with activities of daily living, socialization programs, as well as financial and legal planning (e.g. banking, trusts). A care plan tailored for specific circumstances is prepared after a comprehensive assessment has taken place, and is continuously monitored and modified as needed. A comprehensive geriatric care assessment is thorough and can take anywhere from 2 to 5 hours in length, this of course is broken down into 2 or 3 assessment visits with the patient/family members. The comprehensive assessment is really a compilation of smaller individual assessments with the first one being a primary intake assessment which includes demographic type data as well as a health history, social history, and legal/financial history. From there, a medication profile assessment is included, as well as an assessment of ADLs (Activities of Daily Living) and IADLs (Instrumental Activities of Daily Living). In addition other assessments may include; Falls risk assessment, Home safety assessment, Nutritional assessment, Depression assessment, Pain assessment, Mini Mental State Exam (MMSE), MiniCog Clock Drawing Exam (Cognitive Assessment), Balance assessment, and Gait assessment(ability to walk). If the comprehensive geriatric care management assessment is being conducted by a Registered Nurse, then a physical assessment can be included such as vitals signs recording temperature, pulse, respirations, blood pressure, oxygen saturation, and sometimes FBS or RBS (Fasting or Random Blood Sugar) checks for diabetics. In addition, physical assessments in areas such as cardiopulmonary, gastrointestinal, musculoskeletal, genitourinary, eyes/ears/nose/ throat, integumentary(skin), lower extremities inspection, as well as a modified neuro assessment and medication compliance assessment.

Geriatric Care Managers

Geriatric care managers typically have prior training in nursing, social work, gerontology or other health service areas. They are expected to have extensive knowledge about the costs, quality, and availability of services in their communities. In some countries and jurisdictions, they may obtain certification from various professional associations, such as the *National Association of Professional Geriatric Care Managers* in the United States.

Professional care managers help individuals, families and other caregivers adjust and cope with the challenges of aging or disability by:

- Conducting care-planning assessments to identify needs, problems and eligibility for assistance;
- Screening, arranging, and monitoring in-home help and other services;
- Reviewing financial, legal, or medical issues;
- Offering referrals to specialists to avoid future problems and to conserve assets;
- Providing crisis intervention;
- Acting as a liaison to families at a distance;
- Making sure things are going well and alerting families of problems;
- Assisting with moving their clients to or from a retirement complex, assisted living facility, rehabilitation facility or nursing home;
- Providing client and family education and advocacy;
- Offering counseling and support.

Depending on the country and health care organization, professional fees for the services of geriatric care managers may be billed privately on a fee-for-service basis. In the United States, they are not covered by Medicaid, Medicare nor by most private health insurance policies. However, clients may be able to bill some services to long term care insurance, depending on the history of the individual case.

References

- White F (2015). "Primary health care and public health: foundations of universal health systems". Med Princ Pract. 24: 103–116. doi:10.1159/000370197

- Frenk J (2010). "The global health system: strengthening national health systems as the next step for global progress". PLoS Med. 7: e1000089. doi:10.1371/journal.pmed.1000089. PMC 2797599. PMID 20069038
- Mertig, Rita G. (2012). Nurses' Guide to Teaching Diabetes Self-management. Springer Publishing Company. p. 240. ISBN 0826108288. Retrieved 30 August 2013
- "Mirror, Mirror on the Wall: An International Update on the Comparative Performance of American Health Care". The Commonwealth Fund. 15 May 2007. Retrieved 7 March 2009
- Bodenheimer, Thomas (2002-11-20). "PAtient self-management of chronic disease in primary care". JAMA. 288 (19): 2469–2475. doi:10.1001/jama.288.19.2469. ISSN 0098-7484
- Handler A, Issel M, Turnock B. A conceptual framework to measure performance of the public health system. American Journal of Public Health, 2001, 91(8): 1235–39
- Ziguras, Christopher (2013). Self-care: Embodiment, Personal Autonomy and the Shaping of Health Consciousness. Routledge. pp. 14–15. ISBN 1134419694. Retrieved 31 August 2013
- Organisation for Economic Co-operation and Development. "OECD Health Data 2008: How Does Canada Compare" (PDF). Retrieved 9 January 2009
- Peters, David; Sara Bennet (2012). "Better Guidance Is Welcome, but without Blinders". PLoS Med. 9 (3): e1001188. doi:10.1371/journal.pmed.1001188. PMC 3308928. PMID 22448148. Retrieved 18 May 2012.
- Palo Stoller, Eleanor (1998). Ory,, Marcia G.; DeFriese, Gordon H., eds. Self-care in Later Life: Research, Program, and Policy Issues. Springer Publishing Company. pp. 24–25. ISBN 0826196950. Retrieved 28 August 2013
- "Mortality amenable to health care" Nolte, Ellen. "Variations in Amenable Mortality—Trends in 16 High-Income Nations". Commonwealth Fund. Retrieved 10 February 2012
- Adamiak, E. Chojnacka, D. Walczak, Social security in Poland – cultural, historical and economical issues, Copernican Journal of Finance & Accounting, Vol 2, No 2, p. 23
- Laurin, Jacqualine (1994). "Commentary". In Kikuchi, June F.; Simmons, Helen. Developing a Philosophy of Nursing. Sage. p. 27. ISBN 0803954239. Retrieved 31 August 2013
- Jimmy, B; Jose, J (2011). "Patient medication adherence: Measures in daily practice". Oman Medical Journal. 26 (3): 155–159. doi:10.5001/omj.2011.38
- Sommers, B.D. (2012). "New physicians, the affordable care act, and the changing practice of medicine.". JAMA. 307: 1697–98. doi:10.1001/jama.2012.523
- "OECD.StatExtracts, Health, Health Status, Life expectancy, Total population at birth, 2011" (online statistics). stats.oecd.org/. OECD's iLibrary. 2013. Retrieved 2013-11-24
- Kandula, N.R.; Malli, T; Zei, C.P.; Larsen, E; Baker, D.W. (2011). "Literacy and retention of information after a multimedia diabetes education program and teach-back". Journal of Health Communication. 16: 89–202.
- "The Pharmaceutical Industry in Figures" (pdf). European Federation of Pharmaceutical Industries and Associations. 2007. Retrieved February 15, 2010.
- Judah, G; Gardner, B; Aunger, R (2012). "Forming a flossing habit: An exploratory study of the psychological determinants of habit formation". The British Journal of Health Psychology. 18: 338–353.
- Braveman, Paula; E. Tarimo (1994). Screening in Primary Health Care: Setting Priorities With Limited Resources. World Health Organization. p. 14. ISBN 9241544732. Retrieved 4 November 2012
- Bentley, JM; Nash, DB (1998). "How Pennsylvania hospitals have responded to publicly released reports on coronary artery bypass graft surgery?.". The Joint Commission Journal on Quality Improvement. 24 (1): 40–9

Permissions

All chapters in this book are published with permission under the Creative Commons Attribution Share Alike License or equivalent. Every chapter published in this book has been scrutinized by our experts. Their significance has been extensively debated. The topics covered herein carry significant information for a comprehensive understanding. They may even be implemented as practical applications or may be referred to as a beginning point for further studies.

We would like to thank the editorial team for lending their expertise to make the book truly unique. They have played a crucial role in the development of this book. Without their invaluable contributions this book wouldn't have been possible. They have made vital efforts to compile up to date information on the varied aspects of this subject to make this book a valuable addition to the collection of many professionals and students.

This book was conceptualized with the vision of imparting up-to-date and integrated information in this field. To ensure the same, a matchless editorial board was set up. Every individual on the board went through rigorous rounds of assessment to prove their worth. After which they invested a large part of their time researching and compiling the most relevant data for our readers.

The editorial board has been involved in producing this book since its inception. They have spent rigorous hours researching and exploring the diverse topics which have resulted in the successful publishing of this book. They have passed on their knowledge of decades through this book. To expedite this challenging task, the publisher supported the team at every step. A small team of assistant editors was also appointed to further simplify the editing procedure and attain best results for the readers.

Apart from the editorial board, the designing team has also invested a significant amount of their time in understanding the subject and creating the most relevant covers. They scrutinized every image to scout for the most suitable representation of the subject and create an appropriate cover for the book.

The publishing team has been an ardent support to the editorial, designing and production team. Their endless efforts to recruit the best for this project, has resulted in the accomplishment of this book. They are a veteran in the field of academics and their pool of knowledge is as vast as their experience in printing. Their expertise and guidance has proved useful at every step. Their uncompromising quality standards have made this book an exceptional effort. Their encouragement from time to time has been an inspiration for everyone.

The publisher and the editorial board hope that this book will prove to be a valuable piece of knowledge for students, practitioners and scholars across the globe.

Index

www.ingramcontent.com/pod-product-compliance
Lightning Source LLC
LaVergne TN
LVHW080921210926
848485LV00004B/699